Other books

Also by Arnold Fox, M.D. and Barry Fox, Ph.D.:

The Beverly Hills Medical Diet
DLPA To End Chronic Pain and Depression
Wake Up! You're Alive
Making Miracles
Immune For Life
Beyond Positive Thinking
The Healthy Prostate

Alternative Healing

By
Arnold Fox, M.D., and Barry Fox, Ph.D.

CAREER PRESS
3 Tice Road
P.O. Box 687
Franklin Lakes, NJ 07417
1-800-CAREER-1
201-848-0310 (NJ and outside U.S.)
FAX: 201-848-1727

ALTERNATIVE HEALING
ISBN 1-56414-227-2, $14.99
Cover design by The Hub Graphics Corp.
Cover photo provided by Image Bank
Printed in the U.S.A. by Book-mart Press

To order this title by mail, please include price as noted above, $2.50 handling per order, and $1.00 for each book ordered. Send to: Career Press, Inc., 3 Tice Road., P.O. Box 687, Franklin Lakes, NJ 07417.

Or call toll-free 1-800-CAREER-1 (NJ and Canada: 201-848-0310) to order using VISA or MasterCard, or for further information on books from Career Press.

Library of Congress Cataloging-in-Publication Data

Fox, Arnold, 1928-
    Alternative healing : nontraditional therapies such as
acupuncture, homeopathy, and nutritional healing can help you cope
with illnesses from allergies to ulcers / by Arnold Fox and Barry
Fox.
        p.   cm.
    Includes index.
    ISBN 1-56414-227-2 (paper)
    1. Alternative medicine.   I. Fox, Barry. II. Title.
R733.F73   1996
615.5--dc20   96-4182
                                                        CIP

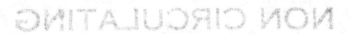

Dedication

To our wives, Hannah and Nadine, who make all things possible.

Acknowledgments

First and foremost, to our wives Hannah and Nadine, for correcting and editing our material, for giving us fresh ideas when we were worn out, and for their love and support.

We are indebted to many people who have helped us gather material for this book, including Robert J. Reo, O.M.D., Ph.D., C.H., who provided us with a great deal of information on Oriental medicine; Murray Clarke, D.Hom., L.Ac., for teaching us about homeopathy; Kathleen Cairns, Psy.D, for her invaluable input on psychology and hypnotism; Ray Sahelian, M.D., one of the nation's leading authorities on melatonin; as well as Arnold Sandlow, D.C., and Craig Ross, D.C., for spending time discussing chiropractic with us. In addition, Louise Taylor of the Healing Arts Center in Woodland Hills, Calif., graciously contributed information on yoga, imagery and energy healing, and Cathryn Hu, Ph.D., O.M.D., provided us with information on Oriental medicine.

We'd also like to thank NatureWorks of New York City for providing us with information on Alpha Lipotene; Wein Products, Inc., of Los Angeles, Calif., maker of the Air Supply personal air purifier; Harris Schnall of JB Harris Company for medical information on Sambucol; Charlie Fox of Wakanaga of America, makers of Kyolic Garlic, for providing us with so much information on garlic and related items; Richard Gash of BioHealth in Irvine, Calif., for information on mare's milk and Equimilk; Terry Lemeroad of Enzymatic Therapies Companies in Green Bay, Wis., for stacks of information on L.72 and other alternative therapies; Abe Chaplan, M.D, for his expertise on DMAE; John Shimanski of Optio of Los Angeles, Calif., for the stacks of information he provided on the medical benefits of green tea; and of course, Earl Mindell, R.Ph., Ph.D., one of the foremost experts on supplements and health; and finally, a special "thank-you" to Jeff Davidson, DTM.

Contents

Preface

As proud as we medical doctors are of modern medicine, the truth is that we are simply not able to keep people as healthy and happy as they would like to be. We can do quite a bit for our patients and can sometimes work miracles, but we have our limits. We also, unfortunately, have turned a blind eye to many useful alternative therapies offered by a variety of healing artists.

As a medical doctor, an internist and cardiologist with more than 40 years of experience on the "front lines" of crisis medicine, I can tell you that it is time to revolutionize health care, it's time to open our minds and our arms to chiropractors, Oriental medicine doctors, nutritionists, naturopaths and other alternative healers in our quest to help people live long, healthy and happy lives.

It's also time for us to "catch up" to the public, which is already embracing alternative therapies. As a survey in the Jan. 27, 1993 *New England Journal of Medicine* showed, tens of millions of American are already relying on chiropractic, acupuncture, herbalism, homeopathy, self-help groups and other alternative approaches.

Many people ask me about alternative healing; in my offices, when I'm lecturing and on my radio program. I tell them that there are many paths to good health and happiness. The key is education, making yourself aware of the numerous possibilities and deciding which is best for you.

Alternative Healing helps you make your choices by examining more than 30 major diseases. We'll look at their causes and consequences, at traditional and alternative treatments. But please remember: This book is meant as an overview on alternatives—not as medical advice. If you suffer from any of the conditions described in the book, be sure to see a doctor. The object is not to toss away your crutches and pills, but to look more to natural approaches and substances. I believe that in the future, all medical doctors will realize that many healers have a role in healing, and will welcome all ideas.

—Arnold Fox, M.D.

Note to the reader: Although this book is the result of a close collaboration between the Foxes, for convenience and clarity we use the "I" voice of Arnold Fox, M.D., throughout.

An overview

Numerous alternative therapies are offered in this book, ranging from the widely accepted chiropractic to less-accepted practices, such as crystal healing. Some of the alternative modalities are based on ancient traditions, other have been developed more recently. Some are able to support at least part their claims with scientific proof, others rely more on faith.

This introduction briefly examines the major alternative therapies that you will find in the book. These are not necessarily the "best" of the alternative approaches. Rather, I chose them because they are either widely practiced or they represent interesting ideas worthy of discussion. You'll see my own approach to treating the various diseases at the end of each chapter.

Acupuncture

As a part of the larger system of Oriental medicine, acupuncture prevents and treats disease by balancing the flow of energy within the body. Everyone is born with a certain amount of energy. The events of daily life "subtract" from the energy stores, while food and air replenish what has been lost. Disease is the result of an energy imbalance in all or part of the body.

The body's energy constantly flows through 12 major "meridians," or tiny channels. Like the blood vessels, these meridians are believed to be tube-like structures filled with fluid, that have smaller, subsidiary meridians branching out from the main ones. At various designated points, meridian branches touch the surface of the skin. The body's energy flow can be influenced by manipulating these areas— known as "acupuncture points"—with needles, manual stimulation, heat or electricity. The 12 main meridians are:

- The *Lung Meridian,* which runs from the top of the chest down the inside of the arm to the thumb, and may be used to treat lung and other ailments.

- The *Large Intestine Meridian,* which runs from the tip of the index finger up to the eye, and may be used to treat head, nose, ear, teeth, neck and other ailments.

- The *Stomach Meridian,* which runs from the head down to the foot, and may be used to treat stomach, intestinal, head and other ailments.

- The *Spleen Meridian,* which runs from the foot up to the chest, and may be used to treat disease of the reproductive, urinary and gastrointestinal systems.

- The *Heart Meridian,* which runs from the chest down the arm to the hand, and may be used to treat heart, nervous system and other ailments.

- The *Small Intestine Meridian,* which runs from the hand to the head, and may be used to treat head, face, shoulder and other ailments.

- The *Bladder Meridian,* which also runs from the head to the foot, and may be used to treat head, spine and other ailments.

- The *Kidney Meridian,* which runs from the foot to the chest, and may be used to treat urinary and reproductive disorders.

- The *Heart Constrictor Meridian,* which runs from the chest to the hand, and may be used to treat heart, stomach, nervous system and other ailments.

- The *Triple Heater Meridian,* which also runs from the hand up to the head, and may be used to treat heart and other ailments.

- The *Gallbladder Meridian,* which runs from the chest down to the foot, and may be used to treat problems with the limbs, chest and other parts of the body.

- The *Liver Meridian,* which also runs from the foot up to the chest, and may be used to treat problems with the liver, gallbladder, reproductive and urinary systems.

In addition to carrying energy throughout the body, the meridians run close to the nerves at various points in the body. Thus, the meridians and nerves can sometimes be stimulated simultaneously.

Very thin acupuncture needles are inserted at the acupuncture points to stimulate the flow of sluggish energy, or to disperse stagnant energy. In addition to or instead of needles, the acupuncturist may use techniques such as:

- Acupressure. Hands-on manipulation of the body points.

- Auriculotherapy ("ear acupuncture"). Using acupuncture points on the ear that correspond to various points in the body. To help locate points in the ear, French doctors devised the upside-down-person system. The bottom part of your ear, your ear lobe, contains the points for your head. As you move up your ear, you come to points representing lower and lower parts of your body.
- Moxibustion. The burning of an herb called *moxa* at designated acupuncture points on the body.

Diagnosis of disease is a subtle process, with the acupuncturist asking many questions about the patient's symptoms, personal and family history, appetite, bowel habits, etc. He or she will study the patient's skin, tongue, eyes, fingernails and other parts of the body, as well as the urine and stool. The acupuncturist will also listen to the sounds made by the patient's speaking voice, breathing and bowels, and will pay careful attention to the pulse.

Although acupuncture was brought to the United States by Chinese immigrants in the 1800s, it was not until President Nixon initiated the "opening" with China that American doctors began studying the healing art. The World Health Organization has listed more than 100 conditions that are treated by acupuncture, including asthma, pain, ulcers, headaches and osteoarthritis. More than 30 states now license acupuncturists. Other health specialists, including physicians and chiropractors, may also use acupuncture.

Aromatherapy

Aromatherapy uses aromatic substances called essential oils to treat a wide variety of physical and emotional ailments. The essential oils, which are primarily taken from plants, are usually inhaled, rubbed on the skin or used in a bath. In some cases, the essential oils are ingested or injected. Among the many essences used in aromatherapy are basil, bergamot, black pepper, camphor, cedarwood, chamomile, fennel, frankincense, hyssop, jasmine, juniper, lavender, melissa, patchouli and rose.

Proponents argue that aromatherapy is useful for treating acne, arthritis, asthma, bronchitis, burns, colds, constipation, depression, diarrhea, fever, flu, gas, headaches, herpes, indigestion, insomnia, memory loss, nausea, poor circulation, premenstrual tension, skin problems, stress, toothaches, wounds and other problems.

About 4,000 years ago, the ancient Egyptians were using fragrant oils to heal the mind and body. Closer to our Common Era, the Greeks used oils from plants as medicines. Roman soldiers carried lavender with them as they conquered the known world, using the plant to disinfect wounds. Various plant oils were used throughout the Middle Ages for many mental and physical diseases and for treating wounds.

Aromatherapy began to be systematized in the sixteenth century by William Turner, who classified plants by their effects on the body. By the end of the eighteenth century, 13 standard preparations had been described in an aromatherapy text. However, the rapid advance of chemistry and pharmacology in the nineteenth and twentieth centuries swept aromatherapy aside.

No one quite knows how aromatherapy works. There are several theories, including:

Unique smell. Each essential oil has a unique smell, which unleashes various physical and emotional responses in the patient's body and mind. According to this theory, smelling something that reminds us of the beach, for example, will cause us to relax as our brains call forth memories of relaxing at the beach.

Physiologic. Essential oils contain esters, alcohols, aldehydes, ketones and many other chemicals that interact with substances in the body, just as medicines do. And certain plants have antibiotic, antiseptic, anti-inflammatory, stimulating and other effects. Where or how the essential oils work on a physiologic level is unknown.

Nervous system effects. At least part of aromatherapy's benefits come from the oil's ability to balance the relationship between the sympathetic and autonomic divisions of the human nervous system.

Once the mainstay of ancient Egyptian medicine, and for centuries a major part of many traditional healing systems, aromatherapy is slowly making its way into Western medicine. There is, however, no standardized course of training for aromatherapists; indeed, no training of any sort is required for people to call themselves aromatherapists. Neither are there widely accepted treatment protocols, so treatment will vary from practitioner to practitioner. Many chiropractors, acupuncturists, masseuses and other therapists are incorporating aromatherapy into their practices.

Ayurvedic healing

Ayurvedic medicine is the medical branch of the Vedic system, an ancient Indian form of philosophy and approach to life. (Astrology and yoga are other prominent branches of the system.) Begun in India perhaps some 5,000 or 6,000 years ago, Ayurvedic healing spread throughout Southeast Asia and to China to the east, and as far west as ancient Greece.

Ayurvedic medicine is based on the belief that three primal forces link every person with the universe: The life breath *(prana)*, the spirit of fire or light *(agni)*, and love and harmony *(soma)*. All matter is composed of varying combinations of air, fire, earth, water and ether (a nontangible substance that fills the empty spaces).

According to Ayurvedic theory, there are two primary causes of disease: 1) An imbalance of the three body humors and 2) karmic disturbances, such as failure to fulfill one's spiritual purpose in life, poor relationships or errors in a past life.

The three body humors, or life forces, are *Vata, Pitta* and *Kapha*. Vata, the "air" humor, sits in the empty spaces in the body and is centered in the colon. Pitta, the "fire" humor, oversees metabolism and perception. It is centered in the small intestines. Kapha, the "water" humor, constitutes most body tissues and is centered in the stomach. Of the three humors, Vata is the most important, for it has overall responsibility for all physical processes.

The symptoms of diseases vary according to the humor in which they manifest themselves. High blood pressure in the Vata humor is seen as blood pressure that moves up and down erratically, with nervousness and insomnia. In the Pitta humor, high blood pressure leads to headaches, nosebleeds, anger, redness of the eyes and face, and sensitivity to light. But if it manifests in the Kapha humor, high blood pressure makes one tired, obese and swollen with fluids.

Treatment for all diseases depends upon the patient's constitutional makeup and which humor is primarily affected, and includes both physical and spiritual elements. Diet, exercise, herbs, internal cleansing, massage, meditation, prayers, changes in lifestyle, colors, gems, metals, crystals, baths, inhaling of aromas and other practices are among the therapies used.

Ayurvedic healing is recognized by the World Health Organization. Thanks in large part to the prolific author and speaker Deepak Chopra, M.D., the healing art is also becoming known in the United States. At this time, there are no state or federal boards licensing Ayurvedic healers. Some medical doctors, naturopaths, chiropractors and other healers, however, are incorporating Ayurvedic ideas and therapies into their practices.

Chiropractic

The modern practice of chiropractic was developed in 1895 by Daniel Palmer, who believed that the body had "innate" healing powers centered in the central nervous system and running along the spine. Palmer felt that disease arose when the nerves were pressured or otherwise interfered with by the spinal vertebrae. When a nerve is interfered with, the organ(s) it serves will become damaged or diseased. The cure for illness, therefore, is to remove the stress on the nerves by manipulating the spine.

The spinal imbalances or dislocations that interfere with nerves are called "subluxations." Subluxations may be caused by trauma or injury, poor posture, improper lifting, lack of exercise, stress, not enough rest or inherited spinal problems. Because the subluxation itself is often very minor and not painful, we don't realize that nerves are being damaged or subjected to interference. Hence, we don't usually connect a pain in the kidney, for example, with a slightly misaligned spine.

Chiropractors employ a "hands-on" approach to diagnosing and correcting spinal problems. Using their fingers, chiropractors will carefully feel along the spine, looking for misaligned vertebra, muscle tension, swelling or any other signs of spinal trouble.

Modern chiropractic is divided into two groups, the "straight" and the "mixed." Straight chiropractors adhere to the original principles of chiropractic, believing that disease is caused by subluxation and other problems with the spine. This spinal misalignment can lead to physiologic, neurologic and musculoskeletal problems throughout the body, and can interfere with the body's ability to heal itself. Straight chiropractors treat disease by manipulating the spine in order to correct any misalignments, and they then allow the body to heal itself.

Mixed chiropractors feel that a properly aligned spine is very important, but that more is needed to help the body heal itself. Thus, mixed chiropractors incorporate a variety of other healing arts, including nutrition, stress reduction, body work, therapeutic exercise and homeopathy into their practices.

Chiropractic is perhaps the most widely accepted of the alternative therapies. Chiropractors are licensed by the various states and, in many states, are allowed to admit patients to hospitals and treat them there. Many physicians will occasionally refer patients to chiropractors, and treatment is covered by many insurance plans.

Color therapy

Color therapy, also known as color healing and chromotherapy, uses light to detect, prevent and treat disease. Color therapists believe that all diseases, bacteria, viruses, organs and other objects give off light of particular wavelengths. Disease comes about when the body is strained and certain parts cannot vibrate at the proper frequencies to give off their normal lights. Disease is fought by applying the proper light to the body.

Many cultures have utilized color healing. It's believed that the ancient Egyptians had rooms and windows built in special ways so as to break up the sun's rays into the colors of the spectrum as they entered the room. This allowed the healers and priests to use the various colors in medical and religious practices.

There is no formalized training or licensing required to become a color therapist. Neither is there a widely accepted school of modern color therapy to set standards for treatment. Thus, beliefs and practices may vary from practitioner to practitioner. In general, however, the color red is considered to be stimulating and good for circulation. The color blue, which is soothing and cooling, promotes growth and vitality. Yellow, a cleansing and purifying color, is the color of joy.

To diagnose disease, the color therapist will look at the color and condition of the skin, urine, stool, eyes and nails, listen to the patient speak and observe how he or she behaves. The patient may be asked how he or she feels mentally, emotionally and physically when certain colors are discussed, or when colored objects are held next to him or her. Special cameras or other devices may be used to look at the patient's aura.

Once the problem has been diagnosed, the color therapist will attempt to heal the patient by either supplying the deficient color or by using other colors to counteract the problem. The appropriately colored light(s) may be shined on various parts of the body, or the wearing of colored clothes or threads may be prescribed. The patient may be asked to eat or drink foods or liquids of certain colors (beets are a red food, for example, and carrots an orange food). Colored gems or stones may be touched to specific parts of the body, and the patient may be asked to meditate on certain colors.

Folk medicine

Folk medicine is "homemade" medicine. It consists of an incredibly diverse array of remedies that people from all over the world have devised over untold centuries. Folk medicine uses foods, herbs, prayers, rituals and many other items and approaches to cure disease. Eating roasted fox liver, chewing honeycomb, drinking whiskey mixed with onions and wearing a necklace made of corn cobs are all examples of folk medicine.

Some folk medicines have proven to be very effective. The modern heart medication called *digitalis* originally came from the foxglove plant, which was used as a folk remedy for heart and other problems. American Indians used preparations made from willow bark to quell pain. Today we know that the willow bark contains a form of aspirin. Chicken soup, the Jewish mother's staple remedy for many ailments, has been found to contain good amounts of potassium and other nutrients that help to improve overall health.

Herbal medicine

Herbal medicine uses herbs to heal a variety of ailments—from hemp for treating glaucoma to fringe tree bark for liver disease. For medicinal purposes, herbs are considered to be anything taken from a plant, such as the leaf, stem, bark, root, or any other part. The herb may be made into a powder, tablet, capsule, extract, tea, essential oil, ointment, balm or tincture.

Herbal healing goes back at least as far as the dawn of recorded history. Ancient Egyptian writings indicate that garlic and other herbs were used medicinally as early as 1800 B.C.E. Hippocrates, the Greek physician and father of modern medicine, classified herbs and foods according to their "hot," "cold," "damp" or "dry" qualities. Herbal healing played a major role in Roman and Arabian medicine, and continues to play a prominent role in Oriental, Ayurvedic, Native American and other healing arts.

Herbal medicine was swept aside by the rise of Western medicine in this country, but has never been completely stamped out. In one sense, herbal healing has been wildly successful, as many powerful Western medicines are based on old herbal remedies. As many as one-fifth of all today's medicines may have originally been derived from plants. And because only a small percent of the world's plant species have been thoroughly investigated for medicinal properties, there may be a wealth of healing potential hidden away in forests, deserts and jungles. Unfortunately, since herbs cannot be patented, the major pharmaceutical companies are unlikely to invest the millions of dollars necessary to research, locate and test each herb.

Many herbs are used today by herbologists, doctors of Oriental medicine, naturopaths, Ayurvedists and other healers. Which herbs, the amounts, and the ways in which they are used depends upon the healer. Some common herbs include apple, borage, burdock, chicory root, comfrey, elder, Feverfew, flax, golden rod, honeysuckle, hyssop, juniper, lavender, lemon balm, lobelia, lungwort, marigold, mint, motherwort, mulberry, myrrh, nutmeg, tarragon, walnut, white birch and wormwood. Depression has long been treated with an herb called St. John's Wort. Recently, an extract of elderberry called Sambucol has demonstrated an ability to prevent the influenza virus from entering body cells.

There is neither a widely accepted school of herbology to set standards, nor a body or board that certifies or licenses herbologists. As a result, herbal treatment may vary from practitioner to practitioner.

Homeopathy

Once a part of mainstream medicine in the United States and taught at more than 20 homeopathic medical schools in the early 1900s, the use of homeopathic medicine declined as the pharmaceutical industry was developed and funding for the homeopathic medical schools was withdrawn.

Homeopathy, which means "similar suffering," was developed by Dr. Samuel Hahnemann in the eighteenth century. Concerned that he was harming more patients then he was helping with the standard medical cures of the day, the German physician began experimenting with Peruvian bark and other herbal preparations. He eventually discovered that substances that cause mild symptoms of disease in a healthy person could cure a person with the full-fledged disease. For example, if a small portion of a substance that caused loose bowels in a healthy person was given to a patient with diarrhea, the problem would clear up.

In time, Dr. Hahnemann devised the "Law of Similars," a basic homeopathic principle that states that "like cures like." Thus, rather than trying to suppress patients' symptoms with drugs, homeopaths attempt to stimulate the body's natural healing powers by giving tiny doses of the very thing that can cause symptoms in healthy people. (This is somewhat similar to the use of vaccines in traditional Western medicine.)

Homeopaths believe that ailments are merely signs that the body is attempting to heal problems afflicting patients on physical, mental and emotional levels. Thus, they look far beyond the physical symptoms when assessing patients. Attempting to get to the "essence" of patients, homeopaths will ask what they like to eat and drink, what they're afraid of, what they dream of, when and how they sleep, whether they're a day or night person, whether they prefer warm or cool weather, what diseases run in their families, how they react and respond to different stressors presently and previously in their lives and so on.

As part of this investigation, the homeopath will ask many questions about the patient's ailment, including: When did it begin? How long has it been going on? What previous treatments have you had? What was happening in your life before the symptoms began? What other diseases did you have recently? Have you been depressed? Anxious? Overtaxed at work or school? Have you lost a loved one? Have you had any difficulty concentrating or sleeping?

If the problem is pain, the homeopath will ask questions such as: When does it hurt? Is it a sharp pain? A throbbing pain? An ache? Is the pain constant, or does it come and go? Does the pain radiate? What makes the pain better or worse? Is the pain worse with movement? Is it better in the morning, afternoon or evening?

The purpose of these and many other questions is to get to the essence of the problem, the fundamental "glitch" in the patient's physical/mental/emotional state that allowed the problem to blossom. Once that has been done, the homeopath can select the most effective "constitutional remedy" for the patient.

The concept of the constitutional remedy is vital to successful homeopathy. Rather than simply prescribing a homeopathic "remedy" (medicine) for an *ailment*, the homeopath selects the single remedy that best captures the *essence* (the true character) of the person. Each of the 2,000-some homeopathic remedies carry "portraits" of a person's temperature, sleep patterns, food likes and dislikes, fears, anxieties, patterns of behavior and personality, and symptoms likely to be manifested. Not any "pain" remedy will do for a pain patient, for example. The portraits of the patient and remedy must be closely matched if the remedy is to be effective.

Although it is a basic principle of classical homeopathy to use only one remedy at a time, there is a trend among modern homeopaths toward using multiple remedies at once. Using the absolute minimum number of doses necessary is another principle of classical homeopathy. A second dose should not be given until the first has ceased to act, and no more remedies should be given once the body begins to heal. (The patient's symptoms, which may grow worse before they improve, should clear up in the reverse order that they appeared.) If the right remedy is used, two or three days should be enough to begin many long-term curative processes. If not, a different remedy ought to be selected.

Homeopathic remedies are derived from plants, minerals and (to a lesser degree) animals. Each remedy has been highly diluted in liquid until there is as little as one part per million of the original substance left in the remedy. During the dilution process, the remedy is repeatedly "succussed" (shaken and struck in a special way). The more the remedy is diluted and succussed, the more "potentiated" and stronger it is.

The process of diluting remedies has drawn a great deal of criticism. Many non-homeopaths believe that none of the original substance is left in the remedy after it has been diluted, and, therefore, the remedy is useless. Homeopaths argue that the remedy retains its power through successive dilutions.

Today, the National Center for Homeopathy and other organizations offer courses and certifications in homeopathy. Medical doctors (M.D.s), doctors of osteopathy (D.O.s), doctors of naturopathy (N.D.s), dentists and veterinarians can be licensed to administer homeopathic remedies. Acupuncturists and chiropractors are similarly licensed in some states. Homeopathic remedies for home use can be purchased at some health food and vitamin stores. Homeopathy is practiced throughout Europe. Even the Queen of England uses the services of a homeopathic physician.

Hypnotherapy

Originally known as "mesmerism," hypnosis is an artificially induced state of intense concentration. Mysterious as it sounds, hypnosis only seeks to copy similar states we all achieve naturally, perhaps several times a day.

Although shamans and other healers undoubtedly used hypnosis unknowingly, it was not until Franz Mesmer, a German physician, began "mesmerizing" patients in the 1700s that the phenomenon began to be studied. By the mid-1800s, hypnosis was being used to relieve pain, and as an anesthetic for surgery. And Sigmund Freud used it to treat psychological conditions, such as convulsion hysteria, long before he discovered psychoanalysis. The American Medical Association has approved of the use of hypnosis since 1958, and today some 15,000 medical doctors use hypnotherapy as an adjunct to their more traditional therapies, as do numerous licensed psychologists. Hypnosis is used to help treat a variety of conditions, ranging from obesity to chronic pain.

Medical doctors, psychologists, dentists, chiropractors and other healers may use hypnosis in their practices, but certified hypnotherapists specialize in hypnotherapy alone. There are numerous ways to induce a hypnotic trance, but most hypnotherapists use some form of the "talking induction." With the patient seated or lying down comfortably in a quiet office, the hypnotherapist simply talks in a calm voice, suggesting that the patient feels very relaxed and his or her eyes are heavy, or that he or she is drifting away to a favorite place, or that he or she is slowly going down into "nothingness" on an escalator. Many variations of the "talking induction" are effective.

Hypnotherapists speak of "conscious" and "unconscious" minds. The critical, analytical conscious mind tends to reject suggestions. The less-critical subconscious mind tends to accept what it is told as reality. Getting to the subconscious mind, it is reasoned, allows healers to implant healing suggestions where they will do the most good.

Hypnosis is similar to guided imagery and other forms of therapy that involve "seeing what you want to be." People cannot be hypnotized against their wills. Neither do they "lose control" or do anything they would not want to do. Hypnosis is entirely dependent upon the cooperation of the patient. Most people can be put into at least a light trance; a smaller number will reach deep, somnambulistic states.

Hypnosis is believed to help fight off illnesses via the mind/body connection. "Positive thinking" helps the body to heal itself. (See the section in this introduction on Psychoneuroimmunology.) Many of us find it especially difficult to be positive and optimistic in the face of serious illness, however. That's where hypnosis comes in. It can help keep the mind focused on the positive, thereby strengthening the health-promoting aspects of the mind/body system.

Because illness can make one fearful, anxious or otherwise emotionally upset, and because emotional distress, acting through the mind/body connection, can weaken the immune system, hypnosis can also be used to help reduce the patient's negative thoughts. One technique is to have the patient describe a place that he or she considers to be peaceful and beautiful. It may be a tropical island, a waterfall, a rolling plain or his or her own backyard.

Under hypnosis, the patient would be asked to imagine being in this beautiful place, feeling very calm and healthy, enjoying good health. Post-hypnotic suggestions would help the patient to mentally "return" to this wonderful place several times a day. This helps to drive some of the negative, fearful thoughts that have been harming the immune system from the patient's mind.

Patients can also be taught relaxation techniques, and can then be hypnotized. While hypnotized, they can be given post-hypnotic suggestions telling them that when they feel themselves slipping into negativity, fear or anger, they will automatically enter into the relaxed states they achieved while practicing the relaxation techniques. In other words, the hypnotic suggestions will direct their minds from negative feelings toward the calm, relaxed state.

Some hypnotists may attempt to change their patient's physiology. They may suggest, for example, that cancer is actually shrinking. There are no studies showing that this works, although it is related to what one attempts to achieve in biofeedback.

There is no agreed-upon length of time before hypnosis brings results, if any are to be found. Several factors affect the length of treatment: how open to hypnotizing the client is, the rapport developed between the hypnotist and the client and the severity of the problem. Many people have been helped in just one session. For some, several sessions are required.

Nutritional therapy

Food has been considered a medicine throughout the ages. However, as drugs and surgeries came to dominate medicine, the idea that food had much value—beyond that of filling the belly and providing calories—fell into disrepute. Even as vitamins and minerals were "discovered" during the past century, it was felt that they were only good for preventing overt vitamin deficiency diseases, such as scurvy, rickets or beriberi.

Fortunately, the past several decades have seen an outpouring of evidence indicating that foods and certain substances in them do have medicinal value, and can also go a long way toward preventing many illnesses. The past 10 or 20 years have seen the discovery of many previously unknown food substances (called "phytochemicals") that appear to strengthen the immune system and help to prevent a wide variety of diseases. Some of the vitamins, minerals and other substances that do this include:

- *Beta carotene* is the "plant form" of vitamin A, which may prevent cancers of the breast, mouth, colon, rectum, bladder, stomach, esophagus, cervix and lungs. It also guards against heart disease and stroke, and slows the appearance of the signs of aging. The vitamin's many "powers" come from its ability to prevent oxidation and quench free radicals. Although two recent (1996) studies have questioned the value of beta carotene, hundreds of other studies have shown positive results. Without doubt, beta carotene and the other carotenes are superb antioxidants and free-radical quenchers. They have shown beneficial effects in laboratory and animal studies, and are included in most nutritional and anti-aging programs.

- *Folic acid* is a member of the B-family of vitamins, which may help to prevent cervical cancer. It has been proven to reduce the incidence of certain birth defects of the spine if taken by pregnant women at the time of conception and through at least the first trimester. Folic acid helps to ward off heart disease by counteracting the effects of homocysteine, an amino acid metabolite (byproduct) that can damage the walls of the vital coronary arteries.

- *Niacin* may help to prevent heart attacks by lowering the total cholesterol and the LDL ("bad") cholesterol.

- *Vitamin C* appears to strengthen the immune system and guard against heart disease by helping to strip cholesterol from the artery walls. It also helps to regulate the liver's production of cholesterol, protect cells from the potentially cancer-causing effects of oxidation, relieve the symptoms of asthma, improve the motility of the phagocytic cells of the immune system and perform many other health-enhancing duties in the body.

- *Magnesium* can help prevent the unnecessary blood clots that trigger heart attacks, lower the total cholesterol and harmful LDL cholesterol while raising the helpful HDL cholesterol, effectively treat certain heart irregularities, lower blood pressure and even increase the chances of surviving a heart attack.

- *Calcium* helps to keep the bones and teeth strong, and the blood pressure at proper levels. This mineral also lowers the risk of cancer of the colon.
- The mineral *selenium* is an antioxidant and works with vitamins A, C and E to prevent the oxidative damage to the body that can cause heart attacks and cancer. Selenium boosts vitamin E, making the vitamin more effective.
- The *ajoene* found in garlic is a potent blood thinner and guards against heart disease and stroke. Also, garlic's *allicin* is a natural antibiotic.
- *Capsaicin,* found in hot chili peppers, may help to clear away mucus blocking the breathing tubes of people suffering from respiratory ailments. Surprisingly enough, this "hot stuff" may also protect against stomach ulcers, and is used in anti-pain ointments. One of these ointments is used for the severe pain that follows attacks of "shingles" (*Herpes Zoster*).
- The *ellagic acid* found in cherries, strawberries and grapes may protect healthy cells from certain cancer-causing carcinogens.
- The *indoles,* which are found in broccoli, cabbage and other members of the "crucifer" family of vegetables, protect against cancer.
- *Lycopene,* which is found in watermelon, pink grapefruit and tomatoes, may help to prevent cancers of the prostate, bladder, colon and cervix.
- The *phenols,* found in fruit, garlic and green tea, apparently protect against heart disease and cancer, and have antiviral properties.

The nutritional healer uses a variety of vitamins, minerals, amino acids, phytochemicals and other substances to prevent and treat disease. Medical doctors, chiropractors, naturopaths, Ayurvedic healers and others may use nutritional therapy in their practices.

When selecting a nutritional healer, remember that there is no widely recognized school of nutritional therapy, no standards or agreed-upon training for nutritional healers. Some nutritional healers are licensed physicians with a special interest in nutrition. Others are naturopathic physicians, chiropractors or homeopaths. Still others may not have completed any approved training and are not licensed or certified at all. Only Registered Dietitians receive a standardized nutritional education and must pass an examination. Registered Dietitians, however, tend to be conservative in their recommendations.

Oriental medicine

Also called traditional Chinese medicine, Oriental medicine is an ancient and comprehensive system that incorporates acupuncture, herbology, nutrition and other disciplines.

The philosophical underpinnings of Oriental medicine focus on two opposing yet balancing forces called *yin* and *yang*. The female yin is dark and cold, while the male yang is light and hot. If yin and yang become unbalanced within the body, disease will arise. The *chi*, or life energy that flows through the body's meridians, is primarily yang in character. The chi must be kept flowing evenly throughout the body, for a lack of chi in any part of the body, or an excess, can lead to disease.

Oriental medicine further classifies body organs according to the Five Phase Theory.

1. The heart is the yin organ and the small intestine the yang organ, related to fire.
2. The spleen is the yin organ and the stomach the yang organ, related to earth.
3. The lungs are the yin organ and the large intestine the yang organ, related to metal.
4. The kidney is the yin organ and the bladder the yang organ, related to water.
5. The liver is the yin organ and the gallbladder the yang organ, related to wood.

Not only must yin and yang be balanced, but the relationships between fire, earth, metal, water and wood must also be harmonious.

In making a diagnosis, the Oriental medicine doctor will ask many questions about the patient's symptoms, personal and family history, appetite, bowel habits and other issues. He or she will study the patient's skin, tongue, eyes, fingernails and other parts of the body, as well as the urine and stool. He or she will also listen to the sounds made by the patient's speaking voice, breathing and bowels, and will pay careful attention to the pulse. Rather than looking for the "germ" that may have caused the disease, the doctor searches for the cause of the disharmony within the patient that allowed disease to arise.

Having found the cause of disharmony, the Oriental medicine doctor uses herbs, acupuncture, massage, nutrition and other means to help the patient. Diet plays an important role in Oriental medicine. Foods are selected depending upon their flavors, organic actions and other qualities, including energies. There are five food energies: hot, warm, neutral, cool and cold. (The energy has to do with the quality of the food, not its temperature. For example, foods with "hot" energy, such as ginger and black pepper, increase the sensation of heat in the body, even when eaten cold.)

Because Oriental medicine stresses the value of prevention, rather than waiting until disease is full blown and damaging, the practitioner will also spend time educating the patient, so as to prevent a further breakdown of bodily harmony.

Psychoneuroimmunology

Psychoneuroimmunology (psycho-neuro-immune-ology) is simply the modern name for what has commonly been called "positive thinking." This new branch of medical science studies the effect of the mind (*psyche*) upon the brain (*neuro*) and the immune system.

The idea that unhappy, negative people tend to be less healthy is an ancient one, but could never be proven. Western medicine turned a deaf ear to the concept, firmly arguing that the human mind and body were absolutely separate entities, that what happened in one had no influence on the other.

The strict separation of mind and body was attacked with the development of the "Type A, B and C Personality" concept in the 1960s and 70s. This concept argued that there were three personality types. The Type As were hard-driving, often angry and unhappy people who tended to develop ulcers and heart disease. Type Cs were quiet, introspective, often frustrated people who swallowed their anger and were at greater risk of cancer. Both As and Cs had many negative, unhappy thoughts floating around in their minds, and these thoughts predisposed them to their characteristic diseases. The third type, the Type Bs, were in the middle—not too hard-driving, not too hard on themselves, praising themselves for their successes and accepting their failures. The Bs were less likely to develop the ulcers, heart disease and cancer that afflicted the As and Cs.

Although the Type A, B and C theory has been criticized and revised, it has also opened the door to "reconnecting" the mind and body and recognizing that thoughts can influence health, for better or worse. With modern laboratory instruments and techniques, we can show that thoughts are "translated" by the body in ways that encourage health or disease. In a landmark study conducted at UCLA, a group of actors were told to act out happy and sad scenes. These were method actors who tried to "become" the people they were portraying and to actually feel just as happy or sad as their characters were supposed to be. The researchers found that when the actors were acting happy, the immunoglobulin A (IgA) in their mouths increased, indicating that their immune systems had grown stronger. But when they pretended to be sad, their immune systems weakened perceptibly and the IgA decreased. Here was proof that mind and body are intimately connected, that thoughts in the head are converted into chemical or other kinds of messages that travel throughout the body, encouraging health or disease (depending upon whether the original thoughts are positive or negative.)

In a sense, negative thoughts are "germs" that weaken the immune system and other parts of the body, creating conditions that encourage disease. Positive thoughts are "medicines" that strengthen the body's natural resistance to disease and innate healing powers.

Psychoneuroimmunology seeks to harness the tremendous power of the human mind for the better. To help them replace negative thoughts with their positive counterparts, patients are instructed to repeat short, positive statements called *affirmations* over and over throughout the day, out loud and to themselves.

Although the mind/body connection is an ancient concept, the modern discipline of psychoneuroimmunology is less than 20 years old. There is no school or licensing for this art, which may be practiced by physicians, chiropractors, naturopaths and other healers. Psychoneuroimmunology is related to many other healing arts, including guided imagery and hypnosis.

For more on affirmations and psychoneuroimmunology, see two of our other books, *Beyond Positive Thinking* (Hay House, 1991) and *Immune For Life* (Prima, 1989).

Reflexology

Reflexology, the application of pressure to the feet, helps to relieve tension, improves the circulation, stimulates the nerves and normalizes the functioning of the organs and glands through a series of pressures, stretches and general movements of the feet.

Reflexology is an ancient healing art that has antecedents in many massage techniques practiced in cultures around the world. The modern art of reflexology was developed by Dr. William Fitzgerald of Connecticut in the early 1900s.

According to the theory developed by Dr. Fitzgerald, the body is divided into 10 longitudinal zones running up and down the body. Each zone runs from one toe all the way up the body, and then down an arm to the corresponding finger. Thus, a zone runs from the left big toe up the center of the body to the head, and then down the left arm to the thumb. The zones are numbered one through five on the right, and one through five on the left. Applying pressure in one part of a zone can relieve pain in another part of the same zone. The theory was later refined to include three latitudinal zones that cut across the body lengthwise: one at the shoulders, one at the waist and one at the bottom of the pelvis. There are three corresponding "lengthwise" zones on the feet. With the body divided into zones, all the organs, bones and other body parts can be precisely "mapped out."

This mapping of the body is important, for it is believed that there is a corresponding pattern of "reflex" areas on the feet and hands. That is, if the kidneys are in zones two and three on the left and right, there are corresponding kidney reflex points in zones two and three of the feet. Furthermore, manipulating the kidney zones in the feet is believed to help heal diseases of the kidneys.

Thus, the reflexologist treats disease by manipulating the proper reflex points on the feet. (The hands are used to a lesser extent.) As there is no accepted school or licensing for reflexology, methods of diagnosis and treatment may vary from practitioner to practitioner.

Water therapy

Water therapy is an ancient form of treatment that emerged in its modern form in Europe in the early 1800s. The therapy uses hot and cold water, ice and steam to prevent and treat a variety of ailments. The therapy is based on the theory that stimulating the body with water can change its energies in specific ways.

Water is believed to improve the circulation, help to detoxify the body, increase energy, restore circulation, cool a fevered body or warm a chilled one, improve digestion, act as a sedative, cleanse and purify, encourage perspiration, help flush out excess fluids, encourage elimination, expel unhealthful substances from the stomach and relieve some forms of pain and cramps.

Water is used as a liquid, as steam and as ice. It may be applied locally or to the entire body via full body showers and baths, sitz baths (that bathe everything from the perianal area upwards to the groin), hot and cold compresses, friction rubs, hot blanket packs, wet sheet wraps, saunas and other techniques.

Water therapists are not licensed, and there are no educational requirements necessary to become one. Thus, the educational backgrounds and approaches to healing will vary.

Other exciting approaches

In addition to the many well-defined and well-rounded alternative therapies discussed above, there are numerous other intriguing methods of fighting disease. I've called them "other exciting approaches" because they do not fit into any of the standard categories.

Some of them, including Revici Therapy for cancer, are highly controversial. Some, like Moerman's anticancer diet, are designed for specific diseases, while others, including chelation therapy, have multiple applications. Some approaches, such as Biostim to treat AIDS, are new responses to a "young" disease. Others, such as having sex to relieve some forms of arthritis pain, are based on older theories.

Some therapies, like music healing, naturopathy and shiatsu, are long-standing healing arts that emphasize treating the entire body. Let's take a brief look at these three approaches.

Music healing combines relaxation techniques, guided psychological "searching" and the body's physical response to music in order to help the body heal itself. The music healer serves as an educator and facilitator, rather than as a "doctor."

The music healer takes the same approach to all diseases and conditions. Since most forms of modern music healing are based on the principles of Oriental medicine, musical selections will be chosen specifically to restore the flow of *chi* (energy) in the afflicted areas.

A typical session begins with the healer and client discussing the client's problems, musical background and tastes. Then the client sits in a comfortable chair or lies on a couch as the music is played.

When helping an asthmatic, for example, the first selection may be Chinese music designed to restore the yin/yang balance of the lungs and kidneys and the flow of chi in the lungs. (See more about these terms in the discussion of Oriental medicine in this introduction.) Various types of music will follow, depending upon the client's tastes and the practitioner's goals. Listening to the music, the client slips into a dream-like state that has been compared to hypnosis, or described as being "just like before you go to sleep." Now the music healer asks the client to describe what he or she is "seeing" or what emotions he or she is feeling. With minimal interruptions and only gentle guidance, the therapist guides the client through these "dreams," looking for troublesome images that may be causing or worsening the client's disease. If any are found, the client is referred to a psychologist or therapist.

Although they do not have standard protocols for treating disease, many music therapists will recommend one to six visits. Each visit lasts about two hours, with 45 minutes devoted to listening to the music. In addition, clients are urged to listen to music at home for at least 15 minutes every day. Because there are no educational or licensing requirements necessary to become a music healer, the treatment may vary from practitioner to practitioner.

Naturopathy, also known as naturopathic or "natural" medicine, traces its philosophic roots back to the Greek physician Hippocrates, who believed that all diseases have natural causes. Like Ayurveda and Oriental medicine, naturopathy is based on the belief that the body has powerful, innate healing powers that should be encouraged, rather than suppressed by powerful drugs. Thus, the healer should first look beyond the symptoms for the root cause of the problem, then help the body heal itself.

To the naturopath, the symptoms of disease are signs that the body is trying to heal itself. A fever, for example, may indicate that the body is attempting to "burn up" bacteria that cannot tolerate high temperatures. The naturopath will search for and treat the underlying disease process that forced the body to resort to having a fever.

Rather than focusing on disease, however, naturopathy is concerned with the maintenance of health. To help promote health, the naturopathic physician should spend a great deal of time educating patients, stressing prevention of disease, and should always treat the entire person, not simply the part of the body that is ailing.

Although naturopaths may prescribe medications and perform minor surgeries, they prefer to use a wide variety of alternative therapies. These include nutrition, herbs, homeopathy, acupuncture, spinal manipulation, stress reduction, lifestyle modification, hydrotherapy, ultrasound, heat therapy, exercise, massage and body work, biofeedback and, of course, health education.

Naturopaths are licensed in many states, where they act as general practitioners or family doctors trained in natural medicine. In order to earn a Doctor of Naturopathic Medicine (N.D.) degree, one must graduate from a four-year course of study in naturopathy.

The Japanese art of *shiatsu* is a form of bodywork designed to improve the flow of energy and blood throughout the body. The practitioner applies pressure and manipulates the body along meridians (channels), as is done in acupuncture, in order to improve the flow of *chi* (energy). Chi will also flow from the practitioner to the patient during the therapy. There are many forms of shiatsu, some limiting themselves to manipulating the body, others encompassing diet and lifestyle as well.

When working with the patient's body, the practitioner uses various movements to attract chi to certain areas of the body (such as the lungs or kidney in asthmatic patients), or to disperse unmoving chi that has stagnated in an area of the body. The practitioner will pay special attention to various meridians or parts of the body, depending upon the patient's ailments.

The calming effects of shiatsu may help to relieve some symptoms of various diseases almost immediately. Ongoing treatments may also help to reduce the severity and frequency of future problems.

These "other exciting approaches" offer us a wealth of ideas. Add them to the existing therapies offered by the more standardized alternatives, plus the techniques of traditional Western medicine, and we have an abundance of powerful tools with which to fight disease and build optimal health.

Now that we've examined a few of the popular alternative therapies, let's see how they're used to treat many of the major diseases afflicting us today.

Chapter 1

Aging

Bernard Baruch, adviser to several presidents, once said that old age was always 15 years older than he. We commonly associate aging with an inevitable decline in physical and mental capabilities. When I was in medical school back in the 1950s, we were taught that certain laboratory blood values automatically changed with advancing age, indicating that the body was failing. For example, two tests that measure the ability of the kidneys to excrete protein are called the BUN (blood urea nitrogen) and the serum creatinine. They're both "supposed" to drift upwards with age, indicating kidney impairment.

I believed that—until I began seeing "old" people with "young" BUN and serum creatinine levels. Although these people were old in years, their bodies and minds were relatively young. Recently, we've learned that there are two "ages": The chronological age, or number of years since birth, and the biological age, also called the functional or physiological age. The biological age is the objective measurement of a person's health status, independent of his or her birth date.

Some people are older than their biological ages, others are younger. The goal is to slow down the biological aging, which is the one that really counts. Norman Vincent Peale, who wrote many books on the power of positive thinking, was a good example of slow biological aging. At 95, he traveled around the country, teaching positivity. He died in his home in New York City at 96, active until the very end.

I think of aging as an ongoing process that gradually reduces the number of healthy cells in the body, primarily through oxidation and free radical damage. As the number of healthy cells in each organ falls, the body is less able to respond to challenges, such as viruses. Eventually, losing healthy cells and assaulted by challenges it can no longer master, the body fails. Serious illness and premature death are the unhappy consequences.

Aging has less to do with counting years than with maintaining the number of healthy cells in the body. Each organ system that contributes to health will be strong as long as we keep its cells healthy and revitalize those that are weakening.

Aging statistics

The only way to avoid chronological aging is to die young. However, with the great advances in hygiene and medical technology, we're living longer than ever. In fact, with the Baby Boomer generation (children born between 1946 and 1964) approaching its fifth decade, we'll soon have more "old" people than ever. The challenge is to keep people biologically young, even as they age chronologically.

Signs and symptoms

- Decline in memory.
- General loss of muscular strength.
- Decline of vision.
- Loss of hearing.
- Thinning and graying of the hair.
- Increased susceptibility to infections.
- Greater risk of osteoarthritis, diabetes, cancer and other diseases.
- Decrease in cardiac output, meaning that one cannot perform aerobic activities as well as before.
- Thinning of the bones (osteoporosis).
- Loss of lean body mass with an increase in body fat.
- Decrease in dexterity of the extremities.
- Decrease in height as spaces between the spinal discs narrow and the muscles holding the head up begin to weaken.

There are many more signs and symptoms associated with aging. The key point I'd like to make is that you should not check the birthdate on your driver's license to see if you're getting older. Instead, consider your mental and physical functioning. Satchel Paige, the great baseball pitcher, explained it perfectly when he asked, "How old would you be if you didn't know how old you was?"

Possible causes

One of the major aging hypotheses, and the one to which I subscribe, is the "Oxidation and Free Radical Theory of Aging." This theory argues that aging is the result of accumulated cellular damage caused by free radicals and oxidation. In other words, our mental and physical abilities are buried under piles of metabolic trash.

Oxidation is the reaction between oxygen and other substances in the body; it's a naturally occurring event. Oxygen is only supposed to interact with certain substances in the body, such as red blood cells. The problem arises when oxygen dallies with forbidden substances.

If you leave a piece of uncovered metal in your backyard, it will rust. In a very loose sense, that's what happens when oxygen reacts with the "forbidden" parts of the body; they become "rusty" and unable to function properly. When too many parts of a cell "rust," the cell weakens. And when too many cells "rust," entire organs can falter.

Naturally, the body has built-in antioxidants, such as SOD (superoxide dismutase), catalase and glutathione peroxidase, which are designed to "keep an eye on" oxygen, preventing promiscuous reactions that can damage the body. Unfortunately, in many cases the antioxidants are not strong enough to prevent the damaging oxidation reactions. Oxidation damage accumulates with time, eventually crippling body cells and weakening entire organs and body systems.

Free radicals are naturally occurring substances in the body; they are "unbalanced" molecules driven to balance themselves by exchanging electrons with other substances in the body. They can't be unbalanced; they must interact with something immediately. Free radicals don't care if "forcing themselves" on an unwilling passerby destroys other molecules, damages DNA, injures the lining of the coronary arteries, leaves a pile of "trash" behind or otherwise damages the body. All they know is that they want to be balanced right now.

Since the body does not have a central heating system, every cell must create it's own energy. That process causes the formation of free radicals. In addition, inflammation due to chronic infection and other normal body processes can lead to the formation of free radicals. Outside sources, such as cigarette smoke, radiation, ultraviolet radiation from the sun, thousands of chemicals in the environment, smog and oxygen (the major source of free radicals) contribute to our load of these unbalanced molecules.

The body has its own array of free radical quenchers to help prevent the unbalanced substances from damaging the body, but natural defenses are apparently not enough to entirely stamp them out. So free radical damage accumulates and the body slowly weakens.

The way to slow down the aging process, therefore, is to help the body control oxidation and quench the free radicals before too much damage is done.

Standard medical treatment

There is no standard Western medical treatment for biological aging. Instead, physicians attempt to treat some of its "symptoms" (such as the hearing loss often associated with aging).

Now let's take a look at some of the many alternative treatments for biological aging. These are not all the possible treatments, for there are too many to investigate in a single chapter. Reading through the alternatives, however, will give you an idea of the many possibilities. This discussion will omit surgery and other cosmetic ways of looking younger. While I'm not necessarily against them, they are not what I mean by slowing biological aging, which takes place on a molecular level. I'm primarily interested in ways of slowing the mental deterioration, degenerative diseases and general loss of energy associated with biological aging.

There's apparently nothing we can do to extend our *lifespan*, which is the maximum number of years that humans are meant to live. (Maximum lifespan is estimated to be 115 to 120 years.) What we can do, however, is to increase the average *life expectancy,* which is the actual number of years that the average person lives. (The life expectancy was about 50 years in 1900. It's roughly 75 years now.)

We'd also like to halt or slow the serious decline of mental and physical health that plagues so many of us in the last 10, 20 or 30 years of life. The goal, as French writer and moralist François Duc de La Rochefoucauld explained, is "to die as young as possible and as late as possible." In other words, we want to live young and healthy to a very old age, full of vim and vigor to the very end.

The information on alternative treatments is meant for educational purposes only. I am not endorsing any treatment or suggesting that you see any alternative practitioner. See your physician before embarking on any anti-aging program, or if you feel ill in any way.

Herbal medicine

There are no herbs that can prevent aging, although some may be used to deal with certain common problems associated with aging, such as insomnia, depression and declining mental facilities. These herbs may be recommended for insomnia:

- Hops (*Humulus lupulus*).
- Jamaican dogwood (*Piscidia erythrina*).
- Passion flower (*Passiflora incarnata*).
- Wild lettuce (*Lactuca virosa*).

Herbs typically used for depression include:

- Basil (*Ocimum basilicum*).
- Borage (*Borago officinalis*).
- Damiana (*Turnera aphrodisiaca*).
- Gentian (*Gentiana lutea*).
- Mugwort (*Artemisia vulgaris*).
- Oats (*Avena sativa*).
- Rue (*Ruta graveolens*).

- St. John's Wort (*Hypericum perforatum*).
- Vervain (*Verbena officinalis*).
- Wormwood (*Artemisia absinthum*).

These herbs may be suggested as an aid to declining mental facilities:

- Amalaki (*Emblica officinalis*).
- Goto kola (*Centella asiatica*).
- Purple sage (*Salvia officinalis purpurea*).

Nutritional therapy

No one can say exactly which nutrients slow the aging process because we don't know exactly why we age. However, one of the major theories of aging, the "Oxidation and Free Radical Theory," argues that aging is the result of accumulated cellular damage caused by free radicals and oxidation. In other words, our mental and physical abilities are buried under piles of metabolic trash caused by oxidation and free radicals.

Using this theory, many nutritional healers recommend the antioxidants and free radical scavengers found in foods and supplements. The antioxidants are a large "family" of substances that "patrol" the body, preventing the oxidants from "rusting" cells and tissue and "dousing" free radicals before they can grab electrons that are needed elsewhere. Many vitamins, minerals, enzymes and other substances have antioxidant or free radical quenching properties, including:

- *Beta carotene*, the "plant form" of vitamin A, which is found in yellow, orange and dark green leafy vegetables such as carrots, spinach, collard greens, mangoes, broccoli and other foods. Almost all of us who are experts in the field of anti-aging medicine believe that the powerful antioxidant and free radical properties of beta carotene (and the other carotenes) slow the aging process and the onset of associated degenerative diseases. Despite recent studies questioning the vitamin's efficacy against cancer, I continue to take beta carotene myself and recommend it to my patients as part of my anti-aging program.
- *Vitamin C*, which is found in green peppers, broccoli, strawberries, spinach, citrus fruits and other foods.
- *Vitamin E*, also known as *tocopherol*, which is found in soybeans, vegetable oils, nuts and other foods.
- *Selenium*, which is a mineral found in whole grains, poultry, meat and fish, and in smaller, variable amounts in vegetables and fruits.

- *Glutathione*, which deactivates free radicals and is found in watermelon, asparagus, avocado, strawberries, oranges, squash, broccoli and other foods.
- *Lycopene*, which is a more recently recognized antioxidant that some researchers believe is more powerful than beta carotene. It is found in tomatoes, watermelon and other foods.
- *Quercetin*, which is a powerful antioxidant and member of the bioflavonoid family, found in many fruits and vegetables, including red and yellow oranges, broccoli, cabbage and Brussels sprouts.
- *Omega-3 fatty acids*, which are found in salmon, mackerel and other fish, help to reduce the incidence of heart attacks, arthritis and other age-related diseases.

The recommended doses may vary from practitioner to practitioner. Other foods that contain large amounts of antioxidants include garlic, onions, cantaloupe and chili peppers.

Here are some other nutritional anti-aging techniques emerging from laboratories and being tested or put into practice by physicians and healers around the world. The science of anti-aging is new, so there hasn't been time to gather long-term data on all of the approaches. However, many show promise and should soon be helping us to remain healthy and vital as we move into our later years.

Acetyl L-carnitine. One of the major problems associated with biological aging is the loss of memory and mental acuity. We call this unhappy process age-associated memory impairment (AAMI). Generally speaking, we lose more than 1 percent of the brain cells called *neurons* every year from age 30 on, thanks to oxidation, free radicals and other processes.

Acetyl L-carnitine, which is closely related to the amino acid carnitine, is a natural compound that helps to keep these important neurons alive. In the past, the amino acid *carnitine* was used to help patients with certain heart and skeletal muscle problems. Doctors began to notice that the carnitine seemed to improve their elderly patients' moods and affects, and began to wonder what it or its relative, acetyl L-carnitine, might do for the brain.

In 1992, Italian researchers published a report on the effects of acetyl L-carnitine on healthy young people. Each was given either 1,500 milligrams (mg) of acetyl L-carnitine or a placebo daily. A month later, those given the acetyl L-carnitine enjoyed improved hand-to-eye coordination and reflexes, and had better attention levels. In some cases, the improvement was 300 percent to 400 percent.[1]

Another study looked at 20 people suffering from the regressive physical and mental symptoms of biological aging. After taking 1,500 mg of acetyl L-carnitine every day for six months, their cognitive abilities and motor skills improved, they were less depressed and more self-sufficient and their social lives had improved.[2] A similar study found that daily doses of 1,500 mg of acetyl L-carnitine led to significantly improved cognitive function, social and emotional behavior.[3]

Acetyl L-carnitine apparently works by helping to prevent cellular debris from "piling up." It is visible in the skin as "age spots." Acetyl L-carnitine helps to reduce a substance called *lipofuscin*, which has long been associated with age-related mental decline.[4] And as an antioxidant, acetyl L-carnitine helps to prevent other damage associated with aging.[5]

Acetyl L-carnitine also appears to increase the metabolism of *acetylcholine*, an important neurotransmitter for both the brain and muscles. A decrease of neurons in the brain that handle acetylcholine has been associated with Alzheimer's disease. Acetyl L-carnitine, in fact, is now being used in the treatment for Alzheimer's. A number of studies have shown that it improves memory and alertness in those with the disease.[6]

Although more studies are needed before conclusive statements can be made, acetyl L-carnitine appears to be a promising remedy for some of the mental deterioration associated with aging. At least one study with laboratory animals has shown that the substance can also help to increase life expectancy.

The largest amounts of the compound are found in beef, chicken, pork and bacon. Smaller amounts are found in whole milk, vegetables, fruits and grains. Acetyl L-carnitine is also available over-the-counter in health food stores.

Alpha-lipoic acid. Although *alpha-lipoic acid* has been known for more than four decades, only recently have medical researchers begun to appreciate its powerful effects against aging and disease. Alpha-lipoic acid is not a vitamin. It is made by the body, but because we don't make enough of it and because the natural production slows with aging, we must get more of it from supplements. So it's called a "conditionally essential" nutrient.

Alpha-lipoic acid has several key functions in the body, including:

- Chelating ("binding up") excess mercury, lead, copper, iron and other dangerous minerals, rendering them harmless so the body can safely excrete them. (Excess iron is deposited in the heart, liver, pancreas and other organs, where it can cause damage. That's why post-menopausal women should not take iron supplements, unless so prescribed by their physicians. Excess iron is not a problem for menstruating women, because they can expel excess iron with the menstrual flow.)
- Helping the body to extract energy from food.

• Acting as a powerful antioxidant.

It also has powerful anti-free radical properties, such as preventing the "cross linking" between DNA and proteins. This cross linking prevents the DNA from manufacturing new working "components" for the body, forcing it to churn out useless "waste products." Alpha-lipoic acid also helps to prevent free radicals from rupturing cellular lysosome membranes and allowing their poisonous materials to escape into the cells, thus damaging them.

Furthermore, alpha-lipoic acid works with other antioxidants, strengthening their combined results. For more than 20 years, European doctors have been using alpha-lipoic acid to treat certain forms of heart disease, control blood sugar and prevent diabetic damage to the eyes. It prevents glycation, which is the damage that elevated blood sugar does to proteins found in the eyes (causing cataracts, macular and retinal degeneration), kidneys (causing kidney failure), heart (causing heart attacks), brain (causing "brain attacks" or strokes), arteries (causing gangrene) and other body parts. Alpha-lipoic acid is currently being studied for use against Alzheimer's and Parkinson's diseases.

Although we have yet to establish the optimal "anti-aging" dosage for alpha-lipoic acid, 300 to 500 mg a day have long been used for diabetic nerve damage. Some researchers suggest that 250 mg per day is a safe and useful range for healthy adults interested in holding aging at bay.

In the United States, alpha-lipoic acid is sold in health food stores as Alpha Lipotene by NatureWorks in New York City.

Coenzyme Q10. Also called *ubiquinone* because it is ubiquitous (everywhere) in plants and animals, *coenzyme Q10* is a natural substance produced by the body. It works with the mitochondria, the "motors" of body cells, to extract energy from food. For years, in fact, cardiologists have been using Q10 to help increase the strength of heart contractions.

Some studies suggest that Q10 has other beneficial effects:

• Aiding in the reduction of high blood pressure.
• Aiding in the reversal of gum disease.
• Assisting in weight loss.
• Revitalizing the immune system and aiding in the fight against infections and biological aging.
• Serving as an adjunct in the treatment of cancer.
• Playing a role in life extension.

Most of these benefits come indirectly, as Q10 "revs up" the body on a molecular level. Coenzyme Q10 is available in health food stores.

DLPA. *Phenylalanine* (PA) is a natural amino acid found in foods, and used by the body for various purposes. Like other amino acids, PA comes in the "right-handed" and "left-handed" forms, which are mirror images of each other, just like your right and left hands. The right-handed form is called DPA while the left-handed form is known as LPA. A 50/50 mix of the two forms produces DLPA.

Exciting studies conducted in the 1970s and 80s showed that DLPA protects the endorphins, the natural morphine-like substances made by the body to block certain forms of pain and depression. By protecting the endorphins from "endorphin-eaters" within the body, DLPA helps to quell some forms of chronic back pain and arthritis, relieve premenstrual syndrome, lift certain types of depression and possibly even strengthen the immune system.

DLPA also increases the levels of a neurotransmitter called norepinephrine, a natural substance that decreases as we age. Lower levels of norepinephrine increase our susceptibility to fatigue, depression, pain and other problems associated with aging. By boosting norepinephrine, DLPA helps to slow the advance of our biological age, even as the chronological age moves ahead.

Phenylalanine is found in eggs, cheese, beef, chicken, fish and other foods. It is also available in health food stores.

Note: I recommend against taking DLPA during pregnancy or lactation. Pregnant or lactating women should not expose the fetus or newborn to anything except their normal diet. Anyone suffering from the genetic disease phenylketonuria (PKU), or on a phenylalanine-restricted diet, should not take DLPA. I do not recommend the use of DLPA for children under the age of 14. For more information on DLPA, go to your library and see our book DLPA to End Chronic Pain and Depression.

DMAE. *DMAE* (dimethylaminoethanol) has been used to treat chronic fatigue and depression. It also seems to help combat the mental deterioration and memory decay that are associated with biological aging, and acts as a mild central nervous system stimulant.

DMAE easily crosses through the blood-brain barrier into the brain, where it plays a role in the formation of a very important neurotransmitter called acetylcholine. DMAE helps to enhance the ability to scan the memory and retrieve information, an ability that often declines with age. It also helps to improve alertness and concentration, to moderate fatigue and depression and to increase energy.

Researchers are currently using doses of about 200 mg a day. Some elderly people have used as much as 1,800 mg per day without problems.

DMAE is available without a prescription. You can purchase it in health food stores as DMAE, or as Pure DMAE from En Guarde

Health Products of Van Nuys, Calif. (DMAE used to be sold as Deaner.)

Ginkgo biloba. *Ginkgo biloba* is made from the leaves of ginkgo trees, common to China. This unique substance contains terpenoid derivatives called ginkgolide A, ginkgolide B and ginkgolide C, plus bilobalide and proanthocyanidins.

We've known for a long time that ginkgo biloba increases the flow of blood to the brain, as well as to peripheral parts of the body such as the hands and feet. Ginkgo helps to prevent blood platelets from sticking together inappropriately to form potentially dangerous clots, and is also a free radical scavenger. In the brain, ginkgo assists in cell metabolism and in the functioning of certain neurotransmitters.

Animal studies have shown that ginkgo biloba extract can improve the memory process and the ability to retrieve what was learned.[7] Studies in healthy humans have shown that extracts of ginkgo biloba can enhance memory and alertness. I have given ginkgo to my patients to help treat the deterioration of memory, attention span and vigilance caused by a lack of oxygen to the brain (cerebral insufficiency).

I've also been using ginkgo myself, as part of my own anti-aging program. One of the beneficial side effects for me is that my previously cold hands and feet have warmed up. Generally, my patients take 50 to 60 mg, two to three times a day. Ginkgo biloba is available over-the-counter in health food stores.

Melatonin. Melatonin is a hormone produced by a tiny part of the brain called the *pineal gland*. When I was in medical school, we wondered about the pineal. We knew that it calcified with age, but we didn't know what it did or what substance it made. Now we know that the pineal gland produces melatonin.

Although melatonin is made in the pineal gland, it is only released when light fails to strike the retina; in other words, when it's dark or we're sleeping. Melatonin secretion is turned off by light, which means (for most of us) it is not released during the day.

One of melatonin's primary functions is to nudge us off to sleep. Melatonin also stimulates the immune system and helps the body to fight infections and cancer. There are hundreds of studies showing its beneficial effects against cancer, with a large number linking *low* melatonin levels to skin cancer (melanoma) and to breast cancer in women. Lack of melatonin has also been associated with immune dysfunction and depression, two important problems of aging.

In laboratory animals, melatonin has extended the lifespan and strengthened the immune system.[8] When middle-aged mice were given melatonin, their fur became thicker, their general health improved and they lived 20 percent longer than did the control mice.[9]

As we get older, melatonin secretion drops off. Indeed, the maximum amount of melatonin released into the bloodstream of the elderly is only half of that of young adults. This most likely is the reason older people have trouble sleeping at night and are tired during the day. Many researchers believe that we should look upon melatonin as one of the many biological markers of aging. They suggest that greater levels of melatonin in the body suggest that one is biologically younger. Melatonin is available in health food stores.

Warning: Melatonin should not be used if you have leukemia, Hodgkin's disease, multiple myeloma or lymphoma. Pregnant or lactating women or those who wish to become pregnant should consult with their physicians before taking melatonin.

When selecting a nutritional healer, remember that there is no widely recognized school of nutritional therapy and no standards or agreed-upon training for nutritional healers, except for Registered Dietitians, who tend to be very conservative in their approaches.

Oriental medicine

Practitioners of Oriental medicine do not consider aging to be a disease. Indeed, aging is an esteemed state and older people have traditionally been revered in Asian countries for their wisdom and understanding.

However, Oriental medicine recognizes that some disease states are more prevalent among the elderly. Thus, everyone is encouraged to remain as healthy as possible by exercising, eating a balanced diet, taking herbal and nutritional supplements, if necessary, and maintaining a positive state of mind. To counteract the onset of disease or declining health, practitioners may recommend the following:

Herbs and spices

Exactly which herbs and spices, and the amount of each, will depend upon the patient and his or her condition. Some herbal formulas that might be used to slow the aging process include *Lu Wei Ba Jing* and *Ren Shen Feng Wang Jaing*.

Diet

In addition to a healthy diet, the Oriental medicine practitioner may recommend these foods to counteract some of the problems that may be associated with aging:

- *Beetroot,* a sweet food that helps improve circulation.
- *Coconut* for premature aging. Coconut is a warm and sweet food that also helps with diabetes, fever and edema (swelling).

- *Lamb,* a sweet, warm food that increases energy, warms the intestines and tones the kidneys and spleen.
- *Maltose,* a warm, sweet food that increases energy and tones the lungs, spleen and stomach.
- *Potato,* a sweet food that increases energy, tones the spleen and counteracts inflammation.
- *Royal jelly,* a supplement that slows the aging process and counteracts fatigue.
- *Shiitake mushroom,* a sweet food that is good for fatigue and anemia.

A basic tenet of Oriental medicine is that there is no reason that one cannot remain healthy and active right up until the end of life, provided that one's chi is balanced and flowing through the body.

Other exciting approaches

Deprenyl (Eldepryl)

I first heard about deprenyl a few years ago from younger doctors who were taking 1 or 2 mg per day as an anti-aging measure. Their interest stirred mine, and I began looking into it. Developed by Professor Knoll of Hungary's Semmelweis University 35 years ago, deprenyl extends the maximum lifespan in animals and "sharpens" the brains of healthy animals, as well. It has been used to treat millions of people suffering from Parkinson's disease.

Parkinson's disease, which leaves its victims with a shuffling gait, tremors, poor coordination and other problems, appears to be a type of accelerated aging caused by the destruction of dopamine-handling neurons (brain cells). When 70 percent or so of these neurons have been lost, we develop Parkinson's. In most of us, there is a sharp decrease in these dopamine-using neurons of the brain starting by the age of 45, with continuing decreases as we age. It's believed that the age-associated decrease in dopamine is responsible for many of the symptoms of aging.

Deprenyl works by protecting a tiny part of the brain called the *substantia nigra,* which contains many dopamine-using neurons. This area of the brain is known to age rapidly. Deprenyl slows the degradation of neurotransmitters and raises the amount of dopamine released. This helps to ensure fine motor control, good immune-system functioning, motivation and possibly a strong sex drive.

Deprenyl has been used in this country since about 1990 for the treatment of Parkinson's disease (and has recently emerged as a promising medication for Alzheimer's disease). I've noticed that when I gave it to my Parkinson's patients—even those in their mid-80s—

they feel physically better and less depressed. In early studies, deprenyl has also extended the lifespan of elderly laboratory animals. And as an added bonus, the chemical configuration of deprenyl is very close to that of PEA (phenylethylamine), which may be one of the most important "chemicals of love."

Although more study is required, deprenyl appears to be a very safe substance when taken in low doses, 10 mg per day being the largest recommended dose. I take 5 mg a day myself as an anti-aging measure. Deprenyl, which is sold in the United States as Eldepryl, is available by prescription only.

DHEA

DHEA (dehydroepiandrosterone) is a natural hormone produced by the adrenal glands and may be the best biomarker of one's biological age. A fair amount of scientific evidence suggests that you can use a person's blood levels of DHEA to predict their odds of getting heart disease, diabetes, cancer and other degenerative diseases, as well as other problems associated with biological aging (the higher the DHEA level, the lower the odds of getting these diseases).

Various studies have linked high blood levels of DHEA to a lower risk of cancer, diabetes, cardiovascular disease, stroke, declining mental abilities, Alzheimer's disease and Parkinson's disease. But DHEA levels fall with age. And between the second and eighth decades of life, production of this hormone falls by 80 percent or more. Keeping DHEA levels high might be a way to delay many of the degenerative diseases and other problems associated with aging and, indeed, to slow the aging process itself.

DHEA, the immune system and cancer. The immune system tends to weaken as we age, increasing our susceptibility to a host of diseases ranging from infections to cancer. This decline is partially connected to a natural body substance called *cortisone*, which increases with age. Cortisone is a "stress hormone" which has the unfortunate effect of suppressing the immune system. DHEA appears to protect the immune system from cortisone-induced damage, thus helping to keep the protective T-cells, B-cells and the "germ-eating" macrophages in action. A stronger immune system will help keep the body healthier and "younger" into the later years. It will also help the body resist cancer, the number-two killer disease in this country. Laboratory studies have given evidence of DHEA's ability to prevent viral-induced breast cancer and chemically induced cancers of the colon, lung and skin.

The "killer T-cells," which are a vital part of the immune system's anti-cancer army, are "trained" by the thymus, a gland that sits behind the breast bone. The thymus shrinks with age, theoretically weakening the killer T-cells' ability to fight cancer. But DHEA slows the shrinkage of the thymus. Keeping the thymus and killer T-cells strong helps to ward off the onset of age-associated illnesses. DHEA is also believed to help keep the immune system strong by regulating the production of interleukon-2.

The DHEA-immune system hypothesis has been tested by deliberately using drugs to suppress the T-cells and B-cells in laboratory animals. Giving the animals DHEA revived their immune systems, despite the presence of the immune-suppressing drugs.[10] And in mice subjected to the potentially fatal brain disease called viral encephalitis, DHEA helped to slow the appearance of symptoms and reduced the death rate.[11]

DHEA and diabetes. Diabetes mellitus Type II is another disease associated with aging. Many of us become "resistant" to our own insulin, resulting in difficulty with storing and utilizing energy. Our bodies are often making enough insulin, but the body can't "get to it." This is one of the reasons both obesity and diabetes strike hard among the older population. In studies with laboratory animals, DHEA appeared to make the body more sensitive to insulin, thus restoring the body's ability to store and regulate energy and to control weight. DHEA seems to work by helping the liver to burn glucose (sugar) and slow its production of new glucose (gluconeogenesis).[12] Some physicians have reported that by giving their diabetic patients DHEA, they reduce the need for insulin injections.

DHEA and obesity. As we age, we tend to lose lean body tissue and to gain body fat. Studies have shown that even when laboratory animals are given unlimited access to food, DHEA helps them to lose weight.[13]

DHEA and the brain. The loss of brain cells due to biological aging can harm memory and the ability to think and reason. In animal studies, small amounts of DHEA both slowed the loss of brain cells and enhanced memory. The ability of mice to remember what they had just learned was improved, even if they were given the DHEA a full hour *after* the training session was over.

In examining the blood of 61 men in nursing homes, researchers found that those with the lower blood levels of DHEA-S (a close cousin of DHEA) were more likely to suffer organic brain damage and to need help with daily activities.[14] These and other findings suggest that DHEA and related compounds may be used to treat Alzheimer's, Parkinson's and other diseases affecting memory and the ability to think.

DHEA and life extension. As humans age, we slowly lose the ability to "stamp out" abnormal cells and to keep the body free of substances that are related to aging (such as serum amyloid-P). Thus, we're more likely to get cancer and other diseases common to old age. Through its ability to strengthen certain aspects of the immune system, DHEA may help us live longer. In at least one animal study, the substance increased lifespan by some 50 percent. Mice given DHEA aged slower, their coats maintaining youthful sleekness and color, while mice who did not receive DHEA began showing the signs of aging. Furthermore, some researchers have reported that men over the age of 50 who died (from all causes) had lower levels of DHEA. This suggests that DHEA, by strengthening the immune system, preventing the accumulation of cellular debris and through other means, may help to keep us living longer and healthier lives.

DHEA has been investigated in many laboratory and epidemiological (population) studies. More information is needed, but this is a promising anti-aging substance. DHEA is available by prescription only.

Diphenylhydantoin or Phenytoin (Dilantin)

Although diphenylhydantoin has been used as an anticonvulsant for many years, only during the past 15 or 20 years have we gradually become aware of its anti-aging properties.

Diphenylhydantoin is especially helpful in combating some of the mental deterioration associated with aging. It helps to:

- Improve concentration by stabilizing the electrical activity of the brain cells.
- Enhance learning ability.
- Strengthen the long-term memory.
- Improve intelligence and verbal performance.

Diphenylhydantoin has been shown to reduce the incidence of tumors and to increase the mean lifespan in mice by 250 percent.[15] We're not sure just how this substance works. It is believed that it extends the lifespan by making a part of the brain called the *hypothalamus* more sensitive to internal balancing signals within the body.[16] (Some researchers believe that the hypothalamus is the key to the body's biological clock.) The doses currently used for anti-aging research (25 to 50 mg per day) are much smaller than those used for epilepsy. Diphenylhydantoin is available by prescription only.

Note: Pregnant women or those with any kind of health condition should not be taking this medication unless under the supervision of a doctor.

Ergoloid mesylates (Hydergine)

I've been recommending *ergoloid mesylates* (EM) for many years to my patients who suffer from senility, confusion and loss of memory.

EM helps to slow, and possibly even reverse, some of the brain deficits associated with aging. It appears to:

- Help protect the brain from free radical damage.
- Reduce the deposition of lipofuscin (a pigment associated with aging) in the brain.
- Protect the brain against damage caused by lack of oxygen. This is especially helpful with strokes and other problems that may cut the flow of oxygen to the brain.
- Increase the flow of blood to the brain and enhance brain metabolism.
- Improve memory, learning and intelligence.

EM is derived from *ergot*, which has long been used to treat headaches. In Europe, EM in the form of the prescription drug Hydergine is routinely used to protect patients suffering from heart attacks, strokes, shock, drowning or other conditions that threaten to interfere with the flow of blood to their brains. By keeping the blood flowing, EM helps to keep the memory and ability to reason intact. In the United States, Hydergine has been approved for use in cases of senile dementia and poor circulation to the brain.

More than 20 European studies have shown that a daily dose of 4.5 to 6 mg of Hydergine significantly helps people suffering from confusion, loss of recent memory, forgetfulness, depression, poor motor skills and other symptoms of senile dementia. And when healthy young people were given 3 mg of the substance four times a day, they were significantly more alert and had improvement in cognitive function. EM is available by prescription only.

Gerovital (GH3)

Gerovital was devised by a Romanian doctor named Ana Aslan, for treating her elderly patients at a geriatric institute in Bucharest. Dr. Aslan "discovered" Gerovital accidentally. She was using injections of procaine, a local anesthetic, to relieve pain in her patients. To her surprise, the patients also reported feeling better overall, which suggested that the procaine was doing more than just blocking pain. She altered and augmented the formula, creating Gerovital-H3, commonly called GH3.

Procaine is believed to break down into two other substances inside the body, one of which is DEAE (diethylaminoethanol), a relative of DMAE. DEAE is also a component of chlorpromazine, which is used to treat cognitive dysfunction.

In animal studies, Dr. Aslan found that Gerovital increased the lifespan of female rats by 6 percent, and of male rats by 21 percent. At the Texas Research Institute of Mental Sciences in Houston, Gerovital increased the survival rate of mice by 33 percent over that of the control animals.

In addition, Gerovital relieves depression and arthritis, improves brain functioning, lowers blood pressure and reduces the levels of the immune-suppressing hormone cortisone. I have been using Gerovital as part of my anti-aging program for my patients in Beverly Hills. The results have ranged from good to tremendous.

Piracetam

Piracetam is perhaps the most important "smart pill" being used by healthy individuals who want to hold off the mental effects of aging, as well as those who already have cognitive difficulties. Piracetam seems to enhance the flow of information between the hemispheres (halves) of the brain, and to improve learning, attention span, understanding and motor mechanisms. Piracetam has been used to treat alcoholism, dyslexia, attention deficit disorder (ADD) and post-stroke problems. Among its many benefits, piracetam is reported to:

- Enhance reaction time.
- Serve as an antioxidant.
- Help prevent unnecessary blood clots that may lead to stroke, heart disease and other problems.
- Strengthen the immune system.
- Alleviate stress.
- Reduce fatigue.
- Improve the flow of blood to the brain.
- Reduce the buildup of the cellular waste (lipofuscin) in brain cells.
- Improve the brain's ability to use glucose (blood sugar) for energy.
- Speed recovery from trauma.
- Protect the brain from certain toxic chemicals.

Interesting studies back up many of the claims. For example, piracetam has helped to significantly improve the age-related dementia of patients in four double-blind, placebo-controlled studies. (Each of which included more than 100 patients.) And in a random, double-blind, placebo-controlled study, people given piracetam had markedly improved performance while driving in real-life traffic conditions.[17]

Piracetam has developed a good reputation in Europe and other parts of the world, although it is not available in the United States. Reports show that it is well-tolerated, but should not be used if you are taking other drugs, including ergot alkaloids (used for migraines), amphetamines, Hydergine and/or caffeine. It generally comes in 400 or 800 mg tablets. Many researchers believe that you should start with an "attack dose," or anywhere from 4 to 8 grams the first day, dropping to levels somewhere around 1,600 mg per day thereafter. Piracetam is marketed as Nootropil by Glaxco.

Advice to aging patients

Many of my patients have had success with the following program. I only use these general guidelines after reviewing a patient's personal and medical history, performing a thorough examination and evaluating the laboratory studies to make sure that the program will be beneficial. Please see your own physician before embarking on any treatment program for aging.

When discussing anti-aging with my patients, I draw a picture of a hand, labeling the thumb and each of the fingers with one of five points in the program. I do this because I want to emphasize, as strongly as possible, that they have within their hands the power to slow the deterioration of their minds and bodies. Each of the five points is important and should not be overlooked.

1. **Good nutrition.** Any anti-aging program must start with proper nutrition. Unless you need a special diet, the best is a low-fat, low-cholesterol diet rich in the complex carbohydrates found in vegetables and whole grains. I like to see my patients eating four to five servings of vegetables a day, at least two to three pieces of fruit, a couple of servings of whole grains, plus some legumes (peas, beans and lentils). I prefer a vegetarian diet myself, but have no quarrel with small amounts of very lean beef or chicken without skin (preferably from animals that were not filled with chemicals and hormones). Low-fat fish is excellent. Some high-fat fish, such as salmon, is also good because it contains the helpful omega-3 fatty acids.

2. **Supplements and medications.** I devise individualized anti-oxidant supplementation programs for my patients, including beta carotene, vitamin C, vitamin E, selenium and alpha-lipoic acid, Coenzyme Q10 and proanthocyanidins. In addition, I've found that Equimilk capsules, made by Biohealth of Irvine, Calif., help to strengthen the immune system. (Equimilk is derived from mare's milk from southern Austria.) As necessary, anti-aging supplements such as piracetam, deprenyl, DHEA, acetyl L-carnitine and the other substances discussed in this chapter can be helpful.

3. **Exercise.** It's vitally important to exercise as much as possible (with your doctor's consent) in order to keep your bones and muscles strong and to strengthen your heart. If all

you can do is walk, that's fine. I encourage my patients to walk 30 minutes a day, at least four days a week. Begin at a comfortable pace, working up, if possible, to two consecutive, 15-minute miles (the old Army pace). And because we tend to lose muscle mass as we age (many of us can hardly hold our backs straight and our heads up), it's very important to do some light weight training for the muscles of the upper body (arms, neck and back).

4. **Optimism and enthusiasm.** A positive, joyful mind-set enables us to handle stress, to get over the "bumps of life." And we know that enthusiastic, optimistic people are generally healthier that those who are unhappy and fear for the worst. Positive thoughts enhance the immune system and encourage us to do all the things necessary to stay young and healthy.

5. **Age with grace.** Although Cicero said that "old age must be resisted and its deficiencies restored," we must remember that with age comes change. We will all benefit by accepting the fact that we're not going to have the body of an 18-year-old forever, and that we all have to make concessions to time. Gypsy Rose Lee showed us how to accept aging with grace and humor when she said, *"I still have everything that I had 20 years ago—except now it's all lower."*

---

[1]   Lino, A., et al. Psycho-functional changes in attention and learning under the action of L-acetylcarnitine in 17 young subjects. A pilot study of its use in mental deterioration. *Clin Ter* (Italy), 149(6):569-73, June 1992.

[2]   Fiore, L., Rampello, L. L-acetylcarnitine attenuates the age-dependent increase of NNDA-sensitive glutamate receptors in rat hippocampus. *Acta Neurologica,* 11(5):346-50, 1989.

[3]   Cipolli, C., Chiari, G. Effects of L-acetylcarnitine on mental deterioration in the aged: Initial results. *Clin Ter,* 132(6 Suppl):479-510, 31 March 1990.

[4]   Amenta, F., et al. Reduced lipofuscin accumulation in senescent rat brain by long-term acetyl L-carnitine treatment. *Arch Gerontol Giatr* 1991; 9(2):147-153.

[5]   Geremia, E., et al. Antioxidant action of acetyl L-carnitine: in vitro study. *Med Si Res,* 1988; 16(13):699-700.

[6]   Cabrero, L., Cortes, B. Current treatment of Alzheimer's disease. *Cienc Med* (Spain) 9(3):82-87, 1992. Cazzato, G., et al. Long-term treatment with acetyl L-carnitine in patients suffering from the dementia of Alzheimer's type. *Neuro Psichiatr Sci Um* (Italy), 10(2):201-15, 1990.

[7]   Winter E. Effects of an extract of gingko biloba on learning and memory in mice. *Prama Biochem Behav,* 1991; 88:109-114.

[8]   Regelson, W., Pierpaoli, W. Melatonin: A rediscovered anti-tumor hormone? *Cancer Investig,* 5:379-385, 1987.

[9]   Maestroni, G.J., et al. Pineal melatonin, its fundamental immuno-regulatory role in aging and cancer. *Annls NY Acad Sci*, 521:140-8, 1988.

[10]   Rasmussen, K.R. Effects of dexamethasone and dehydroepiandrosterone in immuno-suppressed rats infected with Cryptosporidium parvum. *J Protozool*, 1991; 38(6):157S-159S.

[11]   Ben-Nathan, D., et al. Protection by dehydroepiandrosterone in mice infected with viral encephalitis. *Arch Virol*, 1991; 120(3-4):263-271.

[12]   McIntosh, M.K., Berdanier, C.D. Anti-obesity effects of dehydroepinendosterone are mediated by futile substrate cycling in hepatocytes of BHE/cdb rats. *J Nutr*, 1991; 121(12):2037-2034.

[13]   Cleary, M., Zisk, J. Anti-obesity effect of two different levels of dehydroepinandrosterone in lean and obese middle-aged female Zucker rats. *Int J Obes*, 1986;10(3):193-204. Mohan, P., et al. Effects of dehydroepinandrosterone treatment in rats with diet-induced obesity. *J Nutr*, 1990; 120(9):1103-1114.

[14]   Rudman, D., et al. Plasma dehydroepinandrosterone sulfate in nursing home men. *J Am Geriatr Soc*, 1990; 38(4):421-427.

[15]   Dilman, V.M., Anisimov, V.N. Effect of treatment with phenformin, diphenylhydantoin or L-dopa on lifespan and tumor incidence in C3H/Sn mice. *Gerontology*, 1980; 26:241-246.

[16]   Dilman, V., Dean, W. *The Neuroendocrine Theory Of Aging And Degenerative Disease*. Pensacola, Fla: The Center For Bio-Gerontology. 1992.

[17]   Schmidt, U., et al. Arbetis und Forschungsgemeinschaft fur Strassenverkehr und Verkehrssicherheit. *Pharmacopsychiatry* (Germany), 24(4):121-26, July 1991.

AIDS

A young man came to my office in 1982, complaining of fatigue. Within a few months he was hospitalized with pneumonia and a terrible anemia. Within a year, he wasted away and died. Only later did we realize that he had AIDS.

AIDS (Acquired Immune Deficiency Syndrome) is a powerful, puzzling disorder that saps one's ability to resist disease. AIDS cripples the immune system, leaving its victims to suffer from common and uncommon diseases that would normally be brushed aside by the body's defenses.

AIDS was first identified in the United States in 1981, when more than 100 cases were reported to the Centers for Disease Control. Today, AIDS is the number-one cause of death in the United States for people between the ages of 25 and 44. AIDS is not like other infectious diseases that quickly make their presence known. Instead, the virus may sit quietly for years. Then, for reasons not fully understood as of yet, it begins to "flex its muscles," damaging the immune system and prompting the fatigue, weight loss, fevers, decreased resistance to infection, swollen lymph nodes and other symptoms of the condition known as AIDS-Related Complex (ARC). The ARC may remain stable or even decrease for a while. Unfortunately, ARC eventually worsens to become a full-blown case of AIDS.

AIDS is caused by the Human Immunodeficiency Virus (HIV), which destroys the crucial T4-lymphocytes (T4-cells) that play such a major role in the body's defenses. HIV can also infect the macrophages, the giant "cell eaters" that engulf and destroy invading organisms. With the immune system crippled by HIV, one is unable to mount "routine" defenses against pneumonia, tuberculosis and other opportunistic infections that would normally be quelled quite easily. Second-rate infections such as pneumocystis pneumonia and Kaposi's sarcoma become major problems to the HIV-infected patient. The virus can also attack the nervous system, causing brain damage. AIDS is fatal not because the HIV is deadly, but because it strips us of our ability to defend ourselves.

Signs and symptoms

There are no signs or symptoms immediately upon infection with HIV; it may take months or years for the disease to make itself known. Early signs of ARC or AIDS may include:

- Fever.
- Unexplained weight loss.
- Fatigue.
- Diarrhea.
- Night sweats.
- Swollen lymph glands.
- Recurrent skin infections and mouth sores.
- Recurrent respiratory infections.

As the disease progresses, patients are likely to develop a rare form of cancer known as Kaposi's sarcoma, a type of pneumonia caused by Pneumocystis carinii, tuberculosis and/or other problems that can lead to death.

Possible causes

With but a few dissenting voices, the scientific community agrees that AIDS and ARC are caused by the HIV virus. No one knows exactly how or why the virus arose, although most believe that it originated in Africa. The virus is spread from person to person, but not by casual contact such as shaking hands. The contact must include an exchange of bodily fluids. This may occur with, for example:

- Intimate sexual contact.
- Sharing needles used to give injections (especially among intravenous drug users).
- Receiving an infusion of tainted blood (which puts one in intimate contact with a stranger, blood-to-blood).

HIV-infected mothers can pass the virus on to their unborn children. There is even a small possibility that infected patients can inadvertently pass the virus to hospital and laboratory workers who are exposed to their blood, urine and feces.

Standard medical treatment

Current drug treatments include:

- Azidothymidine (AZT), a medicine that can slow the reproduction of the HIV-1 virus in humans, but unfortunately is toxic and not well-tolerated by many patients.

- Dideoxyinosine (DDI), a medicine used in children and patients who cannot tolerate AZT.
- Zalcitabine (DDC), a medicine used in combination with AZT.

Other drugs are used or are being investigated for use in treating Kaposi's sarcoma, P. carinii pneumonia and other ailments associated with ARC and AIDS. Researchers are also working to develop a vaccine against the HIV. Besides medications, physicians recommend that AIDS or ARC patients stay physically active as long as possible and eat a "balanced" diet.

Now let's take a look at some of the many alternative treatments for AIDS. These are not all the possible therapies, for there are too many to investigate in a single chapter. Reading through these alternatives, however, will give you an idea of the many possibilities.

The information on alternative therapies is meant for educational purposes only. We are not endorsing any therapy or suggesting that you see any alternative practitioner. If you have or suspect that you have AIDS, see your physician.

Ayurvedic healing

Ayurvedic healing, a 5,000-year-old system from India, teaches that AIDS is a symptom of low *ojas*. Ojas is the body's *vigor*, the non-tangible essential energy of its vital secretions and reproductive system. It is centered in the heart but spread throughout the body. When the ojas drops low, the body is susceptible to infections, nervous disorders and degenerative diseases. When the ojas is gone, life is gone.

According to Ayurvedic healers, the body's store of ojas is depleted by worry, sorrow, overwork, anger, overindulgence in sex, stress, poor diet, overuse of drugs and other negative emotions, states and substances. Ojas also tends to diminish with age. Rebuilding ojas requires milk and other selected foods, meditation, herbs, a realignment of one's personal and sexual lifestyle and other strengthening practices.

Since ojas is tied to the Kapha (water) humor, low-ojas diseases such as AIDS are generally associated with excesses of the other two humors: Pitta (fire) and Vata (air). To rebalance the humors, the Pitta and Vata must be reduced.

Ojas is also tied to lifestyle. Thus, the Ayurvedic treatment for AIDS requires adopting a *sattvic* lifestyle, while lowering both the Pitta and Vata in order to rebalance the humors.

The sattvic lifestyle

Following a *sattvic* (harmonious) lifestyle helps to strengthen mind and body by purification. All harmful mental and emotional habits, such as pride, anger, gossip and worry, must be set aside. Instead, one should focus on truth, compassion and helping others. Meditation and yoga should be used to help in this pursuit.

Purifying the body requires breathing clean air, practicing soothing exercises, maintaining strict physical cleanliness, using herbs and adopting a vegetarian diet. All aspects of one's physical nature, including eating, sleeping and having sex, should be attended to, but not in excess. In addition, oils, massage, colors and gems should be used to open one's heart to the beauty of the world and to balance the aura.

Some specific measures to aid the ojas include:

- Drinking and eating milk, yogurt, almonds, sesame oil and sesame seeds.
- Taking herbs and tonics such as ashwagandha, bala, ginseng, solomon's seal and sarsaparilla.
- Reducing sexual activity or abstaining. Masturbation and anal sex should definitely be avoided, for they drain energy from the nervous system and sap the vitality.
- Wearing or otherwise utilizing gems such as yellow sapphires and diamonds. Yellow sapphires increase energy and ojas. Diamonds lower Vata and Pitta while increasing Kapha and ojas. Diamonds also confer protection against powerful physical diseases.
- Chanting mantras such as "Om" and "Shrim." "Om" increases ojas while energizing the body and mind. "Shrim" promotes general health and prosperity.

The pro-Kapha regimen

In addition to adopting the general, purifying sattvic lifestyle, the AIDS patient should strive to rebuild his Kapha (water) humor. Or perhaps it is more correct to say that he should work to lower the other humors, Pitta (fire) and Vata (air), allowing the three humors to return to balance.

Anti-Pitta (fire) measures are adopted to "cool" the body. The emphasis in the anti-Pitta regimen is on cooling, cleansing and moderating.

- The diet should be filled with raw foods and juices. The foods should be cool and dry, with many astringent, sweet and bitter-tasting foods. (See Chapter 8 for a further description of the anti-Pitta diet.)
- Herbs are used to strengthen the energy and mind, while aiding elimination and digestion. Herbs typically used include aloe, barberry, cumin, bala, saffron, licorice, marshmallow, sandalwood, rose and betony.

- Yoga and meditation are used to help one exchange fear and anger for calm positivity. "Om," "Som" and "Shrim" are among the mantras used to induce calm.
- Oils, such as coconut and sunflower, are used in massage. Sandalwood, henna and lotus may also be used as incense.
- Laxatives such as rhubarb and psyllium husks are used to help purify the body.
- Gems and colors are important to the anti-Pitta regimen. Jade, blue sapphire and other gems help to cool the body, as do the colors blue and green. Bright colors should be avoided.
- The overall lifestyle should include plenty of exposure to flowers, lakes and other beautiful environments. Cool breezes and water are encouraged, as are forgiveness and other positive attitudes.

To complete the treatment, an anti-Vata (air) regimen is incorporated with the anti-Pitta and pro-sattvic techniques. The anti-Vata therapy emphasizes warmth, calm, grounding and nurturing.

- The diet is based on salty, sour and sweet tastes. The food is warm and heavy, divided into many small meals. (See Chapter 8 for a further description of the anti-Vata diet.)
- Herbs, spices and salts are used to improve the digestion and elimination while strengthening the mind and increasing energy. Rock salt, garlic, ginger, bala, white musali, lycium berries, comfrey root, alamus, nutmeg and basil are among those used.
- Yoga and meditation are used to help calm and "ground" the patient, helping him or her exchange fear and anxiety for hope and optimism. "Ram," "hum" and "hrim" are among the mantras used to reduce fear.
- Oils and scents, such as sesame, almond, wintergreen and musk, are used in massages or incense.
- Licorice, sesame oil and other substances are used to induce purifying enemas. "Nasal therapy" with ginger, basil and other herbs may also be used in the purification process.
- Gems and colors are important to the anti-Vata regimen. Emeralds, rubies and jade are helpful, as are the colors yellow and orange. Avoid dark or very bright colors.

Combining the pro-sattvic with the anti-Vata (air) and anti-Pitta regimens requires a great deal of thought and care.

Herbal medicine

There is no herbal therapy specific to treating AIDS. Instead, herbalists may use these to help strengthen the body in general:

- Aloe vera *(Aloe vera)*.
- Astragalus *(Astragalus membranaceus)*.
- Burdock *(Arctium lappa)*.
- Chinese bitter melon *(Momordica charantia)*.
- Cleavers *(Galium aparine)*.
- Echinacea *(Echinacea angustifolia)*.
- Garlic *(Allium sativum)*.
- Huang Qi *(Astragalus membranaceus)*.
- Hyssop *(Hyssopus officinalis)*.
- Nettles *(Urtica dioica)*.
- Purple coneflower *(Echinacea spp.)*.
- St. John's Wort *(Hypericum perforatum)*.

A report of hyssop suggests that it may be especially useful in combating Kaposi's sarcoma, the cancer that afflicts so many AIDS victims. Test tube studies suggest that the herb *may* prove to have specific, anti-HIV properties. St. John's Wort is also being studied as a potential treatment for AIDS symptoms. In 1988, researchers at New York University noted that the herb appeared to help AIDS patients. The active ingredient in St. John's Wort is apparently hypericin.

Nutritional therapy

There are still few studies on the use of nutrition to treat AIDS and ARC. However, the information we have is encouraging, suggesting that foods and supplements can serve as adjuncts to other treatments.

In general, it is important for the AIDS and ARC patients to eat as nutritiously as possibly, for lack of even a single nutrient can further debilitate the immune system. To complicate the problem, the mere presence of the HIV and other infections can make it harder for the body to absorb nutrients from food, increasing the rate at which the body "uses up" the nutrients that it does have. Many AIDS and ARC patients are deficient in folic acid, thiamin, vitamin C, calcium, magnesium, selenium, zinc and other nutrients. Good nutrition is a must for AIDS and ARC patients to correct the deficiencies and help maintain the immune system.

Some studies have suggested that taking large doses of certain vitamins may be helpful. For example, when vitamin C and HIV-infected T-cells were mixed together in a petri dish, the reproduction of the infected cells was slowed.[1]

In another study, doses ranging from 20 to 200 grams of vitamin C per day were given to more than 250 patients who had tested positive for HIV. The patients were found to be less likely to develop the secondary infections associated with AIDS, and the loss of their vital T-cells was slowed or, in some cases, stopped.[2] In another study, patients were initially treated with very large doses of vitamin C, then given smaller doses. As a result, the "killer T-cells" became more active and Kaposi's sarcoma was suppressed.[3]

Coenzyme Q10, which is made by the body and is found in sardines, mackerel and other foods, has also helped AIDS and ARC patients, who tend to have low levels of Q10. When seven people with AIDS or ARC were given 200 mg of Q10 daily, five reported a lessening of their symptoms and had no opportunistic infections for the next four to seven months. The critical T4/T8 ratio, which is low in AIDS patients, improved in three of the five and normalized in a fourth patient.[4] The T4/T8 ratio compares the number of immune system cells called T4 cells ("helper cells") to the T8 cells ("suppressor cells"). A low ratio, which means there are fewer T4 helper cells to initiate the battle, indicates that the immune system is impaired. I like my patients to have a ratio of about two T4 cells for every one T8 cell.

Alpha-lipoic acid, a "conditionally essential nutrient" made by the body and found in foods, has also shown promise against AIDS. After being infected with HIV, certain important cells belonging to the immune system stop making an antioxidant called *glutathione*. Without this antioxidant protection, these immune system cells are easily weakened by oxidation, making the immune system even weaker. Although alpha-lipoic acid does not cure AIDS, it helps to prevent the oxidation damage to the immune-system cells, helping the body to resist the opportunistic infections that may kill AIDS victims.

When patients with HIV were given 150 milligrams (mg) of alpha-lipoic acid three times daily for two weeks, the immune systems grew stronger in 60 percent of the cases.[5] And in a laboratory study, alpha-lipoic acid prevented HIV from replicating itself. Although more studies are needed, it appears that alpha-lipoic acid may soon be an important weapon in the war against AIDS. (See Chapter 1 for more information on alpha-lipoic acid.)

Other nutrients that may help to stimulate the immune system include beta carotene, vitamins D and E, the amino acids arginine and cysteine and the omega-3 fatty acids found particularly in cold water fish such as salmon.

I have seen a surprising number of HIV-positive people who remain healthy. They credit their good health to a good diet, regular exercise and a positive outlook. Much remains to be learned about the disease, but we do know that what we eat can help to strengthen our immune system, our "doctor within" that plays a vital role in the defense against AIDS and all other diseases.

Psychoneuroimmunology

Psychoneuroimmunology is a science concerned with the mind/body connection. Mind/body healers use positive affirmations to counteract the negative thoughts that have been contributing to the symptoms of AIDS. Affirmations are typically brief, positive statements that focus on how well one feels and on how the disease is being conquered. An affirmation to strengthen the immune system might be worded as follows:

> *"My T-cells are mighty fortresses, safe and strong. My antibodies are 'guided missiles' speeding through my body, sweeping aside any dangers. All the parts of my immune system work together to keep me healthy."*

Patients might be given affirmations such as this to bolster their spirits:

> *"Every day is filled with great people to meet, exciting challenges to overcome and sights to savor. I look forward to bouncing out of bed in the morning and saying, 'Today is a great day!'"*

Patients may also be given affirmations for general health, such as:

> *"I enjoy radiant health, each and every day."*

For more on affirmations and psychoneuroimmunology, see two of our other books, *Beyond Positive Thinking* (Hay House, 1991) and *Immune For Life* (Prima, 1989).

Other exciting approaches

Antineoplaston therapy

Antineoplaston therapy, which was developed by Stanislaw Burzynski, M.D., Ph.D., is based on the principal that there is a second defensive system in the body, in addition to the immune system. This second system, the biochemical system, protects the body against defective or damaged cells.

The biochemical system includes small peptides and organic acids called *antineoplastons*, which reprogram damaged cells. The therapy consists of injections or oral doses of antineoplastons, which were originally made from compounds in human blood and urine. Today, however, they are "factory made" from existing chemicals.

Dr. Burzynski reports that antineoplaston therapy has benefited a small group of AIDS patients treated at the Burzynski Clinic in Houston. He says that their T4 cells (the immune system cells heavily damaged by the HIV virus) improved after four weeks of treatment, and he believes that the antineoplastons "reprogrammed" the genetic material in the HIV-infected cells.

Biostim

AIDS and ARC patients may suffer from a variety of viral, bacterial and fungal infections as their immune systems falter. Anything that helps to energize the immune system will thus be of help in treating AIDS and ARC. As its name indicates, Biostim is designed to "stimulate life" by strengthening the immune system. Although not a cure for AIDS, Biostim may be able to help the body fight off some of the infections associated with ARC and AIDS.

Made from an extract of bacteria, Biostim is reputed to boost the immune system's ability to defend the body against viral, bacterial and fungal infections. It has been used to strengthen the immune systems of cancer patients and to treat chronic bronchitis.

Patients typically take one Biostim tablet, containing 1 mg of the active bacterial extract, daily for eight days, then stop for three weeks. After continuing this cycle for three or four months, they are often able to stop taking the medication, for Biostim's immune-boosting properties are long-lasting. Animal and some human studies have shown that Biostim is generally well tolerated.

Note: People with autoimmune diseases (such as rheumatoid arthritis and multiple sclerosis) should not take Biostim. Neither should pregnant or lactating women, or children. The use of Biostim should be limited to short periods of time.

DHEA

DHEA (dehydroepiandrosterone) is a hormone made by the adrenal glands, which sit atop each of the kidneys. Considered by some to be the best "biomarker" (indicator) of age, DHEA is believed to protect against heart disease, cancer, diabetes, mental deterioration and many autoimmune diseases (such as rheumatoid arthritis). The hormone also increases one's resistance to the viral and bacterial infections that are so often associated with AIDS and ARC.

More importantly, studies have shown that DHEA can help to slow the reproduction of the HIV-1 virus, which is responsible for AIDS and ARC. Low levels of DHEA have been associated with advancement of HIV infection[6] and clinical trials of DHEA's effectiveness as an adjunct treatment for AIDS are currently being conducted.

Although more study is required before definitive statements can be made, DHEA may turn out to fight AIDS on two levels: by preventing the spread of the HIV virus within the body, and by helping to hold at bay the opportunistic infections associated with the disease.

Hyperforat

Hyperforat is based on hypericin, an extract from the herb known as St. John's Wort *(Hypericum perforatum)*. Although it has been used in Germany for several years, it has only recently begun to receive attention in the United States.

Hypericin is being scrutinized in laboratories because it appears to kill the HIV virus, as well as the viruses responsible for genital herpes and the flu. It also seems to increase energy, improve poor mental performance and elevate the mood. Available as tablets or as a liquid, Hyperforat is usually taken in 50 to 150 mg doses, two to three times a day.

Isoprinosine

Isoprinosine is a "combination" drug that appears to be able to strengthen the body's ability to fight off viral infections. Various studies have reported that isoprinosine slows the reproduction of the HIV, as well as the viruses responsible for or associated with Kaposi's sarcoma, herpes simplex, polio and the cold. Not only does the drug appear to slow the replication of certain viruses within the body, but it also seems to slow the rate at which viruses are "shed" into body secretions, which can then be passed on to others.

In a test of the drug's ability to help fight AIDS and ARC, homosexual men suffering from depressed immune systems were given either 3 grams of isoprinosine or a placebo on a daily basis. Four weeks later, the members of the isoprinosine group were more likely to feel better and to enjoy an improved clinical status than those in the placebo group. In another study involving 75 men, isoprinosine helped to reduce Kaposi's sarcoma lesions and restore weight in some men.

In 1989, the Scandinavian Isoprinosine Study Group reported that daily doses of isoprinosine could help to delay HIV infections from becoming ARC or full-blown AIDS.[7] The 831 patients involved in this double-blind study had all tested positive for HIV. They were divided into groups and given either 1 gram of isoprinosine or a placebo, three times a day for 21 weeks. Several times during the study, the men were examined and laboratory tests were performed. Only .5 percent of those who had received isoprinosine developed AIDS, compared to 4 percent of those who had taken the placebo. This suggests that the drug can delay the onset of AIDS in HIV-infected patients, although neither the optimal dose nor the duration of benefits is known.

Although no one is sure how isoprinosine delays AIDS or ARC, it may work by increasing the number of T-cells (which are debilitated by HIV), as well as their activity. Isoprinosine appears to have no serious side effects when taken by healthy people. Some authorities recommend taking isoprinosine on a "cycle" basis (that is, taking it for two months, then abstaining for the next two months before starting again).

Spiramycin

Similar to the common antibiotic erythromycin, spiramycin has been used for decades in France to treat bacterial infections. The drug kills penicillin-resistant bacteria and has been used to treat Legionnaire's Disease, rheumatic fever, dental plaque and other problems.

More recently, researchers have discovered that spiramycin can relieve the cryptosporidosis that may occur with AIDS. The cryptosporidial diarrhea, which may strike people with weakened immunity, can be devastating and deadly, especially for those with AIDS. (Healthy people also get the diarrhea, but their immune systems can defeat the virus that causes the problem.) Early studies show that spiramycin can reduce the severity of the diarrhea, but cannot cure it. The medicine is well-tolerated and apparently has few side effects.

Adult patients may take 1 gram of spiramycin, two to three times a day. The drug has been used in France since 1955, and its major side effects include nausea, vomiting, diarrhea and allergic reactions.

Advice to AIDS patients

Although many of my patients have had success with the following program, I only use the general guidelines discussed below after reviewing a patient's personal and medical history, performing a thorough examination and evaluating the laboratory studies to make sure that the program will be beneficial. Please see your own physician before embarking on any treatment program for AIDS.

The best treatment is prevention. By following these recommendations you can greatly reduce your chances of contracting HIV:

- If you are sexually active, maintain a monogamous sexual relationship.
- Insist upon knowing the "sexual history" of anyone with whom you have sex. Remember that they may not know they are harboring the HIV virus, which can be passed on to you.
- Use condoms for intercourse.
- Do not use intravenous drugs.
- Do not accept transfusions of blood or blood products that have not been properly screened.

If you have already been infected with HIV, don't give up hope. Several years ago, we were speaking at a health conference in Atlanta. Many young men there told us that they had been HIV-positive for years, but were almost symptom-free. When we asked how they remained so healthy, the answers they gave boiled down to a few basic principles:

- Explore all the alternative treatments and discuss their use with your physician.

- Take control of your treatment! This is one of the most important things you can do. Learning, making decisions and actively participating gives you a feeling of control that goes a long way toward combating the helplessness and hopeless that other patients feel.
- Eat the most nutritious diet possible. Fill up on the fresh vegetables, fruits, whole grains and other foods that strengthen the immune system.
- Discuss the use of vitamin, mineral and other supplements, especially large doses of alpha-lipoic acid and other antioxidants, with your physician. Because the demand for nutrients is high with AIDS and ARC, even the best diet may fall short.
- Exercise as often as possible.
- Have fun. Spend time with friends and family, go to the movies, watch the sun set over the ocean—whatever makes you happy.
- Help others. There's nothing like lending a helping hand to make you feel good about life.
- Join a support group that has a positive attitude.
- A positive mental attitude is a powerful medicine.

My son Barry and I have given a seminar around the country called "Immune for Life." We have met large groups of people who are HIV positive, but are following our precepts (good nutrition, supplements, exercise and positivity) and have not developed AIDS. This gives us great hope and expectation that programs such as ours will be helpful supplemental tools in the fight against AIDS.

---

[1]   Harakeh, S., et al. Suppression of human immunodeficiency virus replication by ascorbate in chronically and acutely infected cells. *J Nutr Med*, 1:345-6, 1990.

[2]   Cathcart, R.F. Vitamin C in the treatment of acquired immune deficiency syndrome (AIDS). *Med Hypothesis*, 14(4):423-33, 1984.

[3]   Brighthope, I. AIDS—Remissions using nutrient therapies and megadose intravenous ascorbate. *Int Clin Nutr Rev*, 7(2):53-75, 1987.

[4]   Folkers, K., et al. Biochemical deficiencies of coenzyme Q10 in HIV-infection and exploratory treatment. *Biochem Biophys Res Commun*, 153:888-96, 1988.

[5]   *Arzneimittel-Forschung*, 43:1359-62, 1993.

[6]   Jacobson, M.A., et al. Decreased serum dehydroepiandrosterone is associated with an increased progression of human immunodeficiency virus infection in men with CD4 cell counts of 200-499. *J Infect Dis*, 1991; 164(5):864-868.

[7]   *New Engl J Med*, June 21, 1989, pp. 1757-1763.

Chapter 3

Allergies

A 35-year-old mother of two came to my office with a common complaint: "Dr. Fox, I'm tired all the time." The last time I had seen her, five years before, she had been vibrant and attractive. Now her face was puffy and she had dark circles under her eyes. She described her many symptoms to me: congestion, difficulty breathing, abdominal discomfort and puffiness of the hands, feet and ankles. Then she added: "I get depressed and nervous, don't seem to function well and I sweat on-and-off for no good reason."

It turned out that she had allergies, an odd condition in which an ordinarily neutral or even beneficial substance, such as a pollen or strawberries or tomatoes, is perceived by the immune system to be a threat to the body. Alarmed, the immune system goes on the attack, furiously trying to destroy a harmless substance. But it's the body—the battleground—that suffers. And that suffering is what we commonly call an *allergy*.

The immune system—that wonderful "doctor within"—has special methods of detecting viruses, bacteria, protozoa and other invaders. But in some people, the immune system overreacts. It may mistake food, for example, for a real danger. Not only do we suffer as the battle is waged between our immune systems and the allergen (the food, in this case), but our overall health is compromised because our immune system is wasting energy attacking this harmless substance.

Susceptible people may become sensitized to allergens (things that cause allergic reactions) through what is called a "primary immune response," which gears the immune system up for battle. The B-cells of the immune system become floating factories called *plasma cells*, making antibodies that are "programmed" to seek out and destroy the invaders. One of these antibodies, called Immunoglobulin E (IgE), "latches on" to the allergen. Other parts of the immune system sense the presence of the allergen/IgE complex, and soon the internal warfare is in high gear. You've probably heard of histamine, one of the substances released during the battle. The histamine and other substances act on the small blood vessels and nerves, producing congestion of the mucous membranes, swelling of the eyes or other parts of the body, upsetting of the stomach and producing other reactions that make us miserable.

Signs and symptoms

The signs and symptoms of allergies vary from person to person and according to the allergen. Some of the many reactions include:

- Headaches.
- Diarrhea.
- Flatulence.
- Dizziness or fainting.
- Difficulty in concentrating.
- Anxiety.
- Depression.
- Blurred vision.
- Unsteadiness.
- Muscle aches.
- Skin reactions.
- Sleepiness.
- Rapid heartbeat.
- Hives.
- Sweating.
- Asthma.

Types of allergies

Although the allergic process is generally the same, allergies can affect the body in many different ways. There are gastrointestinal allergies caused by hypersensitivity to certain foods or chemicals. Symptoms of gastrointestinal allergies include vomiting, diarrhea and abdominal pain. Butter, chocolate, citrus fruits, eggs, fish, nuts, peanut butter and wheat are common causes of gastrointestinal allergies.

The skin is frequently susceptible to allergies. There may be an immediate "urticaria" reaction (a stinging, itching skin eruption), delayed dermatitis and even dark colors around the eyes called "allergic shiners." Skin allergies are often caused by eating certain foods or by contact with plants, cosmetics or other substances. Allergies involving the nose may produce rhinitis (runny nose), while those involving the lungs may trigger asthma. Air pollutants, cigarette smoke, dust, pollen and exposure to various plants and animals can cause allergic reactions in either the nose or lungs.

Possible complications and long-term effects

Extreme allergic reactions can lead to a serious condition called "anaphylaxis" (irregular heart beat, lowered blood pressure and difficulty breathing). Allergies that trigger asthma can provoke life-long, potentially serious lung problems, and people have been known to die from allergic reactions to bee stings. Fortunately, most people with allergies will not suffer such extreme reactions. They may be uncomfortable for a while, but they will recover.

I believe that one of the unrecognized "side effects" of long-term allergies is the weakening of the immune system, which is intimately involved in the allergic reaction. It is the immune system, after all, that overreacts to the presence of a harmless substance in the body. When the immune system is busy attacking allergens, the body suffers. The skin, lungs, brain, gastrointestinal tract, kidneys and other "innocent bystanders" may be injured. And how effective can the immune system be when it is busy "saving" us from food or other allergens?

Standard medical treatment

Physicians begin by making a diagnosis. Unfortunately, this is sometimes difficult because allergies often "look like" other disorders. If allergies are suspected, the doctor may run skin and other tests to identify the allergen. Once the diagnosis has been made, treatment usually includes:

- Avoiding the allergens (foods, animals, dust, etc.) that trigger reactions.
- "Allergy shots" to increase tolerance to the allergens.
- Various medications to treat the symptoms, such as antihistamines for runny noses, anti-inflammatory drugs for tissue swelling, medicines for skin rashes and a variety of inhalers, bronchodilators and cortisone to suppress inflammation.

Now let's take a look at some of the many alternative treatments for allergies. These are not all the possible therapies, for there are too many to investigate in a single chapter. Reading through these alternatives, however, will give you an idea of the many possibilities.

The information on alternative therapies is meant for educational purposes only. I am not endorsing any therapy or suggesting that you see any alternative practitioner. If you have or suspect that you have allergies, see your physician.

Acupuncture

The acupuncture that may be used depends on where the allergy has manifested itself.

- If the problem shows up on the skin, acupuncture may be used in points that correspond to the meridians that have an effect on the skin, such as the lung and colon meridians. Points on the hands, wrists and lower arms may be used.
- If the problem manifests itself as a stuffy nose or other respiratory problem, acupuncture points on the face near the openings of the nose and the side of the mouth may be used. In addition, points on the hands, upper chest and upper back at the base of the neck may be used.
- For food allergies, points on the abdomen and lower legs may be used. The point known as Stomach 36 (below the knee, near the skin bone) has a positive effect on the digestive system. Stomach 25, which is near the navel, may also be used.

A study published in the *American Journal of Acupuncture* found that acupuncture provided better relief to patients with allergic rhinitis than did conventional antihistamines.[1]

Color therapy

According to color therapists, bacteria, viruses and other germs, as well as diseases, give off light of particular wavelengths. Disease is fought by applying light of the same wavelength. The color therapist will use colored threads or other means of diagnosing the patient, then apply the appropriately colored light(s). There are no standard protocols for dealing with allergies, but color therapists may choose the colors yellow and green.

Yellow combines the energizing effects of red and the tonic properties of green. It stimulates the lymphatic system, which is crucial to the body's immune defenses, while cleansing the skin and intestines.

Green is a mentally and physically soothing color that disinfects while rebuilding body tissues. It is the color of new life.

There are many ways for the color therapist to apply the proper-colored light to the patient, including through direct light, gems, jewelry, perfume, clothing and colored glass. Patients may also meditate on colors or eat the appropriately colored foods.

- Yellow foods include bananas, banana squash, eggs, yellow cheese, yellow corn, yellow sweet potatoes, pineapples, lemons, grapefruit and butter. Yellow metals and chemicals include platinum and magnesium.

- Green foods include green vegetables, peas, beans and lentils. Green metals and chemicals include barium, chlorophyll, nickel and sodium.

Folk medicine

Folk remedies for the symptoms of allergies are many and varied. There are absolutely no standard protocols or recipes. Some of the folk medicines for allergies include:

- Drinking baking soda mixed in water.
- Swallowing several tablespoons of honey (from local hives) daily.
- Rubbing a mixture of castor oil and garlic on the chest.
- Drinking asparagus and onion juice.
- Eating bananas or licorice (unless you are allergic to them).

Herbal medicine

A great many herbs have been used to treat allergies. There is no standard herbal protocol for treating disease, so the herbs selected will depend upon the herbalist's background and the patient's symptoms. Herbs typically used for food allergies include:

- Agrimony (*Agrimonia eupatoria*).
- Garlic (*Allium sativum*).
- Golden seal (*Hydrastis canadensis*).

For allergies affecting the nose, these herbs may be used:

- Elder (*Sambucus nigra*).
- Eyebright (*Euphrasia officinalis*).
- Golden rod (*Solidago virgauria*).
- Peppermint (*Mentha piperita*).
- Ribwort Plantain (*Plantago lanceolata*).
- Sambucol.

Herbs that may be recommended for allergic skin reactions include:

- Cabbage (*Brassica oleracea*).
- Heartsease (*Viola tricolor*).

To strengthen the immune system in an effort to calm the body's overreaction to allergens, these herbs may be used:

- Astragalus root (Astragalus membranaceus).
- Cayenne pepper (*Capsicum frutescens*).

- Chamomile (*Matricaria chamomilla*).
- Purple coneflower *(Echinacea).*
- Willow bark (*Salix nigra*).

Homeopathy

Homeopathy attempts to cure allergies by helping the body to heal itself. Homeopathic therapy, designed to stimulate the body's defenses, is based on the "Law of Similars," that like cures like; substances that produce symptoms in healthy people will help heal those already suffering from similar symptoms.

The "remedies" (medicines) selected by the homeopath will depend upon the patient's symptoms, plus the physical, mental and emotional state. The homeopath will be looking for the "constitutional remedy" with a "portrait" that most closely matches the patient's portrait (including likes and dislikes, fears, sleep patterns and temperature). Most of the major homeopathic remedies may be used for allergies, depending upon the patient's symptoms. Some remedies include:

- *Allium cepa*, which is indicated when the patient's symptoms are made worse by warm air at the onset of evening, but better by colder temperatures and open air.
- *Arsenicum album,* which is indicated when the patient is chilly, restless and fearful of disease. The slightest exertion tends to tire the patient. He or she may feel better in the middle of the night and in wet or cold weather. Heat and warm drinks make the symptoms worse.
- *Carbo vegetabilis,* which is indicated when the patient is sluggish, obese and fearful during the night. The symptoms are worse at night, in damp or warm weather and after eating fatty food.
- *Euphrasia,* which is primarily used for eye problems. Sunlight and warmth make the patient feel better.
- *Natrum muriaticum,* which is indicated when the patient is weak and weary, depressed and subject to rapidly changing moods. Noise, warmth and mental exertion worsen the symptoms, while open air, irregular meals and pressing against the back relieve them.
- *Pulsatilla,* which is indicated when the patient is timid and has difficulty making up his or her mind. Mild-tempered and given to weeping, the patient feels worse in the heat, after eating and when lying on his or her left side. Open air, cold compresses and moving around make him or her feel better.

Hypnosis

Hypnosis is an interesting adjunct treatment for the symptoms of allergies. The general idea is to give post-hypnotic suggestions so that when the patient notices a symptom, he or she will "tell" himself or herself to allow the problem to slowly ease away.

If, for example, the person has difficulty breathing after inhaling dust, hypnosis may be used to encourage him or her to immediately imagine the breathing tubes being wide open, with the air flowing easily in and out of the lungs. Once the patient has been hypnotized, he or she will be given a post-hypnotic suggestion for easier breathing that might be worded as follows:

> "As soon as you notice any difficulty breathing, imagine that you are standing in your favorite place on a pleasantly cool day. The air is crisp and sweet. Take a deep breath and feel the wonderful air flowing easily through your nose and into your lungs. It feels great. As you exhale, feel the air moving easily back out of your lungs and through your nose. Take another deep breath, feeling the refreshing air sweeping easily into your lungs—and now out.

> "The air flows in and out automatically as you breathe comfortably and relaxedly. Whenever you have trouble breathing, picture yourself in this favorite place, easily breathing the wonderful, cool, refreshing air."

If the patient develops skin rashes as the result of allergies, the hypnotist will give suggestions that the skin is becoming healthy. Under hypnosis, the patient may be guided as follows:

> "Using your mind's eye, look at the rash on your [name of body part]. Notice that it is red and see how large it is.

> "Now with your mind's eye, imagine that you have a cool, golden healing cream on your right hand, and you're gently rubbing that wonderful cream onto your rash. As you gently rub the golden cream in, the redness begins to fade. See how the rash is slowly shrinking, how it's being replaced by healthy skin.

> "As you finish rubbing in the healing cream, the rash is gone. With your mind's eye, see how healthy and glowing your skin is. It feels cool and wonderful."

There is no agreed-upon length of time before hypnosis brings results, if any are to be found.

Nutritional therapy

Nutritional therapy can be used to attack allergies in two ways: first, by eliminating the foods that may trigger allergic reactions and second, by "calming" the body's response to allergens.

The "elimination diet" can help to identify food allergies, if any. The idea is simple: Eat only a few different foods for three or four days. If there are no allergic reactions, introduce more foods into the diet, one by one, until the offending food or foods are identified. The process can be tedious and it can lead to confusing results. For example, if adding cake back to the diet causes an allergic reaction, you can't be sure which ingredient in the cake is to blame. Still, this is a basic and often effective process for identifying food allergens.

Vitamins and minerals that help control allergies

A number of vitamins, minerals and other substances have been found to be helpful in quelling immune reactions:

- *Niacin.* Otherwise known as vitamin B3, niacin may inhibit the release of histamines, which play a major role in the allergic response. When people with hay fever were given injections of a form of niacin called nicotinamide, their symptoms improved.[2] Food sources include almonds, barley and prunes.

- *Pantothenic acid.* When more than 100 patients with allergic rhinitis ("runny nose") were given 250 mg of pantothenic acid twice a day, their symptoms were rapidly relieved.[3] Pantothenic acid can be found in liver, eggs and avocado.

- *Vitamin C.* A study of 437 healthy people found that low levels of vitamin C in the blood are linked to high levels of histamines. (Histamines are produced as part of the allergic reaction.) When 11 volunteers were given 1 gram of vitamin C a day for three days, their histamine levels fell.[4] This finding suggests that vitamin C might block or reduce allergic reactions. Food sources of vitamin C include citrus fruits, asparagus and turnip greens.

  In a test of the vitamin C/histamine connection, 16 people with allergic rhinitis were given 2 grams of vitamin C and a placebo, in either order. Neither the volunteers nor the doctors knew who was taking what or when. The subjects then inhaled histamine. When they had taken only the placebo, the histamine weakened their ability to breathe (maximal expiratory flow). But if they had just been given the vitamin C, there was no such trouble.[5]

- *Vitamin E.* To see if vitamin E could reduce the swelling associated with allergies, volunteers agreed to have histamines injected into their skin. Some were pretreated with vitamin E for five to seven days, some were not. The ones who had received the vitamin suffered much less swelling of the skin at the site of the injection than did the others.[6]

- *Calcium.* Although normally associated with bones and blood pressure, the mineral calcium also plays a role in the allergic response. In one study, 25 people with allergic rhinitis were given intravenous (IV) infusions of calcium and a placebo, in either order. Neither the doctors nor the volunteers knew who was receiving the mineral or the placebo at any time during the study.

  The volunteers were then exposed to inhaled allergens. It took 170 percent as much of the offending substance to trigger an allergic reaction in the sufferers who had received the calcium as compared to the placebo. In other words, calcium reduced the susceptibility to allergies by "raising the threshold" or response.[7]

Other substances have been found to be helpful in reducing the symptoms of allergies, including the minerals molybdenum and zinc and the bioflavonoids catechin and quercetin.

When selecting a nutritional healer, remember that there is no widely recognized school of nutritional therapy and no standards or agreed-upon training for nutritional healers.

Oriental medicine

One of the fastest-growing alternative treatments in the United States, Oriental medicine has a multifaceted approach to treating allergies. The treatment for allergies is not standardized, but depends on where the allergy manifests itself. The first step is to determine the cause of the problem, then work to relieve the symptoms and strengthen the body with a combination of herbs and spices, diet, acupuncture, "ear acupuncture" and other therapies, as necessary.

Herbs and spices

Exactly which herbs and spices and the amount of each will depend upon the patient and his or her condition. Some herbal formulas that might be used include:

- For food allergies, *Hsiao Yao Wan.*
- For hay fever, *Bi Yan Pian* and *Bi Tong Pian.*
- For skin allergies, *Yingchiao Chieh Tu Pien* and *Lien Chiao Pai Tu Pien.*

Diet

Diet plays an important role in Oriental medicine. Foods are selected depending on their flavors, organic actions and other qualities, including energies. There are five food energies: hot, warm, neutral, cool and cold. (The energy has to do with the quality of the food, not its temperature.) In addition to a healthy diet, the Oriental medicine physician may recommend these foods specifically for allergies:

- *Corn silk,* a sweet food that tones the liver and gall bladder and reduces the nasal inflammation seen with some allergies.
- *Hawthorn fruit,* a warm, sour and sweet fruit that tones the liver, stomach and spleen. It also reduces the mucous discharge often seen with allergies.
- *Pumpkin,* a sweet and slightly bitter food helpful with the bronchial asthma that results from some allergies.
- *Tangerine,* a sweet and sour, yet cool fruit that tones the spleen, lungs, stomach and kidneys. It reduces the chest congestion seen in some allergies.

Psychoneuroimmunology

Psychoneuroimmunology (psycho-neuro-immune-ology) is a science concerned with the mind/body connection. Mind/body healers use positive affirmations to counteract the negative thoughts that have been contributing to allergies. Affirmations are typically brief, positive statements that focus on how well one feels, and on how the disease is being conquered. The patient might be given several affirmations.

An affirmation to "calm" the overreacting immune system might be worded as follows:

"My wise immune system always knows when to rise to my defense. All-knowing, all-powerful, it is my eternal protector."

Patients may also be given affirmations to counteract specific symptoms, such as:

"With every breath I take, the air flows easily into my lungs. With each breath, my lungs fill with refreshing, life-giving air."

"My skin is smooth and clear, full of life and health."

"My razor-sharp mind focuses quickly, easily answering all questions and solving all problems that arise."

Finally, they may be given an affirmation for general health, such as:

"I enjoy radiant health, each and every day."

For more on affirmations and psychoneuroimmunology, see two of our other books, *Beyond Positive Thinking* (Hay House, 1991) and *Immune For Life* (Prima, 1989).

Reflexology

Reflexology, the application of pressure to the feet, helps to relieve tension, improve the circulation, stimulate the nerves and normalize the functioning of the organs and glands through a series of pressures, stretches and general movements of the feet. The treatment regimen will depend on the type of allergies and their symptoms.

To treat food allergies, for example, the reflexologist will manipulate the direct reflex points for the stomach and the large and small intestines, which are found between the balls and heels of both feet.

In addition, the associated reflex areas for the spleen, pituitary and adrenal glands will be treated to strengthen the body. The spleen reflex area is about halfway down the left foot below the little toe. The pituitary gland reflex area is in the center of the pad of the big toes. The adrenal gland reflex areas are at approximately the middle of the feet, slightly to the inside.

Advice to allergy patients

Although many of my patients have had success with the following program, I only use the general guidelines discussed below after reviewing a patient's personal and medical history, performing a thorough examination and evaluating the laboratory studies to make sure that the program will be beneficial. Please see your own physician before embarking on any treatment program for allergies.

Although there is no single "cure" for allergies, there are simple, general measures that help to prevent allergic attacks.

1. Avoid the allergens that trigger the allergic response. Pets, dust, foods, feather pillows, various plants, household and workplace chemicals are common allergens. It may even be the detergent used to clean the bed sheets that's causing the problem.

2. Drug reactions are very common, so carefully review all the medications that you are taking with your physician. There are about 55,000 drug products containing perhaps 2,000 different active chemical agents. Find a physician who will

look at *all* the medicines and other substances that have been
prescribed for you by your various doctors and healers, as
well as those that you began taking on your own. Reducing
the number of substances used or switching to different ones
can help many people.

3. Try using air filtering devices and negative ion generators to
help "cleanse" your environment. (Wein Products, Inc., of Los
Angeles, Calif., makes the Air Supply, a personal air purifier
that can be worn around the neck or set on a desk.)

4. Antioxidants, such as beta carotene, vitamins C and E and
the mineral selenium, can be helpful. Twenty years ago, an
"old" and experienced physician showed me how intravenous
vitamin C (the ascorbate form) could quickly terminate an
acute asthma attack. Regularly taking vitamin C orally can
help reduce the frequency of asthma attacks by suppressing
the formation of histamine.

5. Immunotherapy, which we used to call hyposensitization, is
helpful. Small amounts of the offending substance are
injected into the body, allowing the patient to develop
resistance to the allergen.

Allergies can be frightening. I remember how terrified my wife
and I were as our young son Barry began suffering from allergic
asthma. Many times she rushed him to the emergency room, or I
treated him myself right at home. The good news is that with careful
prevention and treatment, most allergies can be managed.

---

[1]   Chari, P., Sehgal, S. Acupuncture therapy in allergic rhinitis. *Am J
Acupuncture,* 16(2): April-June 1988, 143-45.

[2]   Dainow, I. Recherches clinquies sur certaines proprietes anti-allergiques
de la nicotinamide. *Z Vitaminforsch,* 15:245-50, 1944.

[3]   Martin, W. On treating allergic disorders. Letter. *Townsend Letter for
Doctors*, Aug/Sept 1991:670-1.

[4]   Clemeston, C.A. Histamine and ascorbic acid in human blood. *J Nutr,*
110(4):662-68, 1980.

[5]   Bucca, C., et al. Effect of vitamin C on histamine bronchial
responsiveness of patients with allergic rhinitis. *Ann Allergy*, 65:311-14, 1990.

[6]   Kamimura, M. Anti-inflammatory activity of vitamin E. *J Vitaminol*,
18(4):204-9, 1972.

[7]   Bachert, C., et al. [Decreased reactivity in allergic rhinitis after
intravenous application of calcium. A study on the alternation of local
airway resistance after nasal allergen provocation.] *Arzneimmittelforsch,*
40:984-7, 1990.

Chapter 4

Arthritis

Arthritis is not a single disease. In fact, the name simply means an inflammation of one or more joints; its causes and consequences are many and varied. The inflammation is often accompanied by pain, swelling, redness and motion limitation. However, x-rays may show horrifying damage to the joints of people who feel no pain at all, or they may show relatively little damage in people who feel great pain.

Signs and symptoms

As a first-year medical student, I learned the four "cardinal signs" of inflammation: 1) pain, 2) swelling, 3) redness and 4) limitation of motion. All four don't have to be present at once, although they may be. Other possible warning signs of arthritis include:

- Early morning stiffness.
- Warmth in a joint.
- Weakness combined with joint pain.
- Increased pain when the weather changes.
- Unexplained fever.
- "Cracking" sounds when moving joints.

Types of arthritis

There are many illnesses that are referred to as "arthritis." There's osteoarthritis, rheumatoid arthritis, gouty arthritis, psoratic arthritis, juvenile rheumatoid arthritis, bursitis, systemic infectious arthritis, arthritis associated with a venereal disease and many others. ("Arthralgia," which means joint pain, is not necessarily arthritis.)

Let's take a brief look at the three major forms of this disease.

Osteoarthritis. The most common type of arthritis is sometimes called degenerative joint disease or "wear and tear" arthritis. It is caused by a breakdown of the cartilage that normally protects the ends of the bones. Cartilage sits at the ends of the bones like rubber caps on canes. It acts as a buffer, preventing bone ends from rubbing against each other, wearing one another away and causing pain. Unfortunately, the cartilage can thin, become rough or uneven or break down, allowing the bones to grind together. Naturally, the body tries to repair the cartilage, but often makes things worse by allowing the bones to "overgrow." Then they easily rub together, causing the pain and aggravation of osteoarthritis.

Osteoarthritis of the knees—the joints we use so much in walking, running and jumping—is common. In some cases, the cause of the problem is obvious. For example, after kneeling behind home plate for many years, catchers often develop arthritis of the knees. And all the fastballs that have smacked into their gloves make them susceptible to osteoarthritis of the fingers. But there's also *idiopathic osteoarthritis,* a wearing away and overgrowth of bone for no known reason.

A lack of blood flow to a joint can produce *ischemic necrosis* and osteoarthritic damage to the bones. Arthritis can be found in association with diabetes, an overactive pituitary or a low thyroid condition. Excessive iron in the blood (hemochromotosis) and other metabolic problems can also cause arthritis. And mechanical problems such as obesity, joint misalignment, unequal lower extremity length or a turning in or turning out of the foot can cause arthritis.

Osteoarthritis may first announce itself as an ache in a joint. There may be stiffness, especially in the morning. The joint may thicken. Inflammation may appear. Later, the joint can become unstable (wobbly), hurt even when at rest and refuse to respond to regular medical treatment.

Osteoarthritis can strike the hands, feet, knees, hips and even the spine. The majority of the population over the age of 50 will show some form of arthritic changes. For some people, arthritis is a living hell. For others, it is only a minor problem. I've seen people with bulging spinal discs who should have been confined to bed, but felt fine and had no pain or other symptoms.

Rheumatoid arthritis. The second most common type of arthritis is rheumatoid arthritis (RA). When you think of RA, don't think only of joints, but rather a "systemic inflammation," a chronic disease that involves the joints, muscles, ligaments, tendons and the coverings of the muscles (fascia). It may even get into the lungs or the bones.

RA appears to be an autoimmune disease, a disorder in which the body attacks itself. It affects all racial and ethnic groups, attacking more women than men.

Rheumatoid arthritis may strike first not with joint pain, but with marked malaise, fatigue and muscle aches. Only later do the four cardinal signs of inflammation (pain, swelling, redness and limitation of motion) develop. RA is usually symmetrical, which means that it attacks the same joints on both sides of the body (the fingers on both hands, both wrists, etc.). The symptoms include stiffness, difficulty in walking, climbing steps, opening jars, sewing, opening doors and performing other routine activities and motions. Since RA is a systemic disease, the patient will often lose weight, run a low-grade fever and may become depressed. This is usually a slow process, taking many months or even years, although some people are hit all at once. RA progresses to deforming and disabling conditions of the hands, wrists, elbows and other parts of the body.

Gouty arthritis (GA). Usually called simply "gout," this form of arthritis has been known for 2,500 years. Gout accounts for only 5 percent of the arthritis cases doctors see, striking less than half of 1 percent of the population in the United States and Europe.

Gout comes about when the levels of uric acid, a substance normally found in the blood, rise. Some of the uric acid crystallizes ("hardens"), depositing itself in joints. This leads to joint damage and often a great deal of pain. Gout is largely a disease of adult males. When it does occur in women, it is usually after menopause.

When someone mentions "gout," we usually think of swollen toes on swollen-bellied gluttons. About 60 percent of cases do, in fact, develop in the toes. Usually the person goes to bed feeling fine, but awakens in the middle of the night with severe pain. Practically 50 to 60 percent of first attacks involve the large toe, but the problem may later move to other joints.

GA used to be very common among the wealthy in England, who consumed lots of mutton and port wine. GA has been associated with a rich diet for some time, and World Wars I and II showed us how strong the diet/GA link is. During these wars, GA was *not* common in Europe, probably because people could no longer afford to eat the standard high-protein, high-fat diet. After the wars, when people went back to this diet, GA increased. The disease used to be uncommon in Japan, where people ate a diet relatively low in animal protein. But as the Japanese have begun to eat more animal protein, GA has become more common.

Possible complications and long-term effects

Arthritis can lead to severe pain, loss of joint mobility, joint deformation, shrinkage of muscles that are unused because of pain and sometimes an inability to perform daily activities as simple as getting dressed. Arthritis of the spine can cause pain in the upper back, neck, head, arms and chest. And the drugs used to treat arthritis may have side effects as well, some of them severe.

Proper diagnosis is important, so be sure to see a physician before beginning any treatment.

Standard medical treatment

Standard Western medical treatment for arthritis consists of:

- Nonsteroidal anti-inflammatory drugs (NSAIDs), such as aspirin, Advil (ibuprofen) and Orudis (ketoprofen).
- Oral steroids, such as prednisone and hydrocortisone.
- Powerful painkillers, such as codeine, and synthetic narcotics, such as Vicodin.
- Antirheumatic medications, such as gold injections, an immune system suppresser named Methotrexate and an antimalaria drug called Plaquenil.
- Physical therapy.
- Ultrasound.
- Heat therapy.
- Surgery to "clean up" ends of bones.
- Surgical replacement of severely damaged joints.

There is no cure for arthritis, especially if the bone or cartilage has deteriorated. While arthritis medications may help many people, they can have severe side effects, including immune system suppression, intestinal bleeding, nausea, abdominal pain, diarrhea, depression, headaches and elevated blood pressure.

Now let's take a look at some of the many alternative treatments for arthritis. These are not all the possible therapies, since there are too many to investigate in a single chapter. Reading through these alternatives, however, will give you an idea of the many possibilities.

The information on alternative therapies is meant for educational purposes only. I am not endorsing any therapy or suggesting that you see any alternative practitioner. If you have or suspect that you have arthritis, see your physician.

Acupuncture

The acupuncture points used will depend on the "type" of arthritis and where the symptoms are felt. If the arthritis is in the shoulder joints, points called the Large Intestine 15 and Triple Heater 14 might be used. (You can find this point by the little "dimples" that appear on the shoulder when you raise your arms straight out from the side of your body.)

If the arthritis afflicts the elbows, Large Intestine 11 (by the bend in the elbow) may be used. The Large Intestine 4, or "Joining of the Valleys" point on the hand may also be used. (To find this point, push your thumb against your forefinger. As you do, you'll notice a small mound of flesh popping up at the base of your thumb. The highest area on the mound is the point.)

If the arthritis is in the hip, Gall Bladder 30 (in the buttocks) may be used. If the problem is in the knees, the acupuncturist may use the "Eyes of the Knee" points. (If you put your fingers on the bottom of your kneecaps and slide them off, they'll fall into a little indentation right below the kneecap. The acupuncture needle will be placed there and directed under the knee cap.)

If the arthritis is plaguing the foot, acupuncture points located where the toes meet the feet will be used. For any arthritic problems with the face or head, Large Intestine 4 (the Joining of the Valleys point) will be used. In some areas, such as the ankle, spine and jaw, local points right by the problem areas are used.

Acute arthritis calls for daily treatment. For chronic problems, treatment may be given every other day. In addition, patients are encouraged to move their troubled joints as much as possible.

Aromatherapy

Aromatherapy uses the aromatic essences of flowers and plants to influence the mind and body. Aromatherapy treatments for arthritis vary widely because there are no standard therapy guidelines in this field. Generally speaking, the treatment will attempt to relieve pain by strengthening the body's ability to heal itself. Essential oils used for arthritis may include:

- Benzoin (*styrax benzoin*).
- Chamomile (*matricaria chamomilla*).
- Camphor (*cinnamomum camphora*).
- Cypress (*cupressus sempervirens*).
- Juniper (*juniperus communis*).
- Lavender (*lavandula officinalis*).
- Hyssop (*hyssopus officinalis*).
- Rosemary (*rosmarinus officinalis*).

The patient may be instructed to inhale the vapors from these oils as they rise from a bowl of water, to mix them in a base oil and use in massage, to wear as a perfume or to mix with the bath water. Treatment length will vary from practitioner to practitioner and according to the patient's condition.

Ayurvedic healing

The treatment of arthritis recommended by this 5,000-year-old system of healing from India is based on the tenet that arthritis is primarily an *ama* disease caused by poor digestion and a weakened colon, resulting in the accumulation of undigested food and the buildup of waste matter. (Undigested food is referred to as *ama*.) Poor digestion allows toxins to accumulate in the body, and problems with the colon allow the toxins to reach the joints.

Ama is the opposite of *agni*, the digestive fire that normally burns away toxins. Hence, the general treatment for arthritis consists of stimulating the digestive fire and suppressing the ama. (Ayurveda notes that arthritis may also be caused by injury or an immune system gone awry that attacks the body.)

Arthritis may manifest itself in any of the three primary life forces, or humors, in the body.

- Arthritis in the Vata (air) humor produces throbbing pain of varying intensity. The pain may move about. The joints feel stiff, make cracking sounds on movement and the bones may become deformed. Other possible symptoms include dry skin, nervousness, fear, insomnia, lower back pain, constipation and intestinal gas. The pain is made worse by cold. Gout is a Vata-type of arthritis.

- Arthritis of the Pitta (fire) humor produces pain, swelling and inflammation and possibly fever. The pain is often described as "burning." Other possible symptoms include diarrhea, irritability, a feeling of "heat" throughout the body, sweating and flushing. The pain is made worse by heat.

- Arthritis of the Kapha (water) humor produces a dull and aching pain as well as swelling of the joints. Other possible symptoms may be an accumulation of mucus in the respiratory system and mucus in the stool. The pain is made worse by cold and dampness.

The Ayurvedic treatment for all forms of arthritis, regardless of their humors, includes increasing the intensity of the digestive fire in order to burn up the toxins that are harming the body. Hot, spicy foods and herbs, including galangal and cayenne, may be used. Arthritis often calls for a three- to five-day detoxification diet. Vegetables, juices, spices and herbs are taken during the fast, which lasts until the body shows signs that the digestive fire is burning strong. These signs include a return of the appetite, a feeling of lightness and a clear coating to the tongue.

Enemas and other means of cleaning the colon are often used to help detoxify the body. At least one or two colonics are believed to be good for just about everyone, unless the patient is weak or fearful.

Ruby, garnet or other "hot" gems set in gold are used for all three types of arthritis. Various oils may be applied to the skin in order to help the body clear toxins, relieve pain and restore mobility. Heat therapy may also be used. The patient may be asked to sit in a sauna, or may have steam applied directly to the afflicted areas.

A variety of herbs, spices and bitters are applied externally or ingested in order to cleanse the body and to relieve pain and stiffness. These include mint, ephedra, golden seal, gentian, nirgundi, eucalyptus leaves, prasarini, quassia, coptis, scute, phellodendrom, aloe, guggul, du huo, ligusticum, Siberian ginseng, myrrh and yucca.

Treating Vata-type arthritis

In addition to the general treatment, Vata-type arthritis often calls for a three- to five-day detoxification diet and an anti-Vata diet. This diet includes warm, heavy and moist foods that give one strength. Frequent small meals, mildly spiced and with only a few different types of foods per meal are recommended. One should not eat when nervous or worried. Your meal should be cooked for you, and you should eat with friends. (See Chapter 8 for a complete description of the anti-Vata diet.)

Treating Pitta-type arthritis

In addition to the general treatment, Pitta-type arthritis often calls for a five- to seven-day detoxification diet and an anti-Pitta diet. Specific herbs for Pitta arthritis include guggul, sandalwood, aloe, saffron and chaparral. Ice packs are also used for this arthritis of the fire humor.

The anti-Pitta diet consists of cool, slightly dry and heavy foods. The foods should be raw and relatively plain-tasting, not cooked in lots of oil or heavily spiced. Three regular meals, with no eating late at night, are suggested. (See Chapter 8 for a complete description of the anti-Pitta diet.)

Treating Kapha-type arthritis

In addition to the general treatment, Pitta-type arthritis often calls for a one- to two-week detoxification diet. The anti-Kapha diet is light, dry and warm. Cold, oily and heavy foods should be avoided. Three meals a day should be eaten, with lunch being the main meal. Breakfast may be skipped and weekly fasting is helpful. Most or all of the daily food should be consumed between the hours of 10 a.m. and 6 p.m. (See Chapter 8 for a complete description of the anti-Kapha diet.)

Chiropractic

Modern chiropractic is divided into two groups: "straight" and "mixed." The straight chiropractors believe that disease is caused by subluxation and other problems with the spine, which can lead to physiological, neurological and musculoskeletal problems throughout the body. Spinal subluxation, which infringes upon the nerves running from the spine to the limbs, may itself be the cause of arthritis. Straight chiropractors treat arthritis by manipulating the spine to correct subluxation and other imbalances, thus allowing the body to heal itself.

Mixed chiropractors believe that good spinal maintenance is necessary, but they also subscribe to a variety of other alternative therapies, including nutritional therapy, herbalism and physical therapy. Thus, the mixed chiropractor will likely treat arthritis with a combination of spinal manipulation and other therapies.

Mixed chiropractors will carefully evaluate a patient in order to determine the cause of the arthritis. In some cases, the problem may be related to an injury that happened many years ago. Suppose, for example, that your spine is damaged in a car accident and three vertebra in the center of the spine fuse together. Your back may hurt for a little while, and you may take some pain pills or have physical therapy. Unfortunately, you may unknowingly compensate for the fused vertebra by holding your body in an unusual way, or perhaps walking with a slightly wider step. This can put stress on parts of the spine above and below the fused area, causing pain, degeneration and an arthritis-like condition many years later. When viewed with X-rays, the area originally damaged looks fairly healthy, except for being fused. But the areas above and below, which have taken the brunt of the "funny" compensatory walk, may show degenerative changes.

The mixed chiropractor cannot cure the degeneration, but he or she will manipulate the spine in order to: 1) "free" the fused vertebra and 2) realign the damaged areas above and below, allowing the spine to operate properly in the future.

Mixed chiropractors may also call for physical therapy, nutritional supplements to help you rebuild your back muscles and overall health, stretching and strengthening exercises and spine maintenance education (how to walk, sit, lift, etc.).

Color therapy

There are no standard protocols for dealing with arthritis, but color therapists may use a combination of blue, green and orange light.

- *Blue* is soothing. It is used for rheumatism.
- *Green* is calming to both mind and body; it cools and soothes. Green is the color of hope and energy.
- *Orange* combines the healing power of red and yellow light. It is used in gout, rheumatism and other conditions involving abnormal growths in the body. Orange releases energy in the body and encourages a general sense of well-being.

There are many ways for the color therapist to apply the proper color of light to the patient, including through direct light, gems, jewelry, perfume, clothing and colored glass. Patients may also meditate on colors or eat the appropriately colored foods.

- Blue foods include plums, grapes and blueberries. Blue metals and chemicals include copper, lead, oxygen and tin.
- Green foods include green vegetables, peas, beans and lentils. Green metals and chemicals include barium, chlorophyll, nickel and sodium.
- Orange foods include oranges, cantaloupe and mangoes. Orange metals and chemicals include aluminum, antimony and rubidium.

Folk medicine

Folk remedies for the symptoms of arthritis are many and varied. There are absolutely no standard protocols or recipes, but some of the folk medicines for arthritis and arthritis-related symptoms include:

- Drinking raw potato juice.
- Drinking apple cider vinegar.
- Drinking blackstrap molasses mixed with water.
- Rubbing raw garlic and/or ginger on the afflicted joint areas.
- Applying compresses made of castor oil, potatoes, mustard and other substances to the arthritic area(s).

Herbal medicine

Herbs have been used to treat joint pains for centuries. There is no standard protocol for treating arthritis, so which herbs are selected will depend on the herbalist's background and the patient's symptoms. Herbs typically used for arthritis include:

- Angelica (*Angelica archangelica*).
- Black cohosh (*Cimicifuga racemosa*).
- Bladderwrack (*Fucus vesiculosus*).
- Bogbean (*Menyanthes trifoliata*).
- Burdock (*Arctium lappa*).
- Celery (*Apium graveolens*).
- Meadowsweet (*Filpendula ulmaria*).
- Prickly ash (*Zanthoxylum americanum*).
- Willow (*Salix alba*).
- Yarrow (*Achillea millefolium*).

Homeopathy

Most of the major homeopathic remedies may be used for arthritis, depending upon the patient's symptoms. Some remedies include:

- *Actea spic,* which is indicated when the arthritis is centered in the hands and feet and the joints are painful and swollen.
- *Arnica montana,* which is indicated when the patient denies that anything is wrong and prefers to be left alone. Nervous and overly sensitive, he or she may be suffering from rheumatoid arthritis related to cold, damp conditions. Soreness and bruising are problems.
- *Belladonna,* which is indicated when the pain strikes suddenly. The patient may not like stimulus of any kind. The afflicted joints are swollen and red. The pain is "sharp" and related to chills or getting wet.
- *Calcarea carbonica-ostrearum,* which is indicated when the patient is fearful and perhaps confused. The patient has rheumatoid arthritis affecting the shoulders and upper back, which is made worse with wet or damp conditions.
- *Chamomilla,* which is indicated when the patient is angry and restless. The pain is severe.
- *Cimicifuga racemosa,* which is indicated when the patient is overly talkative and restless, appearing to be alternately happy and miserable. The pain appears in the muscles more so than in the bones.
- *Rhus toxicodendron,* which is indicated when the patient is apprehensive and depressed, particularly at night. Lack of movement causes pain and stiffness.

For gouty arthritis, these or other remedies may be prescribed:

- *Aconitum napellus,* which is indicated when the patient is anxious, with a good imagination that can picture many terrible things. The joints are swollen and painful. The pain is worse at night and with warmth, but better with fresh air and rest.
- *Bryonia alba,* which is indicated when the patient is often angry and irritable and worries about the future. Afflicted joints may swell to large proportions. The pain is worse with movement, heat or upon being touched, but better with pressure to the area, rest and cold.
- *Sabina,* which is indicated when the patient is depressed. There is gouty pain and nodules may develop at the afflicted joint. Movement and heat make the pain worse; cool fresh air makes it better.

Hypnosis

Hypnosis has been effectively used as an adjunct treatment to help control the pain of arthritis as well as for any accompanying depression or negative feelings. A typical hypnotic session might include suggestions such as:

"Concentrate on the pain in your [name of joint]. With your mind's eye, see a large red ball. This is your pain. It's big, it hurts. With your mind's eye, see yourself picking up your pain ball and holding it with one hand on each side. See yourself squeezing on the ball. It slowly shrinks as you continue squeezing. Little by little the pain ball shrinks, and little by little the pain in your [name of joint] diminishes. Feel the pain fading away as you continue squeezing the pain ball down to nothingness."

Some hypnotists will attempt to change their patient's physiology. They may suggest, for example, that swelling in the hypnotized patient's joints is being reduced. Some hypnotic suggestions for this might include:

"Feel the heat of inflammation in your [name of joint] fading away. With your mind's eye, see the redness fading away, the swelling disappearing, as a wonderful sensation of coolness floods your [name of joint]."

There are no studies showing that this approach is effective, but it is related to what one attempts to achieve in biofeedback.

Nutritional therapy

The low-fat, low-cholesterol diet filled with the complex carbohydrates found in vegetables and grains has been shown to be very helpful in dealing with many cases of arthritis. This type of diet reduces the fat in the tiny arteries that supply blood to the joints, allowing more oxygen and other nutrients to nourish them.

In addition to a good low-fat diet, a number of vitamins, minerals and other nutrients may be recommended for arthritis, including:

Vitamin E, like the nonsteroidal anti-inflammatory drugs used for arthritis, inhibits the prostaglandins that play a role in pain. When 50 patients were given either 400 IU of vitamin E or a placebo, the vitamin E group reported greater pain relief and had to use less pain medication.[1] In another study, 29 patients were given either vitamin E or a placebo for 10 days. Then the groups were switched without their knowledge, so that the vitamin E group was getting a placebo and the placebo group the vitamin E for an additional 10 days. The vitamin E produced "good" pain relief in 52 percent of the patients, compared to 1 percent for the placebo.[2] Vitamin E is found in wheat germ, nuts and tomatoes.

Boron, a relatively "unknown" mineral, plays a major but largely unrecognized role in bone health. It helps the body regulate calcium, keeping this important mineral from leaving the body and weakening the bones. Although its role in arthritis is not well-understood, epidemiological studies from several countries have shown that in areas where the soil contains more boron and people are presumably eating boron-rich foods grown in that soil, there is less osteoarthritis.[3] When boron supplements were given to hospitalized arthritis patients, some 90 percent reported "complete remission" of symptoms.[4] Good sources of boron include apples, nuts and green leafy vegetables.

Selenium, sulfur and zinc levels may also be reduced in arthritis patients. Therefore, nutritional healers may check the levels of these nutrients and suggest supplements, if appropriate. You'll find selenium in almonds, barley and oranges. Sulfur is in meat, milk, poultry and fish. Zinc is in turnips, corn and oysters.

Other substances of value for arthritis include:

Omega-3 fatty acids, found in many fish, have shown promise in fighting arthritis. Some 26 osteoarthritis patients ranging in age from 52 to 85 were given either an omega-3 fatty acid called EPA (eicosapentaenoic acid) or a placebo. Six months later, those who had received the EPA had less pain and were better able to perform normal activities, as compared to the placebo group. The results in this study were small but encouraging.[5]

Superoxide dismutase, a controversial supplement known as SOD, has also shown promise as an arthritis fighter. When 253 people with noninfectious joint inflammation were given a supplement containing SOD, 228 of them reported decreased pain and swelling, along with increased mobility of the afflicted joints.[6] The results of this unpublished study, as well as those of other studies, have generated a great deal of debate. SOD is made in the body and is also available as a supplement. New forms of SOD supplements are more easily absorbed by the body than were the older ones.

Yucca plant extracts have been used to treat inflammation and to boost the immune system. The yucca is found in deserts in the southwestern United States and in Mexico. Yucca is ingested as a supplement, but the plant itself can also be eaten.

Beche-de-Mer (sea cucumber), perna canaliculus (New Zealand Green-Lipped Mussel) and *primrose oil* have also been examined. More studies are necessary before we can say whether or not they will be of significant value in treating arthritis in the future. All three of these substances are taken as supplements.

Here are other nutritional-related approaches to treating arthritis:

DLPA. In 1972, scientists at the Johns Hopkins University School of Medicine discovered that the human brain produces chemicals that closely resemble morphine, the most powerful painkiller known. They named these newly discovered substances *endorphins*, which means "the morphine within." Studies with laboratory animals found that the endorphins were incredibly effective. An endorphin called *beta-endorphin* was 18 to 50 times stronger than morphine. And *dynorphin* was apparently 500 times more powerful! Scientists quickly theorized that the human body makes these tremendous natural painkillers to "mask" routine or unnecessary pain, among other things.

There are two broad categories of pain. Acute pain (the powerful pain that strikes when we hit our thumbs with hammers, for example) is necessary. The pain tells us that we're doing something wrong, and to stop doing it immediately. But chronic pain that lingers for days, months, even years, serves no useful purpose. Researchers believed that the endorphins were responsible for masking this "useless" chronic pain.

The theory made a lot of sense, but left open the question of why millions of people were suffering from chronic pain. Why weren't the endorphins doing their jobs?

Like everything else in the body, the endorphin system is balanced. The body makes endorphins, and "endorphin-eaters" to destroy them. Apparently, the endorphin-eaters get the upper hand in many people. They do their job too well, destroying too many endorphins and preventing the internal painkillers from masking chronic pain.

Fortunately, a way to protect the endorphins was quickly discovered. The substance was a simple nutritional amino acid called *dl-phenylalanine* (DLPA). DLPA is not a drug, and it does not block pain. Instead, it protects the endorphins from the endorphin-eaters, helping to restore the body's ability to deal with pain. Phenylalanine is found in fish, chicken, eggs and other foods.

Studies have shown that DLPA effectively blocks arthritis pain and joint inflammation in many patients. It is much safer than the standard arthritis medications and considerably less expensive in the long run. Best of all, it is long-lasting. Whereas standard anti-pain and anti-arthritis drugs last for several hours, DLPA can continue quelling pain for up to four or five days.

I've had a great deal of success using a combination of DLPA and other therapies with my patients. Although DLPA is available without prescription in health food and vitamin stores, I urge you to discuss the matter with your physician before treating yourself with the amino acid. (See "Advice to arthritis patients" on page 93 for more on how I use DLPA for my patients.)

Note: I recommend against taking DLPA during pregnancy or lactation. Pregnant or lactating women should not expose the fetus or newborn to anything except their normal diet. Anyone suffering from the genetic disease phenylketonuria (PKU), or anyone on a phenylalanine-restricted diet should not take DLPA. I do not recommend the use of DLPA for children under the age of 14.

Shark cartilage. Researchers investigating the use of shark cartilage to treat cancer also experimented with arthritis patients. The theory was that some percentage of arthritis cases were at least partially caused by the growth of new blood vessels in the cartilage. (Cartilage, which keeps bones from scraping together at the joints, is not supposed to have its own blood vessels.) It was believed that shark cartilage, which contains a substance that discourages the growth of new blood vessels, might help relieve arthritis pain in many patients.

Arthritis patients suffering from severe pain were studied in the early 1970s. Following three to eight weeks of cartilage injections, of the 28 patients in the study, 19 reported "excellent" improvement, six rated their improvement as being "good" and three did not respond to the treatment. Furthermore, the relief lasted from six weeks to more than a year, and there were no toxic effects.[7] A later study involved 10 patients bedridden with osteoarthritis. Following three weeks of receiving shark cartilage orally, eight of the 10 were able to leave their beds and move around with relative ease.[8]

In a larger-scale study, 147 patients were given either cartilage extract or a placebo. Those who received the placebo were also encouraged to use various medicines when their pain flared up. Five years later, the cartilage group reported a drop of 85 percent in pain scores, compared to a 5-percent drop in the placebo group. The cartilage group also had less joint deterioration and lost less time from work due to pain.[9]

The results of various studies suggest that shark cartilage may help to reduce or relieve pain in 60 percent or more of those suffering from osteoarthritis and rheumatoid arthritis. People with other forms of arthritis have also benefited. Although there are no firm guidelines regarding length of treatment, one should begin to notice a lessening of pain and/or swelling within two to three weeks after beginning the shark cartilage. In cases where symptoms are not reduced within four to five weeks, the cartilage will probably not be effective.

Dosage levels have not been tested and confirmed. As a rule of thumb, many healers suggest 1 gram of dried shark cartilage be taken daily for every 15 pounds of body weight. The dosage is often dropped to 1 gram for every 40 or so pounds of body weight when the cartilage has begun taking effect.

Although shark cartilage is available in health food and vitamin stores, I urge you to discuss the matter with your physician before treating yourself.

When selecting a nutritional healer, remember that there is no widely recognized school of nutritional therapy and no standards or agreed-upon training for nutritional healers.

Oriental medicine

Oriental medicine has a multifaceted approach to treating arthritis. The first step is to determine the "type" of arthritis, such as:

- *Xing Bi.* With this "migratory" arthritis, the pain moves around the body. It's caused by wind, dampness and cold invading and obstructing the chi (energy) and blood circulation. The patient is often thin, dislikes wind and has a white coating to the tongue.
- *Tong Bi.* In this "painful" type of arthritis, severe pain stays in place at one or more joints. It's caused by excessive cold, which slows the circulation of chi and blood. It's made worse by cold and lack of movement, but feels better with heat. There is typically no inflammation or redness at the afflicted joint.
- *Zuo Bi.* This is a "fixed" type of arthritis characterized by dampness and internal stagnation, in which the afflicted parts of the body become heavy and numb. The tongue typically has a greasy white coating, and the pain is worse on rainy and cloudy days.
- *Re Bi.* Caused by the conversion of pre-existing problems into heat, this "hot" arthritis produces swelling, tenderness and sharp pain in one or more joints. The patient's tongue is typically covered with a dry yellow coating, and the pulse is "slippery" and fast.

Having determined the "type" of arthritis, the Oriental medicine doctor then works to relieve the symptoms and strengthen the body with a combination of herbs and spices, diet, acupuncture, "ear acupuncture" and other therapies, as necessary.

Herbs and spices

Exactly which herbs and spices and the amount of each will depend upon the patient and his or her condition. One of the herbs used for arthritis is *dried ginger,* a hot substance that warms the intestines while toning the stomach, lungs and spleen.

Herbal formulas that might be used for arthritis include *Chen Pu Hu Chien Wan, Feng Shih Hsiao Tung Wan* and *Guan Jie Yan Wan*.

Diet

In addition to a healthy diet, the Oriental medicine physician may recommend these foods specifically for arthritis:

- *Black soybean*, a sweet food that increases blood circulation and is useful for rheumatoid arthritis.
- *Cherry,* a warm and sweet fruit used for rheumatism.
- *Grape,* a sweet and sour fruit that increases energy while strengthening the lungs, spleen and kidneys.
- *Papaya,* a sweet fruit that helps with rheumatoid arthritis.
- *Royal jelly,* a supplement used to treat rheumatoid arthritis.

Psychoneuroimmunology

Mind/body healers use positive affirmations to counteract negative thoughts. Affirmations are typically brief, positive statements that focus on how well one feels and on how the disease is being conquered. The patient might be given several affirmations. For example, an affirmation to help counter arthritis might be worded as follows:

"My joint is feeling better all the time. With my mind's eye, I can see my immune system restoring my joint to health. Every day, in every way, I feel better and better."

Patients may also be given an affirmation for general health, such as:

"I enjoy radiant health, each and every day."

For more on affirmations and psychoneuroimmunology, see two of our other books, *Beyond Positive Thinking* (Hay House, 1991) and *Immune For Life* (Prima, 1989).

Water therapy

Water therapy offers many treatments for arthritis. The main thrust of the treatments is to rid the body of the toxins that are thought to be causing the joint pain and inflammation.

- Colonics are used to wash toxins out of the colon and to stimulate the kidney and other parts of the body.
- Drinking distilled water throughout the day is encouraged to flush toxins out of the body.
- Brief cold showers or baths and massages with cold towels may help to increase the circulation.

- Saunas, steam rooms or hot baths are used to produce sweating.
- Cold compresses are used to relieve local pain.

There are no widely accepted protocols for water therapy, so each practitioner will have his or her own methods.

Other exciting approaches

Sex

Although I'm not aware of any large-scale studies on the effectiveness of sexual activity as an arthritis remedy, some people have told me that their pain and inflammation is temporarily relieved following sex. Sexual activity encourages the production of endorphins, norepinephrine, dopamine, adrenaline and other substances in the body that help to lift the mood, temporarily reduce inflammation and pain, and otherwise make one feel good. In addition, the pleasurable aspects of sex can take one's mind off of other problems, at least temporarily. For these reasons, sex can be quite helpful.

Advice to arthritis patients

Although many of my patients have had success with the following program, I only use the general guidelines discussed below after reviewing a patient's personal and medical history, performing a thorough examination and evaluating the laboratory studies to make sure that the program will be beneficial. Please see your physician before embarking on any treatment program for arthritis.

This is the seven-point program that has been successful for many of my arthritis patients:

1. Slim down, if necessary.
2. Strengthen the body with good nutrition.
3. "See" your joints move.
4. Keep your joints flexible.
5. Relieve pain with DLPA.
6. Use other medications as necessary.
7. Remain positive!

Let's take a closer look at these points.

1. Slim down, if necessary

Although obesity does not cause arthritis, it certainly doesn't help painful, inflamed joints in the hips, knees or ankles if they are forced to carry excess weight. Take a load off your joints by slimming down to your ideal body weight.

2. *Strengthen the body with good nutrition*

Adopting a healthful diet based on fresh vegetables and fruits, plus whole grains and small amounts of protein and dairy products is a good way to begin strengthening the body. I often suggest nutrient supplements to my arthritis patients in order to help build their general health and strength. The regimen may include:

- **Beta carotene.** Plenty of beta carotene, the plant form of vitamin A, from yellow and orange vegetables and fruits and green leafy vegetables. I recommend at least one serving of a beta-carotene-rich food every day.
- **B complex.** Contains 50 mg of the major B vitamins, twice a day. B vitamins can also be found in whole grains, dried beans and legumes such as split peas and lentils.
- **Niacin.** 25 mg of this form of vitamin B3, three times a day. Niacin has helped to reduce joint stiffness in some patients. If you develop a flushed face or other unpleasant reactions, reduce the dosage until the symptoms disappear. Some severe cases have been helped by 500 mg of niacinamide, a form of B3, three times a day. Food sources include barley, buckwheat, split peas and whole grains.
- **Vitamin C.** Up to 1,000 mg three times a day with meals, to start. Good sources of vitamin C include citrus fruits, cantaloupe, broccoli and Brussels sprouts.
- **Vitamin E.** 400 mg of vitamin E in the form of D-alpha tocopherol with breakfast, and the same with lunch. Vitamin E can also be found in wheat germ, nuts and green leafy vegetables.
- **Selenium.** 200 micrograms a day. Selenium is also found in almonds, barley and oranges.
- **Zinc.** 220 mg of zinc sulfate a day. Take twice a day if arthritis is flaring up. Sources of zinc include turnips, corn and oysters.

3. *"See" your joints move*

Use the power of the mind/body connection to "see" your pain go away. Arrange matters so that you will not be disturbed for at least 20 minutes. Sit down in a comfortable chair in a quiet room. Look at your arthritic joint(s). Think about how they feel. Now close your eyes and picture those joints as being healthy, pain-free and mobile. Imagine yourself easily moving the joint(s). With your mind's eye, see yourself using the joint(s) in daily activities, in hobbies and sports. Notice that there is no pain or discomfort.

Practice "seeing" yourself healthy for 20 minutes, three times a day.

4. *Keep your joints flexible*

I urge all my arthritis patients to move about and exercise as much as possible. It's very important to maintain as much joint mobility and general strength as possible. The exercises can be as simple as walking or riding a bicycle. Other simple exercises include lifting your arms above your head several times to the front and several times to the sides, rotating your arms in circles at your sides, twisting at the waist from side to side and reaching over to touch your knees or toes. Many simple but beneficial exercises can be done while sitting in a chair or lying in bed. Yoga also helps to improve flexibility. The point is not to set Olympic records, but to keep moving as much as possible.

5. *Relieve pain with DLPA*

The first four steps of this program are designed to strengthen overall health. This step, DLPA, is designed to relieve the pain and inflammation. I often have my patients begin with 750 mg of DLPA at breakfast and at lunch. Later, if necessary, a third dose at mid-day may be added. For some patients, I recommend DLPA with aspirin, since the two work well together. Taking one coated aspirin (325 mg) in the morning helps to strengthen DLPA's effects.

It takes anywhere from two days to three weeks for DLPA to take effect, so I encourage my patients to stay positive.

Note: I recommend against taking DLPA during pregnancy or lactation. Pregnant or lactating women should not expose the fetus or newborn to anything except their normal diet. Anyone suffering from the genetic disease phenylketonuria (PKU), or anyone on a phenylalanine-restricted diet should not take DLPA. I do not recommend the use of DLPA for children under the age of 14.

6. *Use other medications as necessary*

I carefully review the medications my patients are taking, reducing or eliminating those that are unnecessary, that conflict with other medications or that exhibit unnecessarily strong side effects.

7. *Remain positive!*

Western medicine has no cure for arthritis, and the disease often becomes progressively worse. The side effects of many common medications may also compound patients' woes. It's no wonder that many arthritis sufferers become depressed, angry or frustrated. These are natural reactions, but not the most helpful. Difficult as it may seem, it's best to remain as positive as possible. You see, pain is a subjective phenomenon, often made worse by fear, anger or other negative feelings. While positive feelings, such as joy and optimism, cannot eliminate pain, they often make it much more bearable. Positive thinking is a medicine for pain.

[1]   Blankenhorn, G. [Clinical effectiveness of Spondyvit (vitamin E) in activated arthroses. A multicenter placebo-controlled double-blind study.] *Z Orthop*, 123(3):340-43, 1986.

[2]   Machtey, I., Ouaknine, L. Tocopherol in osteoarthritis: A controlled pilot study. *J Am Geriatr Soc,* 26:328, 1978.

[3]   de Fabio, A. Treatment and prevention of osteoarthritis. *Townsend Letter for Doctors,* Feb-Mar 1990:143-48.

[4]   Newnham, R.E. Arthritis or skeletal fluorosis and boron. Letter. *Int Clin Nutr Rev,* 11(2):68-70, 1991.

[5]   Stammers, T., et al. Fish oil in osteoarthritis. Letter. *Lancet*, 2:503, 1989.

[6]   Rothschild, P.R., et al. Effect of oral antioxidant enzyme supplementation upon musculoskeletal inflammation. Unpublished study. Biotec Food Corporation, Honolulu, Hawaii, 1989.

[7]   Prudden, J.F., Balassa, L.L. The biological activity of bovine cartilage preparations. *Semin Arthritis Rheum,* 3(4):287-321, 1974.

[8]   Described in *Sharks Don't Get Cancer* by I.W. Lane and L. Comac. Garden City Park, N.Y., Avery Publishing Group, 1992. p. 113-114.

[9]   Rejholec, V. Long-term studies of anti-osteoarthritic drugs: an assessment. *Semin Arthritis Rheum,* 17(2) (Suppl 1):35-53, 1987.

Chapter 5

Asthma

Asthma is a respiratory disease in which the bronchial tubes and smaller airways in the lungs become narrow, making breathing difficult. Allergies are the most common cause of asthma. According to the Asthma and Allergy Foundation of America, 50 percent of older adults, 70 percent of young adults and 90 percent of children with asthma also have allergies.[1]

Asthma attacks may be brief or may last for several days. They can build up slowly or hit suddenly. Three separate events may be involved in an asthma attack:

1. The muscles surrounding the airways constrict (tighten), squeezing down on the airways.
2. Cells lining the inside of the airways secrete a thick, sticky mucous that coats the airway walls, leaving even less space for the air to flow through.
3. Irritated by the constricted muscles and excess mucous, the tissue on the inside of the air passages may swell, further reducing the airspace.

Imagine breathing through a rubber tube the width of a garden hose it's easy. Now put some thick mud into the tube, stuff in some cotton, squeeze down hard on the middle and try breathing through it again. It's not so easy anymore.

Asthma statistics

No one knows exactly how many Americans have asthma, but most authorities agree that some 10 to 12 million Americans of all ages and races are affected. Asthma is the most common of chronic childhood diseases. According to the American Medical Association, it cost just under $6.5 billion to treat asthma in 1990 alone. Nearly 3 million workdays are lost to asthma each year.

There has been an alarming increase in asthma in recent decades. During the 1970s and 80s, the number of Americans with asthma rose from 3 to 4 percent of the total population. Hospitalizations for asthma increased 10 percent between 1987 and 1991, from 450,000 to 490,000 hospitalizations per year. And every year, emergency rooms across the country treat 1.8 million cases of asthma.

The severity of the disease seems to be increasing, as well. Whereas approximately 2,000 people per year died of asthma in the late 1970s, close to 5,000 are now dying of this same disease every year.

Signs and symptoms

There are many signs and symptoms of asthma. Some asthmatics may experience many of them, others but a few. The signs and symptoms one experiences before and during an attack may change over time, but usually include:

- Tightness of the chest.
- Shortness of breath.
- Rapid, shallow breathing.
- Easier breathing when sitting up.
- Wheezing (a whistling sound with breathing).
- Nonproductive coughing (dry cough).
- A chronic cough, even when resting.
- Tightness of the neck muscles.
- Fatigue.

As an attack becomes more severe, signs and symptoms include:

- Breathlessness.
- Difficulty talking.
- Exhaustion.
- Bluish/grayish skin, lips and nail beds.
- Restlessness.
- Confusion.
- Chest retractions.

Possible causes

The substances and situations that trigger an asthma attack are many and varied, both emotional and physical as well as internal and external. Asthma triggers include:

- Allergies to such things as animals, pollen, feathers, dust, molds, foods, food additives, cockroaches and fungi.
- Irritants and pollutants, including cigarette smoke, paint, household and workplace sprays, cleansers, ozone, carbon dioxide, nitrogen dioxide and auto exhaust.
- Medicines, including aspirin and penicillin.

- Infections, including common colds and influenza.
- Stress.
- Emotional upheaval.
- Excitement.
- Vigorous exercise.
- Nonspecific causes, including cold air and sleep (nocturnal asthma).

Asthma triggers may cause an attack, worsen an existing attack or lower one's resistance to other triggers.

Possible complications and long-term effects

People who suffer from repeated asthma attacks may develop lung infections, pneumothorax (lung collapse), respiratory failure, permanent lung damage or COPD (chronic obstructive pulmonary disease). Airways narrowed over and over again during asthma attacks may become permanently narrowed.

A serious bout or several bouts with asthma may weaken the immune system and general health, leaving the sufferer vulnerable to other diseases. The most serious outcome is, of course, death, and some 5,000 Americans die of asthma every year.

Standard medical treatment

Standard Western medical treatment for asthma consists of:

- Removing the triggering agent(s). For example, cleaning every day to make sure your home is dust-free, getting rid of the dog or cat, throwing out the feather pillow, etc.
- Hyposensitization—lessening sensitivity by exposure to larger and larger "doses" of the triggering agent through injections.
- Medications—bronchodilators to relax the airways, corticosteroids to reduce inflammation of the airways, antibiotics to treat infection, allergy shots to reduce sensitivity to triggers, etc.

In brief, Western medicine aims to reduce sensitivity to triggers and to treat symptoms with medicines.

Now let's take a look at some of the many alternative treatments for asthma. These are not all the possible therapies, for there are too many to investigate in a single chapter. Reading through these alternatives, however, will give you an idea of the many possibilities.

The information on alternative therapies is meant for educational purposes only. I am not endorsing any therapy or suggesting that you see any alternative practitioner. If you have or suspect that you have asthma, see your physician.

Acupuncture

The type of treatment used depends on the type of asthma. For example, with "cold asthma," the acupuncturist seeks to warm up the lungs and help the body remove the phlegm. With "hot asthma," the acupuncturist seeks to dispel the excess heat and remove the phlegm.

No matter which type of asthma, the overall goal is to restore normal movement of the chi, or the life energy, and the yin/yang balance. Thus, the acupuncturist carefully places needles in the lung, urinary bladder, stomach and other channels to reduce the phlegm and wheezing; in the kidney, urinary bladder and renal channels to strengthen the kidney; and in the liver and gall bladder channels to get the stagnant chi moving and to strengthen the lung and kidney. *Moxibustion* and *cupping*—techniques for applying heat to the skin— might be used to help reduce the frequency and severity of attacks. Exercise may be recommended to help keep the chi circulating, along with yoga or similar activities to reduce stress.

Aromatherapy

Aromatherapy uses the aromatic essences of flowers and plants to influence the mind and body. Aromatherapy treatments for asthma vary widely, since there are no standard therapy guidelines for the field. Essential oils used for asthma include:

- Benzoin (*Styrax benzoin).*
- Chamomile (*Matricaria chamomilla).*
- Eucalyptus (*Eucalyptus globulus).*
- Frankincense (*Boswellia thurifera).*
- Hyssop (*Hyssopus officinalis).*
- Lavender (*Lavandula officinalis).*
- Marjoram (*Origanum marjorana).*
- Valerian (*Valeriana officinalis).*

Basil, fennel and thyme may also be used. The patient may be instructed to inhale the vapors from these oils as they rise from a bowl of water, to mix them in a base oil and use in massage, to wear as a perfume or to mix with bath water. Treatment length will vary from practitioner to practitioner and according to the patient's condition.

Some aromatherapists caution against having asthmatic patients inhale the vapors from the oils, as asthmatics often have allergies that may then be worsened. Some of the symptoms of asthma may be immediately relieved, at least partially, as the essence of these oils help the patient relax and breath easier. Some aromatherapists also claim that long-term therapy can strengthen the lungs and the body in general, thus helping to prevent future attacks.

Chiropractic

Straight chiropractors who offer supportive treatment for asthma may manipulate the spine to correct subluxation and other imbalances, thus allowing the body to heal itself. There is no specific mixed spinal adjustment for asthma. However, some mixed chiropractors report that asthma is often associated with a misalignment of the center and/or upper part of the spine, and that the problem gets better when the spine is adjusted. It is believed that injuries, poor posture or other problems with the spine may upset the neurological and physical functioning of the lungs, contributing to breathing problems such as asthma.

Color therapy

Although there are no standard protocols for dealing with asthma, color therapists may choose the colors red, green, orange, lemon-yellow and turquoise.

Red increases circulation and energy and reduces nervousness. Red should not be used if there is already too much red in the patient (indicated by an overly reddish face, fever, easy excitability or red hair).

Green is considered a master-healer, good for all conditions and for helping the body rid itself of toxic substances. Green also helps quiet one down, which is useful in dealing with the emotional components of asthma.

Orange is often used in asthma to normalize body functions and to reduce spasms of the bronchial tubes.

Lemon-yellow helps reduce mucus.

Turquoise is a relaxing, cooling color and a powerful tranquilizer.

There are many ways for the color therapist to apply the proper color to the patient, including through direct light, gems, jewelry, perfume, clothing and colored glass. Patients can also meditate on the colors or eat the appropriately colored foods.

- Red foods include radishes, beets, tomatoes, red cabbage, red currants, red plums, watermelon, whole wheat, liver, red wine and grapes. Red metals and chemicals include barium, cadmium, copper, nitrogen, iron, neon, oxygen, potassium and zinc.
- Green foods include green vegetables, peas, beans and lentils. Green metals and chemicals include barium, chlorophyll, nickel and sodium.

- Orange foods include oranges, cantaloupe and mangoes. Orange metals and chemicals include aluminum, antimony and rubidium.
- Yellow foods include bananas, banana squash, eggs, yellow cheese, yellow corn, yellow sweet potatoes, pineapples, lemons, grapefruit and butter. Yellow metals and chemicals include platinum and magnesium.

The time it takes to see results is not known with any certainty.

Folk medicine

Folk remedies for the symptoms of asthma are many and varied. There are absolutely no standard protocols or recipes. Some of the folk medicines for asthma and asthma-related symptoms include:

- Fox liver in red wine or roasted fox liver. Used by Russian shamans.
- Smoking cigarettes made from dried stramonium leaves, then slowly eating rock candy dipped in apple brandy. Used by Cherokee Indian medicine men.
- Chewing honeycomb. Used by New England folk healers.
- A syrup made of honey, lemon juice and lemon rinds. Used by gypsies all over the world.
- A poultice of fried onions applied to the chest. Used by Hungarian gypsies.
- Stringing corn cobs around the neck. Used by Indian healers in the Amazon region.
- A drink made from whiskey, raw onions and brown sugar. Used by Irish folk healers.
- Chicken soup. Used by Jewish mothers and grandmothers.
- Eating garlic by itself or mixed with either vinegar or honey.
- Granules of bee pollen.
- Wrapping strips of cloth, which have been soaked in vinegar, around the wrists.
- Wearing animal furs inside out, with the furry part touching the bare chest.
- Taking one tablespoon of roasted egg shells mixed with molasses or honey.

Herbal medicine

Herbalists use a variety of herbs to treat many diseases and symptoms. There is no standard herbal protocol for treating disease. Much depends upon the herbalist's background. Herbs typically include:

- Black cohosh (*Cimicifuga racemosa*).
- Blood root (*Sanguinaria canadenis*).
- Boneset (*Eupatorium perfoliatum*).
- Cayenne (*Capsicum minimum*).
- Chickweed (*Stellaria spp.*).
- Coltsfoot (*Tussilago farfara*).
- Cowslip (*Primula veris*).
- Elecampane (*Inula helenium*).
- Ma huang (*Ephedra sinica*).
- Eucalyptus (*Eucalyptus globulus*).
- Garlic (*Allium sativum*).
- Gum plant (*Grindelia camporum*).
- Hyssop (*Hyssopus officinalis*).
- Lobelia (*Lobelia inflata*).
- Mullein (*Verbascum thapus*).
- Plantain (*Plantago major*).
- Skullcap (*Scutellaria laterifolia*).
- Sundew (*Drosera rotundifolia*).
- Thyme (*Thymus vulgaris*).
- Valerian (*Valerianan officinalis*).

These herbs are believed to help remove mucous from the lungs, reduce wheezing and shortness of breath, open the air passages, tone nerves in the chest and ease spasmodic coughing.

Homeopathy

Homeopathy attempts to cure asthma by helping the body to heal itself. Most major homeopathic remedies may be used for asthma, depending upon the patient's symptoms. Some remedies include:

- *Aconitum napellus*, which is indicated when the patient is cold in temperature, fearful and impatient and imagining terrible things to come. The attacks come on suddenly and are worse at night and in a warm room, but are better with rest and fresh air.

- *Arsenicum album*, which is indicated when the patient is anguished, restless and cold in temperature. Symptoms include fear and weakness and are worse at night.
- *Bryonia alba,* which is indicated when the patient is irritable and angry, thirsty and warm. There is little phlegm, and the wheezing noises sound "dry." The symptoms are worse in the morning and in warm weather and are better with rest, cold drinks and cool temperatures.
- *Chamomilla,* which is indicated when the patient is irritated and whiny or if the asthma attack begins when the patient is or has recently been angry.
- *Ipecacuanha,* which is indicated when the patient is pale, feeble, irritable and miserable. A great deal of phlegm has accumulated in the chest, symptoms are severe, the patient coughs frequently, is nauseated and vomits. Dampness and warmth make the symptoms worse.
- *Kali bichromicum,* which is indicated when the patient is obese, flabby and cold. The tongue may be yellow-coated or red, dry and cracked. Heat helps to relieve the symptoms, which are worse with cold and at night.
- *Natrum muriaticum,* which is indicated when the patient is weak, depressed, grieving, frightened or angry. Dampness worsens the asthma, which is often associated with early morning diarrhea.
- *Phosphorus,* which is indicated when the patient is sensitive and perceptive, yet fearful. Although often lazy, the patient is given to bouts of great mental or physical exertion, which leaves him or her exhausted. He or she may suffer from burning chest pain and difficulty in breathing. The symptoms are worse in the evening or with physical or mental exertion. Rest and cold foods and drink provide some relief.
- *Pulsatilla,* which is indicated when the patient is timid, emotional and gentle. His or her wheezing begins or worsens at night and is often worse after eating (especially after eating rich or fatty foods).

Relief from symptoms of an asthma attack may begin to occur within 30 minutes to an hour. According to classical homeopathic theory, two or three days should be enough to begin the long-term curative process, assuming the right remedy has been used. If not, another remedy is selected. Thus, the length of treatment will depend on how well the homeopath analyzes the patient's "portrait" and determines the proper treatment.

Hypnosis

Hypnosis has been effectively used as an adjunct treatment for asthma. Many studies have shown it to be very helpful in treating patients who have asthma caused by substances (allergens), infections and/or emotional upset.

Whether or not the asthma attack is triggered by emotional factors, once it starts, the patient may become restless, anxious or fearful. Hypnosis can help control this fear (which often worsens the asthma), thus preventing the attack from progressing. In many cases, hypnosis and post-hypnotic suggestions can help reduce the severity of the attack and improve breathing.

The hypnotist's primary goal is to help the patient relax and remain calm before and during an attack. Patients are taught relaxation techniques and are then hypnotized. While hypnotized, they are given post-hypnotic suggestions so that when they feel an attack coming on or are in the midst of an attack, they will automatically enter into the relaxed state they achieved while practicing the relaxation techniques. In other words, the hypnotic suggestion will direct their minds away from the fear of the attack and toward the calm of the relaxed state. This helps keep the attack from worsening and may even reduce its severity. A typical suggestion might be:

> "Feel how easily you are now breathing, how effortlessly and easily the air flows in and out of your lungs. {Pause.} As you inhale, the air gently moves into your nose, down your windpipe and into your lungs. As you exhale, the air is gently squeezed out. {Pause.} Concentrate on your easy breathing. {Pause.} Imagine that you are on a mountaintop, at the beach, in your backyard or wherever it is that the air is sweet and clear and easy to breathe. {Pause.} If you feel an asthma attack beginning, you can think of this beautiful place where it is so easy to breathe. You can think of this place and relax. Keep thinking of this wonderful place as you feel your body relaxing. Your breath will flow freely, and the problem will fade away."

If a patient's asthma is triggered by stress or other emotional factors, hypnosis can be used to "desensitize" the patient to his or her negative feelings. A standard approach is to have the patient and hypnotherapist write out a list of situations and emotions, from least stressful to most stressful. Then under hypnosis, the patient is directed to remain calm in those situations.

A study published in the *Journal of the Royal Society of Medicine*[2] found that hypnosis-assisted relaxation worked in 16 chronic asthma patients who had continuing difficulties despite medication. The number of hospitalizations fell from 44 per year to 13, and the length of each stay was reduced. Six patients were able to get off of medication entirely, while eight patients had their medications reduced.

Some hypnotherapists have attempted to use hypnosis to reverse *bronchospasm* (tightening of the airways). Studies have shown that although hypnotized asthmatics report feeling better after receiving the suggestion that they are relaxed and are breathing easier, lung tests administered on the spot have proven that they are not actually breathing any better. (This can be dangerous for an asthmatic who mistakenly believes he or she is breathing easier and may not know when to take his or her medicine or seek help.) That this direct-suggestion technique has worked in a small number of cases is probably due to the fact that the patients involved were highly hypnotizable. A more effective technique may be to train the patient in proper breathing techniques while under hypnosis, then give suggestions to the effect that he or she will practice these techniques daily under self-hypnosis.

Hypnosis can also be used to help patients discover unknown triggers. An individual may not realize, for example, that his or her attacks are often triggered by smelling a certain flower or by talking with his or her ex-spouse on the telephone. Under hypnosis, patients can be "walked through" the events that precede their attacks, finding possible triggers.

Nutritional therapy

Nutritional healers may recommend a wide variety of vitamins, minerals and other nutrients for asthma. Most commonly, they will select vitamins A, C, E, B6, B12 and the minerals magnesium and selenium.

Vitamin C

Intravenous (IV) vitamin C has been used to treat people in the midst of asthma attacks. Many years ago, a young woman with a full-blown asthma attack came to my office in Beverly Hills. When I told her that I could end the attack with either medicines or vitamin C, she chose the vitamin C. Quickly setting up an IV bottle containing vitamin C mixed in fluid, I watched as the first drops flowed into her blood stream. In no time at all she was breathing easily.

Vitamin C works by suppressing the release of histamine and reducing the effects of leukotrienes, which cause the small bronchial (breathing) tubes to constrict. Vitamin C works best on allergic asthma, but has been used by physicians to treat asthma caused by infection.

For subacute asthma, which strikes once a week or less, nutritionally minded doctors may recommended 2,000 mg of hypoallergenic vitamin C powder, twice a day. The powdered vitamin C is often mixed with calcium, magnesium and potassium. For prevention of occasional asthma, 1,000 mg of vitamin C in tablets (up to six a day) is recommended. Some physicians report that vitamin C used this way can help to reduce the number and severity of attacks. Good sources of vitamin C include cabbage, oranges and strawberries.

Other supplements

The mineral magnesium has been used to help open up the bronchial tubes in hospitalized patients suffering from acute asthma,[3] and large doses of vitamin B12 have also been reported to be helpful. Because low blood levels of the mineral selenium have been associated with asthma, some nutritional healers may recommend blood tests to measure one's selenium levels and supplements if selenium is low. Magnesium can be found in peanuts, bananas and beet greens. Good sources of B12 include meat, fish and milk. Selenium is found in cabbage, carrots and onions.

Vitamin A (beta carotene) and vitamin E are not known to work directly against asthma, but are considered important for general health and a strong immune system. Along with vitamins A, C and E and the mineral selenium, an antioxidant known as alpha-lipoic acid helps to strengthen the body. Good sources of beta carotene include the yellow-orange fruits and vegetables and green leafy vegetables. Vitamin E can be found in broccoli, green beans and wheat germ.

Fluids

To help loosen mucus, drinking two to three quarts of water a day is often suggested. Some nutritional healers believe that milk should be avoided because some people are allergic to milk protein and that allergy may precipitate an asthma attack. Liquids containing caffeine should be avoided because they are diuretics, causing a loss of water.

Oriental medicine

One of the fastest growing alternative therapies in the United States, Oriental medicine has a multifaceted approach to treating asthma. The first step is to determine the cause of the asthma, which may be related to lung, kidney, fluid metabolism or digestive disorders or other problems. Once the cause of the asthma has been discovered, the doctor of Oriental medicine works to relieve the symptoms and strengthen the body with a combination of herbs, acupuncture, diet and other therapies.

According to practitioners of Oriental medicine, asthma is often related to problems with the kidney. The kidney is responsible for converting fluids into substances, which the body can then metabolize. In order to do so, the kidney draws energy from the tremendous fire in the lower part of the body called the "Ming Men Fire." (This is the center of energy in the lower abdomen.) If this fire isn't strong enough to fuel the kidney, body fluids will not be "steamed." Instead, they will settle in the lungs, producing the symptoms of asthma. Furthermore, people with kidney-related asthma are often frightened of the disease, and their fright further afflicts the kidneys. These people often throw themselves into work, family, hobbies or other projects so they don't have to face the disease or their fear.

Having determined the type of asthma, the Oriental medicine doctor treats it appropriately. The type of treatment will vary from doctor to doctor because Oriental medicine is a broad discipline encompassing many healing arts.

Herbs and spices

Exactly which herbs and spices and the amounts of each will depend upon the patient and his or her condition. Some of the herbs used for asthma are:

- Black cohosh (*Cimicifuga racemosa*).
- Blue cohosh (*Caulophyllum thalictroides*).
- Ephedra (*Ephedra sinica*).
- Gentian (*Gentiana lutea*).
- Lungwort (*Pulmonaria officinalis*).
- Pleurisy root (*Asclepias tuberosa*).
- Skunk cabbage (*Symplocarpus foetidus*).
- Thyme (*Thymus vulgaris*).
- Valerian (*Valeriana officinalis*).
- Vervian (*Verbena officinalis*).
- Wild cherry bark (*Prunus serotina*).

Diet

Because foods are believed to have a profound influence on specific organs as well as on the body in general, and because a strong kidney is important in fighting asthma, the patient would be advised to eat foods that strengthen the kidney. These include:

- Blue and black foods, such as blueberries, black beans, blue corn, purple cabbage and fresh figs.
- Salty foods, such as miso, seaweed and vegetables in soy sauce.
- Small amounts of pork and fish.
- Pork kidneys. (Eating an equivalent animal organ strengthens the patient's distressed organ.)

Pork kidneys in black bean sauce (organ meat plus a black food) is an excellent combination of foods to strengthen the kidney and ameliorate kidney-related asthma.

Psychoneuroimmunology

Mounting scientific evidence backs the argument that negative feelings can contribute to the cascade of biochemical events that can cause or worsen asthma. Mind/body healers use positive affirmations to counteract the negative thoughts that have been contributing to the symptoms of asthma. Affirmations are typically brief, positive statements that focus on how well one feels and on how the disease is being conquered. The patient might be given several affirmations.

Affirmations are verbal statements, always framed in positive terms, describing how good one feels. The patient would most likely be given affirmations specific to asthma, as well as general affirmations concerning good health and happiness. An asthma affirmation might be worded as follows:

> *"All day long, I breathe beautiful, fresh air in and out of my lungs. With each inhalation, my lungs fill with health-giving air. With each exhalation, the air flows easily and completely out. With each breath, I become stronger and healthier."*

The general affirmation may be worded as follows:

> *"Every day, in every way, my mind and body are filled with energy and health. Every day is filled with challenges, joy and love. Today's a great day, just waiting to be conquered."*

The patient will be instructed to repeat these and other affirmations several times a day.

Mind/body healing can help reduce the severity and frequency of asthma by countering its emotional component. Benefits may be seen almost immediately or may take several weeks to develop, depending upon the beliefs of the patient.

Reflexology

Reflexology, the application of pressure to the feet, helps to relieve tension, improve the circulation, stimulate the nerves and normalize the functioning of the organs and glands through a series of pressures, stretches and general movements of the feet.

For asthma, direct reflex points for the lungs and bronchi will be manipulated. In addition, the associated reflex areas for the solar plexus, adrenal glands, pituitary gland, thyroid and heart may be manipulated. Corresponding points on the hands may also be utilized.

The lung reflex areas are at the base of the toes, on the tops of the feet and in the center of the balls of the feet. Reflex areas for the bronchi are found on the tops and bottoms of both feet, slightly below the space between the first two toes. The solar plexus reflex areas are below the balls of the feet, in the midline. The adrenal gland reflex areas are at approximately the middle of the foot, slightly to the inside. The pituitary gland reflex area is in the center of the pad of the big toes. The thyroid gland reflex area is at the ball of the big toe in both feet. The heart reflex area is near the center of the ball of the left foot.

Water therapy

Water therapy is based on the theory that stimulating the body with water can change its energies in specific ways. Hot water, cold water, ice and steam may produce reactions that encourage the body to heal itself.

The water therapist may recommend strengthening the body by sitting in a steam room or otherwise inhaling steam and by directing warm shower water to the chest, abdomen and sides of the torso. For an asthma attack in progress, the water therapist may recommend applying damp, hot compresses to the chest area while lying down or holding the compress to the stomach while walking around. Hot foot baths and ice packs to the back of the head may also be suggested.

Advice to asthma patients

Although many of my patients have had success with the following program, I only use the general guidelines discussed below after reviewing a patient's personal and medical history, performing a thorough examination and evaluating the laboratory studies to make sure that the program will be beneficial. Please see your own physician before embarking on any treatment program for asthma.

Asthma is a common respiratory problem in both adolescents and adults, affecting 5 to 8 percent of the population. There has been a rise in the prevalence of asthma, the severity of many cases and an increase in deaths due to asthma. Since I do not treat children, what I have to say about preventing and treating asthma refers to adults.

1. Diagnosis. The first step is to make a correct diagnosis. As we learned in medical school, "all that wheezes is not asthma." Therefore, a careful history must be taken, with the doctor looking for symptoms such as cough, chest tightness, shortness of breath, wheezing, exercise-induced symptoms and more. The doctor should also look for certain conditions that are often associated with asthma, including allergic skin conditions, rhinitis (inflammation of nasal mucosa), sinusitis and even nasal polyps. During the

physical examination, the doctor may hear wheezing while listening to the lungs. If the asthma struck early in childhood, the patient may have developed a deformity called "pigeon chest," in which the chest protrudes outward. Lung tests called *spirometry* are used to document the severity of the disease (and to measure improvement with treatment).

It is very important that the physician rule out other conditions before making the diagnosis of asthma. These include: congestive heart failure, pneumonia, chronic bronchitis, a pulmonary embolus (a blood clot in the lungs), laryngeal ("voice box") dysfunction, mechanical obstruction of the airways and coughs caused by medications, such as ACE inhibitors, used for high blood pressure.

2. *Remove the triggers.* Having made the diagnosis of asthma, it is very important to identify the allergens—the substances that trigger the attacks. Common triggers include cigarette smoke, chemicals in the office or factory, pollens, molds, animal dander, plants, household cleansers, perfumes, house dust and mites. Once you've identified the triggers, the next step is to reduce your exposure to them or avoid them altogether.

3. *Strengthen the "doctor within."* Keeping the immune system, the "doctor within," as strong as possible helps the body to withstand the asthma attacks that do occur. Thus, I encourage my patients to adopt good nutritional habits, exercise as much as they are able, learn to deal with stress and so on.[4]

   I recommend to my patients that they take the "4 ACES": vitamin A in the form of beta carotene, vitamin C, vitamin E in the form of d-alpha tocopherol and the mineral selenium. These 4 ACES are powerful antioxidants that help to strengthen the body's resistance to disease. The newer antioxidants, such as alpha-lipoic acid and proanthocyanidins, are also of value.

4. *Use medications as necessary.* Although I prefer to use drugs sparingly, medicines are often necessary to prevent asthma or to treat attacks in progress. "Allergy injections" may also help by increasing your immunity to allergens.

I know how terrifying it can be when you can't breathe. I've watched many patients, including my own son, suffer through attacks. The good news is that, with careful management, the number and severity of attacks can often be reduced. Many, many asthmatics are able to lead very active and happy lives.

---

[1]   *Asthma And Allergy Answers*. Asthma Foundation of America. Undated, received from the Foundation on June 16, 1994.
[2]   Morrison, J.B. "Chronic Asthma and Improvement With Relaxation Induced by Hypnotherapy." *Journal of the Royal Society of Medicine*, December 1988:81:701-704.
[3]   Moppen, M., et al. "Bronchodilating Effect of Intravenous Magnesium Sulfate in Acute Severe Bronchial Asthma." *Chest,* 1990; 97:373-376. Okayama, Hiroshi, et al. "Treatment of Status Asthmaticus With Intravenous Magnesium Sulfate." *Journal of Asthma,* 1991; 28(1);11-17. Skobeloff, E. *Journal of the American Medical Association,* Sept. 1, 1989; 262(9):1210-1213.
[4]   For more on the "doctor within," see *Immune For Life* by Arnold Fox, M.D., and Barry Fox, Ph.D. Rocklin, Calif: Prima Publications, 1989.

Chapter 6

Cancer

Many years ago, when I was a young doctor with a brand new practice, a woman walked into my office complaining of foot pain. She seemed upset when I asked her to fill out the complete medical history form that all my patients were required to complete, and balked when I asked her to change into a patient gown for the examination.

"It's only my foot," she complained. "Why can't you just look at my foot?"

I explained that it was very important for the doctor to examine the entire body, head to toe. After much discussion, she reluctantly agreed to the full examination. She eyed me warily as I examined her head, her eyes, her nose, her throat, her neck. Suddenly she said, "Stop!" She was adamant; I mustn't look at her chest.

"It's just a sore on my foot," she repeated.

Again, I insisted upon performing a complete examination, and she reluctantly agreed. As soon as she lowered her gown, I saw the biggest, ugliest, ulcerative tumor I had ever seen. It had eaten into her breast, destroying about a third of the normal breast tissue. I was shocked! "Why didn't you tell me?!"

Later, I learned that she was so frightened by the ulcerating lump on her breast that she couldn't bear to face it or to ask for help. Instead, she went from doctor to doctor complaining of foot pain, subconsciously hoping that someone would notice her breast cancer. I happened to be the one to find it. I immediately drove the woman to the hospital, where she underwent surgery the next day. The pathologist later told me that the cancer had been slow to spread. Otherwise, she would certainly have died.

This woman was so frightened of cancer that she could not admit to herself that she might have had it. Even today, decades into the "war on cancer," many people are terrified by the disease.

What is cancer?

Cancer is not a single disease. Instead, it is a group of diseases with common characteristics. Simply put:

1. Cancer is the uncontrolled growth of body cells. One cell divides into two, two become four, four become eight, eight become 16 and so on. As the renegade cells grow, they "forget" the rules of cooperation the body cells are supposed to follow. They forget that they're only supposed to take in so much nourishment. They forget that they're supposed to perform certain functions. They forget that they're but one small part of a whole, working for the good of all cells. Instead, they are only interested in themselves and their continued growth. That's all they care about.

2. Cancer arises in various tissues of the body, including the skin, lungs, liver, colorectal area, breast, pancreas, ovaries and stomach.

3. Cancer takes many forms. Some are aggressive, growing rapidly and spreading throughout the body. Others grow slowly and remain unchanged for a long time. Prostate cancer is usually a slow-growing cancer that may not trouble a man for many years. In fact, many men will die of other causes, never knowing that they had cancer in their prostate glands.

4. Cancer harms or destroys its host by destroying body tissue and interfering with normal function. A tumor growing in the brain can "crush" brain tissue. Skin cancer can "eat" away the skin.

Cancer cells are driven to grow. They *must* grow. Throwing off the genetic instructions that regulate their growth and behavior, they revert to a wild, primitive stage. Feeding and growing are their only concerns.

Although every cancer is an uncontrolled growth, each kind is different. From a medical perspective, cancer is not one disease but many, arising from diverse origins and organs, and for many reasons. In a sense, cancer is a collection of parasitic cells that live off the rest of the body. Eventually, cancer commits suicide by killing its host. Doctors may call the various forms of cancer Hodgkin's disease, mesothelioma, adenocarcinoma, bronchogenic carcinoma or retinoblastoma. The cancer may be slow or fast. It may lie silent for a long time or it may furiously run rampant throughout the body.

Cancer statistics

Cancer is the second leading cause of death in the United States today (heart disease is number one). According to the American Cancer Society, more than one million new cases of cancer will be diagnosed this year. (This figure does not include skin cancer, which will account for an additional 700,000 to 800,000 cases.)

Despite the "war on cancer" that began in the 1970s and the billions of dollars spent since, we suffer from more cancer than ever.

More than half a million of us will succumb to cancer this year. Here are the 10 leading cancers for men and women:

Men	*Women*
1. Lung	Lung
2. Prostate	Breast
3. Colon and rectum	Colon and rectum
4. Pancreas	Ovaries
5. Lymphoma	Pancreas
6. Leukemia	Lymphoma
7. Stomach	Uterus
8. Esophagus	Leukemia
9. Liver	Liver
10. Bladder	Brain

Signs and symptoms

The symptoms can vary quite a bit, depending upon the cancer. They may be vague, intermittent and hardly noticeable, or powerful and constant. Symptoms include, but are not limited to:

- Pain.
- Fatigue.
- Weight loss.
- Listlessness.
- A persistent sore throat.
- Hoarseness.
- A cough.
- Depression.
- Pains in the upper or lower stomach.
- A change in bowel habits.
- Blood in the stool or urine.
- Unexplained or unexpected vaginal bleeding.
- Sores that don't heal.
- Moles that change color or are irregular.
- A feeling of "fullness" in the abdomen.
- Tenderness, hardening or thickening of the breasts.
- A lump under the arm.
- Ulcerated nipples.
- Difficulty in starting or stopping urination.

Don't be alarmed if you have a sore throat or some pain. Most sore throats *are not* cancer. Be aware, however, of any symptoms that seem to last too long or keep coming back. My mother had an annoying cold that wouldn't go away. That cold turned out to be leukemia, a cancer of the blood.

Possible causes

Cancer has been associated with numerous causes, including:

- Viruses.
- Radiation.
- High-fat diet.
- Obesity.
- Genetic errors.
- Asbestos and other substances, such as benzene.
- Exposure to sunlight.
- Smoking and/or chewing tobacco.
- Immune system failure.
- Nutritional deficits.

What causes a normal cell to become cancerous? There are two steps. First, the normal cell must be initiated or damaged in some way so that it ignores its normal instructions. At this point, the initiated cell is not dangerous. It may sit quietly for months, years or even decades. Only when it is activated does it truly become a cancer cell.

Many things can initiate or activate cancerous cells. Some, like excess dietary fat, both initiate *and* activate. Many studies have shown the strong association between a high-fat diet and the "cancers of affluence." Described as such because they hit hardest in the countries where the richest diets are consumed, they include cancer of the breast, ovaries and uterus in women; cancer of the pancreas and prostate in men; and cancer of the colon and rectum in both men and women. The National Cancer Institute believes that about 30 percent of the cancer deaths in men and roughly 60 percent of cancer deaths in women are related to the standard American high-fat diet.

Other initiators and promoters include tobacco, toxic chemicals, ultraviolet radiation from the sun, and x-rays. Even aflatoxin, a poison related to a fungus sometimes found on peanuts, has been cited.

Standard medical treatment

The standard Western approach to cancer consists of trying to remove the cancer surgically or to "kill" it with radiation and/or chemotherapy. Various medicines to relieve pain and other symptoms of cancer are used.

Now let's take a look at some of the many alternative treatments for cancer. These are not all the possible therapies, as there are too many to investigate in a single chapter. Reading through these alternatives, however, will give you an idea of the many possibilities.

The information on alternative therapies is meant for educational purposes only. I am not endorsing any therapy or suggesting that you see any alternative practitioner. If you have or suspect that you have cancer, see your physician.

Ayurvedic healing

According to Ayurvedic theory, cancer is parasitic negative energy that feeds off the reluctant host's body. All three body humors (Vata, Pitta and Kapha) may be involved, as the body's digestive fire loses heat and the body is overwhelmed by toxins. Since emotional stagnation is often the cause of cancer, the emotions must be treated along with the body. Emotional cleansing and rejuvenation should be as important as the physical treatment or the cancer will recur.

The cancer can take different forms, depending on which of the three humors is most involved.

- With the Vata (air) type of cancer, the skin appears brown or gray. Tumors will be hard and dry. Depression, fear and anxiety are common.
- With the Pitta (fire) type of cancer, tumors will be infected. Bleeding and burning sensations are felt. Anger and irritability are common.
- With the Kapha (water) type of cancer, benign tumors may appear at first, later becoming malignant and dangerous. Fatigue and congestion are common.

All forms of cancer, regardless of their predominant humor, are first treated with detoxification and strengthening. Patients will be given herbs to aid in:

- **Destroying toxins.** Herbs for this purpose include goldenseal, aloe, bitter katuka, black pepper, prickly ash and calamus.
- **Strengthening the immune system.** Herbs for this purpose include ginseng, ligustrum, ashwagandha, bala, black musali, white musali, comfrey root and Solomon's seal.
- **Cleansing the blood.** Herbs for this purpose include dandelion, burdock, sarsaparilla and red clover.
- **Stimulating the circulatory system to keep nutrients flowing to body tissues and to carry away toxins.** Herbs for this purpose include saffron, myrrh and guggul.
- **Expelling phlegm and other substances in the breathing tubes.** Herbs for this purpose include seaweed, kelp, Irish moss and fritillary.

Specific herbs will also be given, depending on the humor in which the cancer has manifested.

- For Vata-type cancer, haritake, calamus and other herbs are prescribed.

- For Pitta-type cancer, dandelion, gotu kola, turmeric and saffron are among the recommended herbs.

- For Kapha-type cancer, bhallatak, ginger, guggul, myrrh and cayenne are often suggested.

For all types of cancer, the diet will be vegetarian. This is because cancer thrives in the presence of protein, which must be kept to a minimum. Raw vegetables, plus vegetable and fruit juices are thought to help dispel the negative life energy from the body, while spices are used to help fan the digestive fires.

In addition to herbs and diet, gems may be worn as rings or other jewelry to encourage the reassertion of the positive life force.

- Diamonds, to encourage longevity.

- Diamonds, yellow topaz and yellow sapphire, to strengthen the immune system.

- Blue sapphire, to force the parasitic negative energy that has produced the cancer out of the body.

- Garnet, red coral and ruby, to improve the circulation.

Because it is so important to strengthen the emotions, mantra therapy is also prescribed. Chanting "om" energizes everything and every process or technique. Chanting "ram" is good for the emotionally based disease of cancer, because it promotes peace and calm while evoking protection from the divine light. Chanting "hum" helps to dispel the negative energy and emotions that feed cancer. Chanting "hrim" helps to detoxify the body. (The "i" in "hrim" is pronounced as a long "e.")

Color therapy

There are no color therapy protocols for dealing with cancer. Therapists may choose the following colors to strengthen the body:

- *Orange* stimulates the thyroid gland and respiratory system and is good for breathing. Orange helps to integrate mental and physical energy, promotes a general sense of well-being and promotes circulation. If the cancer is caught in the very early stages, orange may stop it in its tracks.

- *Violet* cleanses the blood and encourages the white blood cells in their fight against cancer. It helps the body maintain the proper sodium-potassium balance, which helps to prevent tumor growth. An overall healer, violet has many positive psychological effects.
- *Purple* helps to reduce pain.
- *Green* is a soothing and cooling color which can help to stabilize the emotions and rebuild the tissues. It also has disinfectant properties, which help to cleanse the body. As the color of energy, hope and new life, it is an appropriate color to treat cancer.
- *Indigo* purifies the blood and strengthens the immune system.
- *Blue,* which helps to keep the blood stream healthy and build vitality, has anticancer properties.

Since depression is so often a result of cancer, the color therapist may use blue to help lift the mood. Blue is a very soothing color, used to relax the mind. The color of the expanding spirit, blue is said to make people "tired" of being depressed. The blue color is applied to the head.

To combat the nausea that often accompanies cancer or cancer treatments, blue may be applied to the stomach.

Skin sores or ulcers that arise out of cancer treatment may be treated with violet.

There are many ways for the color therapist to apply the proper color of light to the patient, including through direct light, gems, jewelry, perfume, clothing and colored glass. Patients can also eat the appropriately colored foods.

- Orange foods include oranges, cantaloupe and mangoes. Orange metals and chemicals include aluminum, antimony and rubidium.
- Green foods include green vegetables, peas, beans and lentils. Green metal and chemicals include barium, chlorophyll, nickel and sodium.
- Blue foods include plums, grapes and blueberries. Blue metals and chemicals include lead, oxygen and tin.
- Violet metals and chemicals include strontium and titanium.
- Purple metals and chemicals include europium and gadolinium.
- Indigo metals and chemicals include bismuth, potassium and strontium.

Herbal medicine

Herbalists use a wide variety of herbs to treat diseases and symptoms. There is no specific herbal treatment for cancer. Instead, many herbs may be used to help strengthen the immune system, which is the body's weapon against all forms of disease. Herbs may also be used to help relieve some of the symptoms of cancer as well as the side effects of some cancer treatments. Herbs typically used to strengthen the immune system or otherwise improve body functioning include:

- Burdock (*Arctium lappa*).
- Cleavers (*Galium aparine*).
- *Huang Qi* (*Astragalus membranaceus*).
- Nettles (*Urtica dioica*).
- Purple coneflower (*Echinacea spp.*).

Cancer patients often feel depressed and anxious and may be subject to panic attacks. Herbs to help with these problems include:

- Basil (*Ocimum basilicum*).
- Damask rose (*Rosa damascena*).
- Damiana (*Turnera diffusa*).
- Lavender (*Lavandula spp.*).
- Lemon balm (*Melissa officinalis*).
- Mugwort (*Artemisia vulgaris*).
- Neroli oil (*Citrus aurantium*).
- Pasque flower (*Anemone pulsatilla*).
- Skullcap (*Scutellaria lateriflora*).
- Wood betony (*Stachys officinalis*).

In addition, aspen, mustard and mimulus may be used for apprehension, gentian for dejection and despondency, gorse for advanced cases of helplessness and wild rose and rock rose for severe fear or panic attacks.

There is no standard herbal protocol for treating cancer. Much depends on the herbalists' individual backgrounds.

Hypnosis

Hypnosis is sometimes used as an adjunct treatment for cancer. The primary goal of hypnosis for cancer patients is not to treat the disease itself, but to strengthen the body's ability to fight off the cancer and to reduce the patient's fear of the disease.

There is no protocol for using hypnosis against cancer, so hypnotists have varying techniques. The basic idea is to put the patient into a hypnotic trance, then have him or her imagine the immune system defeating the cancer. Some images that might be helpful include:

- Imagining immune-system cells as soldiers, tanks, jet airplanes and submarines. With the mind's eye, the patient can see his or her immune system army fighting and easily defeating the cancer.
- Seeing cancer cells as colored balloons that easily pop when the patient pricks them with a pin.
- Visualizing a tumor as a "house of cards" made up of individual playing cards. The patient could then see himself or herself blowing the cancer apart with a gentle breath.

The actual imagery used will depend upon the patient's vision of the cancer. There is no agreed-upon length of time necessary for using hypnosis to help treat cancer. Several factors affect the length of treatment: how hypnotizable the client is, the rapport developed between the hypnotist and the client, and the severity of the cancer.

Nutritional therapy

The medical literature is filled with studies looking at diet, nutrition and cancer. Mounting evidence shows a clear relationship between various nutrients and cancer, suggesting that good nutrition is a powerful preventive strategy, and can play an important role as an adjunct therapy for those who already have the disease.

Vitamins and minerals

Vitamin A. Solid research has shown that vitamin A reduces the risk of many cancers, including cancers of the bladder, esophagus, stomach, lung, prostate, cervix, head, neck, bladder and skin, as well as the cancer of the blood cells known as leukemia.

Vitamin A is an important immune system booster, helping to keep the thymus and lymphoid tissue in good shape. Good amounts of vitamin A are needed to make sure the total number of T- and B-cells (immune-system cells that help fight off invaders) remains high. Vitamin A even helps those who already have cancer respond to treatment. In a study of 37 women about to undergo chemotherapy for breast cancer, researchers found that 87 percent of those with high levels of vitamin A responded to treatment, compared to only 36 percent of those with low levels.[1] Good sources of Vitamin A include liver, cheese and milk.

Beta carotene. Beta carotene, a member of the carotenoid family, is the "plant form" of vitamin A. Some of the beta carotene that we eat is converted by the body into vitamin A.

Consuming large amounts of foods containing beta carotene has consistently been found to offer protection against cancers of the cervix, colon, esophagus, stomach, larynx, lungs and skin. As the *American Journal of Clinical Nutrition* points out, "One of the most consistent epidemiological findings in nutrition research has been an association between beta-carotene intake and status and reduced lung cancer risk..."[2] Preliminary evidence from the 22,000-physician Physician's Health Study indicates that those who are receiving large amounts of beta carotene have only 12 percent of the expected cancers.

Thiamin (Vitamin B1). Low levels of thiamin intake may be associated with a greater risk of prostate cancer.[3] A deficiency of B1 can lead to shrinking of the thymus, the "school" for immune-system cells, as well as a deficiency of T-cells and B-cells. Vitamin B1 can be found in garbanzo beans, split peas and whole grains.

Riboflavin (Vitamin B2). The intake of riboflavin may be inversely correlated with the risk of cancers of the prostate and esophagus.[4] That is, the more riboflavin one gets, the smaller the risk. Lack of B2 can lead to problems in producing antibodies and reduced numbers of T-cells and B-cells. Vitamin B2 sources include broccoli, collards and dried beans.

Folic acid. This member of the B-family of vitamins may help to prevent cancer of the cervix. A test of the folic acid/cervical cancer hypothesis involved 47 young women who were taking birth control pills. They all had mild or moderate cervical dysplasia, a possibly precancerous condition. Some of them were given folic acid, others a placebo, on a daily basis. Three months later, the women receiving the folic acid showed significant improvement.[5] I have given folic acid to women with abnormal cervical pap smears, and their tests have reverted to normal. Good sources of folic acid include broccoli, Brussels sprouts and cauliflower.

Folic acid is necessary in order for future immune-system cells to mature in the bone marrow. A lack of folic acid may lead to a decrease in the numbers of neutrophils (immune system cells that "eat" foreign bodies) and T-cells, and to the shrinking of the thymolymphatico organs (the "base" for much of the immune system). Lack of folic acid has also been associated with an increased risk of rectal cancer.[6]

Vitamin C. Linus Pauling, Ph.D., sparked a tremendous controversy with his suggestion that vitamin C may help to prevent or cure cancer. Although the medical establishment remains firmly set against the double-Nobel-prize winner's theories, mounting evidence suggests that the late Dr. Pauling was right.

We now know that vitamin C makes the immune system's white blood cells more mobile. It stimulates the T-cells, which engage cancer in "hand to hand" combat; the B-cells, which produce "guided missiles" that lock in on cancer cells; and the macrophages, which "engulf" and destroy foreign bodies. Good food sources include cantaloupe, papaya and spinach.

Some 90 epidemiological studies have looked at the use of vitamin C or foods containing it as a means of preventing cancer. Most of those studies concluded that there is evidence that vitamin C protects against cancers of the pancreas, stomach, oral cavity and esophagus. There is strong evidence that the vitamin protects against cancers of the breast, rectum and cervix. And there is newer evidence suggesting that vitamin C plays a major role in preventing lung cancer.[7] In a study of 3,000 men, those with the lower levels of vitamin C were more likely to develop cancer.[8] In a 13-year study of 4,224 men, cancer patients had significantly less vitamin C in the blood than did healthy controls. The lowest levels were found in victims of gastric cancer.[9]

Vitamin C may kill certain tumor cells directly, strengthen the body's ability to handle cancer, prevent cancer-causing oxidation damage and increase the effectiveness of other cancer therapies.[10] One study of 50 cancer patients tested whether vitamin C could strengthen radiation therapy. Some of the patients were given radiation only, others were given radiation plus 5 grams of vitamin C a day. Four months later, 63 percent of those who had received the vitamin showed a complete response to treatment (all known traces of the cancer had completely disappeared) compared to only 45 percent of the radiation-only group.[11]

Vitamin E. Although excessive vitamin E can hamper the immune system, good amounts are needed in order to keep the numbers of T-cells and B-cells up to proper levels. As an antioxidant, vitamin E helps protect the body against the cancer-causing effects of oxidation. Food sources include wheat germ, nuts and green, leafy vegetables.

Good levels of vitamin E in the blood have been linked to protection against cancers of the cervix, stomach, bowels, breast, head, neck, lungs and skin. When blood was drawn from 766 patients before they were diagnosed with cancer and from 1,419 controls, researchers found that low levels of vitamin E increased the cancer risk by one and a half times. In studies on humans and animals, vitamin E has been found to enhance the effectiveness of several chemotherapy agents.

Selenium. Like vitamins A, C and E, the mineral selenium is an antioxidant. As such, it helps to protect the body from the potentially cancer-causing effects of oxidation. A lack of selenium slows the body's ability to produce antibodies when a foreign or dangerous substance appears in the body. Studies have shown that selenium deficiency is associated with increased risk of cancer of the breast, stomach, pancreas, skin and other parts of the body.

It's interesting to note that the amount of selenium in foods depends upon the quantity of selenium in the ground where the food was grown. People living in areas with selenium-poor soil, who are presumably eating selenium-poor foods, are more likely to die of cancer than those living in areas where the soil is rich in selenium. Foods that are high in selenium include onions, garlic and green beans.

Phytochemicals

Phytochemicals are other substances found in foods that help us remain healthy. ("Phyto" refers to "food.") Neither vitamins nor minerals, the phytochemicals are a remarkably large and diverse group of substances with a variety of duties in the body. Some phytochemicals that may help to fight or prevent cancer include:

- *Bioflavonoids.* A group of compounds, such as quercetin and catechin, that have antioxidant properties. As antioxidants, they help to protect body cells from the oxidative damage which can turn normal cells cancerous. The bioflavonoids have also been called "vitamin P." Bioflavonoids are found in orange and yellow citrus fruits (such as oranges, grapefruits and tangerines), green tea and other foods.
- *Ellagic acid.* A substance found in strawberries, grapes and other foods that helps to protect the body against cancer-causing substances.
- *Indoles.* Found in cabbage, cauliflower, broccoli and other "cruciferous" vegetables, these substances have demonstrated powerful anticancer properties.
- *Isoflavones.* Hormone-like substances that may help to prevent the growth of tumors that are normally "spurred on" by the female hormone estrogen. Isoflavones are found in peas, beans and lentils.
- *Lignans.* Found in flax, lignans slow the growth of cancerous and precancerous cells in laboratory animals. Flax oil is consumed by many as a supplement.
- *Limonene.* Found in the oil of citrus fruits, limonene has slowed the growth of tumors in laboratory animals.
- *Lycopene.* An antioxidant and close cousin to beta carotene, lycopene may help prevent cancer of the cervix, bladder and pancreas. Lycopene is found in tomatoes, red peppers and other foods.
- *Monoterpenes.* Powerful antioxidants that help prevent the oxidative damage that can lead to cancer. They are found in various vegetables and fruits.
- *Protease inhibitors.* Substances that interfere with the proteases that can encourage the growth of breast, colon and other cancers. Protease inhibitors are believed to neutralize a host of carcinogens, ranging from radiation to substances in diesel fuel exhaust. They are found in whole grain oats, rice, potatoes, chickpeas, soybeans, kidney beans and other foods.

- *Saponins*. Substances that kill colon cancer cells in laboratory tests. Saponins are found in sunflower seeds, soybeans and other foods.
- *Sulfides*. Natural substances found in garlic and cruciferous vegetables, such as broccoli and cauliflower, that prevent certain carcinogens from acting on healthy cells.

These are just some of phytochemicals that protect against cancer. The point of this review is not to make you an expert, but to give you a glimpse into the exciting new discoveries about food that may revolutionize the nutritional approach to health and cancer.

Specific foods that may aid in treating cancer

Avocado. Avocados contain a cancer-fighting antioxidant called glutathione. Glutathione has shown the ability to block many carcinogens that would otherwise turn normal cells cancerous.

Beans. Eating large amounts of dried, cooked beans may help to reduce the risk of getting breast cancer or dying of cancer of the pancreas. The fiber in beans offers protection against many cancers—the protease inhibitors help to keep cellular DNA from being modified, the lignans slow the growth of tumors and the phytoestrogens help to "dilute" the cancer-causing effects of estrogen.

Citrus fruits. Citrus fruits are filled with antioxidants, carotenoids, coumarins, flavonoids, limonoids, terpenes and other substances that fight cancer. Studies have shown that eating large amounts of citrus fruits is equated with less cancer. One study found that people eating a single citrus fruit every day had less than half the risk of developing cancer of the pancreas as did those eating but one citrus fruit a week.

Crucifers. Cabbage, broccoli, Brussels sprouts, cauliflower and other members of the crucifer family of vegetables contain powerful anticancer agents called the indoles, which help to prevent cancer of the colon and other cancers. Crucifers also contain beta carotene, vitamin C and fiber, all of which strengthen the immune system, plus sulfides to fight cancer directly.

Fish. Major studies have found that eating large amounts of fish protects against cancers of the breast, colon and other parts of the body. It is believed that the omega-3 fatty acids (found especially in cold-water fish such as salmon) slow the growth of tumor cells.

Garlic. This tasty spice contains ajoene, quercetin, DAS (diallyl sulfide) and many other substances that help to control cancer. The DAS in the oil of garlic seems to disarm cancer-causing substances and slow the growth of tumors. Many studies have found that eating more garlic cuts the risk of many types of cancer. Laboratory studies have shown that substances in garlic can reduce the risk of cancers of the breast, colon and esophagus by three-quarters.

Grapes and strawberries. Although their anticancer properties have not been completely studied, we know that grapes and strawberries contain large amounts of ellagic acid. Ellagic acid helps to keep cells from mutating into dangerous forms, and "cleans up" cancer-causing agent like cigarette smoke. Red grapes also contain the powerful antioxidant called quercetin.

Mango. The mango contains large amounts of the cancer-fighting vitamin C and beta carotene, as well as vitamin E and fiber. Together, these four nutrients protect against cancers of the colon, rectum, pancreas, prostate, breast, cervix and stomach.

Mushrooms. Eating shiitake mushrooms can strengthen T-cells and macrophages that engage cancer cells and other antigens in "hand to hand" combat within the body. Mushrooms can also stimulate the body's production of interferon, interleukin-1 and interleukin-2, all three of which help fight off cancer. The button mushroom, popular in the United States, has no known anticancer effects.

Nuts. Various nuts contain protease inhibitors. These substances interfere with the proteases that encourage cancer. In addition, Brazil nuts have good amounts of the cancer-fighting antioxidant selenium, while walnuts contain the antioxidant ellagic acid.

Onions. Onions contain quercetin, sulfur compounds and other substances that help the body to resist cancer. The National Cancer Institute has found that the risk of stomach cancer drops by 40 percent when one eats three ounces of onions or garlic a day.

Soy. Soybeans, as well as tofu, soy milk and other products made from soy, contain a variety of potential cancer fighters. Soy's anticancer armament includes isoflavones, genistein, daidzen, protease inhibitors, phytic acid and saponins. Perhaps one of soy's most effective cancer fighters, however, is the group know as "phytoestrogens."

The phytoestrogens found in soy are estrogen-like substances that may reduce the risk of cancer by "diluting" the effect of estrogen (a natural hormone) in the body. It is believed that estrogen "locks" onto cancer cells and helps them to grow. The weaker phytoestrogens in soy also lock onto cancer cells, but cannot spur their growth. With the weaker phytoestrogens in the way, less estrogen will be able to "connect" with cancer cells.

Researchers have found that people eating large amounts of soy or soy products have less cancer, including less cancer of the breast and prostate. Because breast and prostate cancers are "hormone dependent," (encouraged by the presence of estrogen or testosterone), the lowered incidence of these cancers in people who eat a lot of soy is probably due to the phytoestrogens.

Tea. Green tea contains catechins, polyphenols and other cancer-fighting substances. Drinking green tea has helped to prevent or slow the appearance of cancers of the skin, stomach and lungs in laboratory animals.

These are just a few of the many foods with anticancer properties. Other foods include apples, apricots, asparagus, barley, cantaloupes, carrots, celery, cherries, collard greens, currants, dandelion greens, figs, eggplant, guava, kale, kiwi fruit, lentils, oats, papaya, parsley, pasta, peppers, potatoes, whole-grain rice, seaweed, spinach, tomatoes, turnips, watercress, watermelon and wheat.

Although diet alone is not a cure for cancer, eating the most healthful foods possible can help to strengthen the body's natural defenses. If the cancer has not altered your appetite or ability to eat foods, the best diet would be based on fresh vegetables and fruits, plus plenty of whole grains, with only small amounts of organically grown lean meat, low-fat poultry and dairy products.

Other nutritional therapies

Chaparral. This is a desert shrub, also known as the creosote bush, which is grown in the southwestern deserts of the United States. Native Americans used preparations made from chaparral leaves as a general health booster. Later, chaparral tea was used to treat a variety of diseases. During World War II, researchers at the University of Minnesota identified a powerful antioxidant in chaparral called NDGA (nordihydro-guaiaretic acid). NDGA seems to be a natural chemotherapy agent, attacking cancer cells as well as bacteria, viruses and fungi. Tests with laboratory animals have shown that chaparral can prevent cancer of the skin when a known carcinogen (benzoyl peroxide) is applied. Studies with human cells in test tubes have shown that NDGA may be helpful in treating some cancers of the gastrointestinal tract.

Chaparral is a quinone, a group of chemicals with anticancer properties that are, unfortunately, toxic themselves. That's why taking chaparral can lead to vomiting, nausea and abdominal cramps, and may damage the liver. A number of chaparral-associated cases of hepatitis have been reported by the Centers for Disease Control. I have personally seen a woman who came to me after she developed what was believed to be chaparral-associated hepatitis. Chaparral therapy should always be supervised by an experienced physician.

Essiac tea. This herbal tea is made from burdock root, Indian rhubarb, slippery elm bark and other substances. Although several of the individual ingredients have demonstrated anticancer activity, proponents of Essiac tea argue that the whole is greater than the sum of the parts. In other words, drinking the tea, with its ingredients working together, is better than taking the tea's components one at a time.

Based on a native Canadian recipe, Essiac tea was introduced into Canada by a nurse named Rene Caisse in the 1920s. Although Ms.

Caisse never revealed the Essiac recipe, teas based on what is believed to be her original notes are currently on the market.

Shark cartilage. The seemingly indestructible shark has survived tremendous environmental changes in its 400 million years of existence. Two interesting observations about the shark led to the development of a new treatment for cancer. First, the shark seems to be totally resistant to cancer. Second, the shark has no bones. Instead, its skeleton is made up of cartilage.

Cancer cells are hungry cells. As a tumor grows, it secretes substances that force the body to "build" new blood vessels to support it. Without new vessels feeding it, the cancer could not grow very large. A 1983 article in *Science*[12] suggested that shark cartilage might be an effective treatment for cancer because something in the cartilage inhibits the growth of these blood vessels. Various studies with laboratory animals showed that implanting shark cartilage next to tumors could indeed "starve" the tumors by preventing the growth of new blood vessels. The anti-blood vessel substance turned out to be a macroprotein named CDI (cartilage-derived inhibitor).

In studies on human cancer victims, oral administration of shark cartilage has reportedly helped women suffering from advanced breast cancer as well as patients with other cancers. Shark cartilage is administered either orally or by enema.

The government has allowed the proponents of shark cartilage treatment to administer controlled amounts to those advanced cancer patients who have not been helped by standard therapies, such as surgery, radiation and chemotherapy. According to the advocates of shark cartilage, the preliminary studies show good results against solid tumors (those in the prostate, pancreas, ovaries and uterus). Future studies will reveal more about this and other intriguing nutritional therapies.

When selecting a nutritional healer, remember that there is no widely recognized school of nutritional therapy and no standards or agreed-upon training for nutritional healers.

Psychoneuroimmunology

Mounting scientific evidence backs the argument that negative thinking can harm the immune system, increasing the risk of various types of cancer (and other diseases). Fortunately, the reverse appears to be true: Positive thinking can strengthen the immune system.

The power of the mind/body connection was demonstrated in older Jewish men and elderly Chinese women, whose positive thoughts kept them alive at significant times of the year. Researchers have found that the death rate for older Jewish men drops in the spring, right before Passover. The death rate still remains low throughout the eight-day celebration, then rises above normal immediately afterwards. Passover is a significant holiday, one in which the father or grandfather plays an important role. It may be that men who might otherwise have died are kept alive by joyful anticipation. Their positive thoughts alone may be able to delay death. The same apparently holds true for the elderly Chinese women who eagerly look forward to a holiday that highlights *their* importance, the Harvest Moon Festival.

Mind/body healers use positive affirmations to counteract the negative thoughts that have been contributing to the symptoms of cancer. Affirmations are typically brief, positive statements that focus on how well one feels and on how the disease is being conquered. The patient might be given several affirmations.

An affirmation to resist cancer might be worded as follows:

"Every moment of every day, my body gets stronger and stronger. My immune system easily knocks out invaders, my heart carries health-giving blood to every cell, and I am filled with energy and the joy of life."

An affirmation to fight fear might be worded as follows:

"I look forward to every day and every challenge ahead. I know that I can leap over obstacles and achieve all my goals."

Patients may also be given affirmations for general health.

Water therapy

Although there is no treatment for cancer itself, water therapy may be used to alleviate some of the symptoms of the disease or the side effects of treatment.

- For *pain*, both heat and cold may be helpful. Hot full-body baths, hot footbaths, hot and moist compresses, hot blankets, cold compresses, cold hand baths or footbaths, and drinking ice water are some ways of applying heat and cold.
- For *vomiting*, hold one ice pack to the stomach, another to the midline of the upper back.
- For *loss of appetite*, a bag of ice or cold water held to the stomach before meals helps to stimulate the appetite.
- For *fear or nervousness,* tepid baths, hot footbaths, and applying hot, moist compresses to the spine are recommended.
- For *fatigue*, take long, warm baths followed by a quick burst of cold water (from the shower nozzle is the easiest way). Brushing the feet with a loofa or a brush while bathing helps to stimulate the body.
  Another approach is to alternate very brief, all-body cold showers with slightly longer hot ones, several of each in quick

succession. (The cold showers should last for several seconds, the hot showers a little longer.)

Practices may vary from practitioner to practitioner, because there are no widely accepted protocols for water therapy.

Other exciting approaches

Antineoplaston therapy

Antineoplaston therapy is based on the idea that there is a second defensive system in the body, the biochemical system, which protects the body against defective cells. (Cancer cells are all defective in that they ignore their genetic programming.)

The biochemical system's "soldiers" are small peptides and organic acids called *antineoplastons*. Instead of killing cancer cells, antineoplastons reprogram them. All cells are born with programming that tells them how many times to multiply before dying. This programming "breaks down" in cancer cells, allowing them to multiply forever, but antineoplastons correct the error. Although antineoplastons are found in the human body, they are generally low in cancer patients.

The therapy consists of injections or oral doses of antineoplastons. The type of antineoplaston used depends on the cancer. Antineoplaston "A" works against leukemia, lymphoma, bone cancer and breast cancer. Antineoplaston "L" is effective against leukemia. And antineoplaston "O" is used to treat osteosarcoma.

Chelation therapy

A controversial therapy called *chelation* involves injecting substances, such as a chemical food preservative called EDTA (ethylenediaminetetraacetic acid), into the body that bind with dangerous substances. Once they have bound to the chelating agent, the harmful substances are passed in the urine. The word "chelation" comes from the Greek word meaning "to grasp" or "to claw," like a lobster. Since the late 1940s, standard medical literature has recommended its use to reduce toxic amounts of lead in the body.

Proponents argue that chelation may help cancer patients in several ways. EDTA injected into the body as the chelating agent may:

1. Improve overall circulation, getting more oxygen to all body tissues. Increasing the amount of oxygen in the body also weakens cancer cells, which prefer a poorly oxygenated (anaerobic) environment.
2. Bind to and "disarm" lead, mercury and other toxic metals that *may* be implicated in cancer or a weakened immune system.

3. Remove the protective coating surrounding cancer cells, making them more vulnerable to attack by the immune system.

Physicians using chelation as an adjunct to standard cancer therapy often add various vitamins and minerals to the chelating solution. The solution is administered via an intravenous (IV) drip, and the typical chelation session takes between two and four hours. Patients may receive chelation therapy up to three or four times a week.

DMSO

DMSO (dimethyl sulfoxide) is used as an adjunct to other cancer treatments. A clear liquid, it may be injected into the muscles or veins, taken orally or applied to the skin.

An antioxidant, DMSO protects against the free radicals that alter body fat, cells, proteins and anything else they touch in their search for oxygen molecules. Specifically, DMSO helps to relieve some of the side effects of standard cancer treatment (such as the lip sores and nausea caused by radiation or chemotherapy). It must be used with caution, however, for DMSO itself can cause nausea, headaches, dizziness and skin rashes.

Eumetabolic therapy

"Eumetabolic" simply means "good metabolism." Devised by Hans Nieper, M.D., of Germany, the therapy aims to: 1) strip away the mucous layer that surrounds and protects tumor cells; 2) convert cancerous cells to normal cells by correcting their faulty programming; and 3) correct mineral imbalances in the body.

This treatment for cancer consists of various vitamin and mineral supplements, drugs, laetrile, extracts of certain plants and animals and a near-vegetarian diet consisting of vegetables, fruits, wholegrain cereals, juice and skim milk. In order to stimulate the immune system, patients are given a weakened version of the tuberculin bacillus (BCG). Low doses of radiation or chemotherapy may also be used.

Some of the animal extracts used come from insects. Dr. Nieper uses these because, he notes, although insects have no immune systems, they are immune to viral diseases.

Finally, patients are advised to stay away from certain locations that put out dangerous electromagnetic radiation (geopathogenic zones). A person known as a *dowser* uses a divining rod to identify geopathogenic zones under or near a patient's house, workplace and other areas.

Gerson therapy

One of the oldest alternative treatments, Gerson therapy was devised by Dr. Max Gerson, a German physician who emigrated to the United States in the 1930s.

Gerson's theory of cancer holds that cancer is caused by toxins and electrolyte imbalances in the cells. It is believed that when cells are injured, they lose potassium and are flooded with sodium, upsetting the normal sodium-potassium balance. Treatment consists of a vegetarian diet, plus vegetable and fruit juices. All the food must be organically grown to make sure it contains no toxins. The juices are made only from these organically grown foods. Patients drink juice every hour on the hour for 13 hours a day. Each patient consumes about 20 pounds of food in solid or juice form every day.

To help restore the electrolyte balance, sodium intake is severely restricted and potassium supplements are given. Thyroid extract is given to increase energy production within the cells, helping the cells to pump out waste and heal themselves. Protein intake is limited, for excess protein is believed to inhibit the immune system.

Coffee, which encourages the release of toxic substances trapped by the liver, is given as an enema to help detoxify the body. Several coffee enemas a day may be used to relieve the nausea and other symptoms that are caused by detoxification.

Hyperthermia

Hyperthermia, which means "lots of heat," is based on the idea that cancer cells "can't take the heat" as well as healthy cells. Cancer cells are believed to die at temperatures above 107 degrees—temperatures that normal cells can survive.

High temperatures are generated with microwaves, radio waves or ultrasound. Computerized delivery and monitoring devices make sure that the heat is applied only to specific areas of the body. For some conditions, such as localized prostate cancer, the heat is narrowly focused. When whole-body hyperthermia is called for, the patient is anesthetized and wrapped in special blankets or a suit, then heated to 108 degrees or so. No one knows exactly how hyperthermia works. Researchers have theorized that it:

1. Destroys the blood vessels feeding tumors. A tumor's vessels are believed to be less heat-resistant than normal vessels.
2. Cripples the enzymes that repair cancer cells, making it impossible for cells that have been subjected to radiation therapy to repair themselves.
3. Interferes with the metabolic activity of the cancer cell.
4. Liberates tiny cancer-killing "poison packets" (lysozymes) within the cells.

5. Alters the ability of the cancer cells to manufacture protein, which inhibits the immune system.
6. Makes the walls of cancer cells more permeable, allowing cancer-harming substances to move into them.

Hyperthermia is usually used in conjunction with radiation or chemotherapy, not as a stand-alone therapy. Proponents of hyperthermia argue that the heat treatment makes the other treatments stronger. This means that many patients should be able to cut back on their chemotherapy or radiation, both of which have powerful and debilitating side effects.

Immuno-augmentative therapy

Some 30 years ago, Lawrence Burton, Ph.D., and some of his colleagues injected cancer-ridden mice with a substance that caused the mice's tumors to shrink within hours. Newspapers announced that a "15-minute cancer cure" had been found.

Immuno-augmentative therapy is based on the idea that cancer victims are deficient in one or more of the four *blood fractions* Dr. Burton identified. He labeled these naturally occurring proteins tumor antibody 1 (TA1), tumor antibody 2 (TA2), tumor complement (TC) and deblocking protein (DP). The therapy consists of injecting the patients with the needed fractions, which are taken from healthy blood. Patients are given injections or inject themselves once or twice a day for as long as necessary to rebuild the body's store of all four.

According to Dr. Burton, the therapy does not directly cure cancer. Instead, it restores the body's natural defense mechanisms to their full strength, allowing the body to dispose of the cancer. The four blood fractions are believed to work in a specific sequence to either destroy the cancer cells or to restore them to normal functioning.

The patient's blood is drawn and analyzed once or twice a day during the initial six to eight weeks of intensive treatment. Results of blood tests are used to continually calibrate the blood fraction serum for each individual patient.

Iscador

Iscador is extracted from European mistletoe, a plant long used as a medicine in areas of Northern Europe and Scandinavia. Laboratory studies have shown that substances in the mistletoe increase the body's resistance to disease by stimulating the thymus, increasing the number of white blood cells called granulocytes and encouraging white blood cells to engulf and destroy foreign substances and damaged cells. Other substances in the mistletoe directly attack tumors.

Iscador is primarily used in conjunction with standard cancer treatment. It is sometimes given to patients daily for two weeks before their surgeries to prevent the spread of cancer and may be used after surgery or radiation therapy. It may be injected into the body near the tumor site or taken orally.

Kelley's nutritional-metabolic therapy

A dentist named William Kelley developed a wide-ranging theory of cancer, believing that it could be caused by: 1) a malfunctioning pancreas that doesn't put out enough cancer-fighting and other enzymes; 2) an imbalance of minerals within the body; 3) the body's inability to properly digest and use proteins; and 4) the ability of cancer cells to protect themselves with an electromagnetic force, which weakens the immune system.

To combat cancer, Kelley's nutritional-metabolic therapy analyzes a person's metabolism, assigning him or her to one of 10 categories, depending on the patient's condition and type of cancer. Depending on the category, patients are given a specific diet, as well as supplements of pancreatic enzymes, raw beef concentrates and many vitamins and minerals. The supplements are periodically discontinued to allow the body time to "clear out" the remnants of tumors killed by this therapy. Coffee, which stimulates the liver, is given as an enema to help detoxify the body. In addition, the patient is encouraged to accept the disease as part of the natural life process and to believe that a higher power will assist his or her recovery.

Live-cell therapy

Operating on the principle that fetal cells will stimulate the immune system, live-cell therapy consists of injecting fetal or embryonic cells from calves, sheep, horses, monkeys or other animals into the cancer patient. Live-cell therapy is also believed to strengthen target organs. If, for example, the cancer is in the liver, fetal liver cells would be injected into the patient to help regenerate the cancerous organ.

Because several months may pass before the effects of live-cell therapy are felt, patients are generally treated with diet, detoxification and various supplements during this time. Live-cell injections are given weekly for several weeks, then every three to six months.

Livingston-Wheeler therapy

Believing that cancer was caused by a bacteria, Virginia Livingston-Wheeler, M.D., identified and named the germ *Progenitor cryptocides*, which means "hidden primordial killer."

Dr. Livingston-Wheeler believed that *Progenitor cryptocides,* like many other bacteria, is always present in the human body. It only becomes a problem when the immune system weakens for one reason or another, allowing *Progenitor* to multiply and secrete a hormone that allows cancer to take hold.

Using the blood and urine of cancer patients, Dr. Livingston-Wheeler made special *Progenitor* vaccines for each patient individually. The full Livingston-Wheeler therapy consists of the vaccine, a diet based on raw vegetables and fresh fruits, various supplements and a plant hormone called absicsic acid. Smoking and the use of alcohol are prohibited on the program.

The Livingston Foundation Medical Center Clinic in San Diego, Calif., used to develop a unique vaccine for each patient out of his or her blood or urine. Under orders from state authorities to cease doing so, the center now offers a "generic" vaccine.

Moerman anticancer diet

Devised by a physician named Cornelis Moerman, the diet is a recognized anticancer treatment in the Netherlands. The Moerman diet is based on the idea that poor eating habits disrupt the body's normal functioning, allowing cancer to take hold.

The basic Moerman diet consists of fresh vegetables and fruits, whole grain cereals and breads, buttermilk and natural seasonings. The vegetables and fruits should be organically grown. Instead of water, patients drink fresh vegetable or fruit juice. Small amounts of dairy products are allowed, including egg yolk and low-fat, low-salt cheese. In addition to the foods, supplements of vitamins A, C, E and B-complex, and iron, iodine, sulfur and citric acid are given.

Moerman devised his diet after studying the pigeon, which normally does not get cancer. It's based on the pigeon's natural diet.

Revici therapy

Named for its founder, Dr. Emanuel Revici, this therapy is based on the idea that good health is the result of a dynamic balance between opposing forces or activities within the body. The constructive (anabolic) force makes things grow and build upon each other. The opposing destructive (catabolic) force breaks things down, releasing their stored energy.

According to Revici, the body runs through a four-stage defense procedure when something foreign or dangerous invades it. At each stage, specific defensive substances are manufactured by the body. But if the defense reaction breaks down for any reason, the body remains stuck in the last stage completed, churning out that stage's characteristic substances. The substances build to dangerous levels and cause disease.

Revici's theory holds that cancer is caused by imbalances of either sterols or fatty acids, depending upon which stage the body's defense reaction was in when it was halted. Revici therapy is based on curing the imbalance. If the cancer is caused by excess sterols, the patient is given fatty acids. If excess fatty acids are believed to be the cause,

sterols are given in order to harmonize the body's internal environment. Other substances, including the mineral selenium, are also used.

Urea therapy

In many cultures, the drinking of one's urine has a long history of
use for intestinal distress and as a general tonic. It has also been applied topically for skin problems. In the 1950s, Dr. Evangelos
Danopoulos of Greece reported that the urea in urine also had anticancer properties. Urea apparently disrupts the ways in which cancer
cells group together, killing them by upsetting some of their normal
metabolic activities. It has been used to treat cancers of the skin, cervix, lungs, eyes, breast and liver.

Liquid urea can be injected into the skin around skin tumors or
directly into the tumors themselves. Powdered urea can be applied to
tumors, and it can be taken orally in liquid or pill form.

Wheat grass therapy

Devised by Ann Wigmore, wheat grass therapy is designed to detoxify the body and strengthen its natural defenses against cancer
and other diseases. The program is based on drinking wheat grass
juice, which contains chlorophyll and many vitamins, minerals and
phytochemicals. In addition to the juice, patients are put on a diet
based on sprouted grains, raw vegetables and fruits, nuts and seeds.
Wheat grass juice enemas, exercise, visualization and stress reduction
are also part of the therapy.

Advice to cancer patients

*I only treat cancer patients when working with their cancer special-
ists. Although many of my patients have had success with the following
program, I only use the general guidelines discussed below after reviewing a patient's personal and medical history, performing a thorough examination and evaluating the laboratory studies to make sure
that the program will be beneficial. Please see your own physician before embarking on any treatment program for cancer. Cancer patients
are best served by a team of physicians and other health professionals.*

Cancer is a frightening disease. We continue to suffer from the
scourge, despite the billions of dollars spent on research and treatment. Our strongest weapon against cancer has been, and continues
to be, prevention. Protect yourself by reducing or eliminating your risk
factors with these "Nine Steps for Preventing Cancer":

1. Stop smoking.
2. Be careful with chemicals.
3. Slim down to your ideal weight.
4. Reduce the fat in your diet.

5. Give your "doctor within" all the nutrients and
   phytochemicals necessary to keep it strong.
6. Limit your exposure to the sun.
7. Have regular checkups.
8. Learn to recognize the signs of cancer.
9. Remain optimistic and positive.

Cancer is the number-two killer disease in this country. But if we do nothing more than stop smoking, eliminate most of the fat (especially animal fat) from our diets, reduce our exposure to chemicals and protect ourselves from the damaging rays of the sun, we can cut the rate of cancer in half. Let's take a closer look at the Nine Steps for Preventing Cancer.

1. Stop smoking.

It's been about 30 years since the Surgeon General of the United States began warning that cigarette smoking causes lung cancer. About one-third of the cancers striking us down are related to tobacco, especially to cigarettes and chewing tobacco. There's no good reason to smoke and no "safe" way to do it. It's best to give it up.

2. Be careful with chemicals.

Look at all the chemicals you use or are exposed to—everything from hobby glue to oven cleaners. Some of them are probably reasonably safe, but you don't know which ones may harm you. Ask yourself if you really need to use or be around each substance. If not, throw it out. Some of the dangerous chemicals we knowingly or unknowingly come in contact with are benzene, acrylonitrile, arsenic, benzidine-derived dyes and many solvents.

At work, you can ask to see the Material Safety Data Sheets (MSDSs) that are supposed to be kept for various chemicals. These sheets will tell you if the substances you use or come into contact with are potentially carcinogenic.

3. Slim down to your ideal weight.

Many studies have connected obesity to cancer. For example, males and females 25 percent or more overweight have an increased risk of rectal cancer. Males who are 25 percent or more overweight are also more likely to develop colon cancer. A study of 750,000 men and women found cancer deaths increased in those 40 percent or more overweight. Simply dropping down to your ideal weight will significantly reduce your risk of cancer.

Here's a rough rule of thumb to approximate ideal weight. For men, it's 106 pounds plus an additional five pounds for every inch of height over five feet if they have slim wrist bones, an additional six pounds for every inch of height over five feet if they have medium wrist bones and an additional seven pounds for every inch of height over five feet if they have thick wrist bones.

For women, it's 100 pounds plus an additional four pounds for every inch of height over five feet for women with tiny wrist bones, an additional five pounds for every inch of height over five feet for women with medium wrist bones and an additional six pounds for every inch of height over five feet for women with large wrist bones.

4. *Reduce the fat in your diet.*

According to the National Cancer Institute, about 30 percent of the cancer deaths in men and roughly 60 percent of cancer deaths in women are related to a high-fat diet. I believe the numbers are higher. Everyone now agrees a high-fat Standard American Diet (SAD) is responsible for many cancers, including the "cancers of affluence."

Unwrap a stick and a half of butter. Squeeze it in your fist. Rub that butter between your two hands, spreading it all over your hands and fingers. That's about as much fat as there is in the food the typical person eats in a day. Feel that fat on your hands. Imagine all that fat oozing into your body cells, gumming up the works, initiating and activating cancer cells, turning normal cells cancerous.

You don't have to count the fat grams in your food or worry about the balance between saturated and unsaturated foods. There's an easy way to switch to a low fat diet. Make fresh vegetables and fruits and whole grains the basis for your diet. Limit your intake of meat, poultry and dairy products and always select the low-fat varieties. Instead of burying your salads under mounds of fatty dressings, use vinegar, lemon juice or other low-fat seasonings.

I'll be the first to admit that fat *does* taste good. But you know what? Not too long after you switch to a low-fat diet, you stop missing it. Pretty soon, the fat you used to crave doesn't taste good anymore.

5. *Give your "doctor within" all the nutrients necessary to keep it strong.*

We're learning that many foods, such as cabbage and broccoli, have specific anticancer properties. Others, such as carrots, contain beta carotene or other natural antioxidants that protect normal cells against the potentially cancer-causing damage of oxidation. Still other foods are high in the fiber that helps to guard against cancers of the colon and rectum.

Many exciting studies have shown that nutrients such as vitamin A and beta carotene reduce the risk of all types of cancer, especially cancers of the lungs, larynx, esophagus, stomach, colon, rectum, prostate and urinary bladder. You'll find good amounts of beta carotene in carrots, spinach, sweet potatoes and other vegetables. Other nutrients such as vitamin C, vitamin E and the mineral selenium have also proved helpful in a laboratory setting.

Crucifers, excellent cancer-fighting foods, are a family of vegetables that includes broccoli, Brussels sprouts, cabbage, cauliflower, kohlrabi and kale. Even the conservative National Academy of Sciences agrees that crucifers, along with carrots and spinach, are important cancer fighters, especially in preventing cancer of the colon.

Fibrous foods seem to protect against cancer of the colon, while also lending protection from heart disease. Eating plenty of vegetables and whole grains will help stack the odds in your favor. I've also found high-fiber diets to be useful in combating diabetes (both insulin-dependent and noninsulin-dependent).

Many other nutrients and phytochemicals help to strengthen the body's resistance to cancer, including vitamins B1, B2, C and E, folic acid, selenium, zinc, bioflavonoids, isoflavones, lignans, limonene, lycopene, protease inhibitors, phytic acid and sulfides.

Specific foods that have anticancer properties include apples, apricots, asparagus, barley, beans, broccoli, Brussels sprouts, cabbage, cantaloupe, carrots, cauliflower, currants, dandelion greens, eggplant, garlic, grapefruit, guava, lentils, mangoes, mushrooms, oats, onions, oranges, papaya, parsley, pasta, peppers, potatoes, spinach, strawberries, tangerines, tea, tomatoes, turnips, watercress, whole-grain rice and whole-grain wheat. All of these play a role in the battle against cancer.

For many patients, I recommend taking the 4 ACES (A as beta carotene, vitamins C and E and the mineral selenium), Coenzyme Q10 and the proanthocyanidins. In addition, I strongly recommend the use of green tea and soy products for their cancer-fighting properties.

6. *Limit your exposure to the sun.*

Although the warmth of the sun is pleasant and suntans are considered attractive, too much exposure to the sun can cause skin cancer. It's best to use a good sunscreen when going outdoors and to limit your time in the sun. Hundreds of thousands of us will develop skin cancer this year, and the incidence of melanoma, the deadliest form of skin cancer, is steadily increasing.

7. *Have regular checkups.*

Regular examinations, Pap smears, mammography for women, the PSA (prostate specific antigen) and other tests can help nip some cancers in the bud. But make sure that your physician spends the time it takes to examine you from head to toe, to discuss your risk factors and to answer all your questions. Your doctor should ask you about your diet, your work, your hobbies, your family medical history and much more as part of his or her search for cancer risk factors. If he doesn't spend time with you, consider a new doctor.

8. Learn to recognize the signs of cancer.

Not every cancer advertises its presence, and the symptoms are sometimes easy to confuse with other problems. However, there are symptoms we all can watch for, including:

- A lump in the breast, nipple discharge or changes in the shape of the nipple may be signs of breast cancer.

- Vaginal bleeding between periods, abnormally heavy bleeding during periods and vaginal discharges may be signs of cancers of the cervix, uterus or vagina.

- Changes in bowel habits, continually feeling bloated, bloody stools (or black bowel movements), constipation and diarrhea may be signs of colorectal cancer.

- A cold, flu or feeling of general malaise that seems to last too long may be a sign of leukemia (a blood cancer).

- Persistent coughing, chronic hoarseness, coughing up of blood, difficulty breathing or pain upon breathing may be a sign of lung cancer.

- Painless red or white patches in the mouth or persistent, painful lumpy or swollen areas in the mouth may be signs of oral cancer.

- Dribbling of urine, having to urinate often, difficulty in starting the urinary stream and other changes in urinary habits may be signs of prostate cancer.

- Moles or birthmarks that change size or shape, small sores or bumps that appear for no reason and sores or other wounds that do not heal properly may be signs of skin cancer.

Simple self-examination is a powerful diagnostic tool. Here are some things you can do to watch for signs of cancer:

- Everyone can look at their urine and stools when they use the bathroom. Is there blood? Does your feces look like it was squeezed out of a tube? Have your bowel habits changed for no discernible reason? These may be signs of cancer.

- Many skin cancers are first noticed by the person's spouse.

- It is especially important for women to learn to self-examine their breasts.

- Ask your doctor to show you how to check under your armpits for gland enlargement and how to check your liver (in the right upper part of the abdomen, just below the right rib cage) for lumps.

- Women should learn how to use a mirror to look at their labia (the outside areas of the vagina).
- Men should feel around their scrotums and check their testicles for tenderness or lumps.

Men and women can disrobe and stand in front of a full-length mirror, checking any moles to see if they've grown, looking for skin discolorations or other problems. Be sure to check your back as well as your front. Stand with your back to the full-length mirror. Using a large, hand-held mirror, examine the back of your body from head to toe.

I teach my patients the A-B-C-D method for identifying potentially malignant moles:

A = Asymmetry. *The two sides of the rounded mole are not symmetrical (they don't match).*

B = Border. *The outer border is not smooth or clearly defined. Instead, it looks scalloped or notched.*

C = Color. *Malignant moles may have multiple pigments (colors).*

D = Diameter. *Malignant moles are usually larger than a pencil-top eraser.*

Any abnormal findings, or even a suspicion of one, should be acted upon immediately. It's best to be overly cautious.

9. *Remain optimistic and positive.*

My own observations during 40 years of treating patients have convinced me that optimistic and positive people tend to have stronger immune systems than those who surrender to gloom. I firmly believe that enthusiasm, belief, love, forgiveness and perseverance are powerful medicines.

If you do get cancer...

Through the years, I've seen many cancer patients. I've noticed that the ones who look upon the disease as a challenge, who maintain a positive outlook on life, who continue to smile, love and laugh do much better than those who are filled with gloom and doom.

Our mind has a powerful influence upon our health. Thanks to modern scientific tools, we know that thoughts of joy, hope and love help to realign body chemistry and strengthen the immune system. On the other hand, many studies have shown that feelings of helplessness, hopelessness, anger and alienation predispose us to many diseases. This is not a new idea. Hippocrates, the ancient physician, noted that unhappy women were more likely to come down with breast cancer.

Face your disease (be it cancer or anything else) with determination to survive and thrive. Don't lose sight of your joy and love; in fact, make every effort to double them. Fill your mind with positive thoughts. Think of yourself as being healthy. Walk as if you were healthy, talk as if your were healthy, act as if your were healthy. With your mind's eye, picture yourself healthy. Keep that great thought in your mind all day long. Every thought in your head becomes a "thing" in your body. Positive thoughts become endorphins and other biosubstances that boost the immune system and help tilt the odds in favor of health.

---

[1] Brown, R.R., et al. Correlation of serum retinol levels with response to chemotherapy in breast cancer. Meeting Abstract. *Proc Am Assoc Cancer Res,* 22:184, 1981.

[2] Singh, V.N., Gaby, S.K. Premalignant lesions: role of antioxidant vitamins and beta-carotene in risk reduction and prevention of malignant transformation. *Am J Clin Nutr*, 53:386S-90S, 1991.

[3] Kaul, L., ibid.

[4] Kaul, L., et al. The role of diet in prostate cancer. *Nutr Cancer,* 9:123-28, 1987. Guo, W., et al. Correlation of dietary intake and blood nutrient levels with oesophageal cancer mortality in China. *Nutr Cancer,* 13:121-27, 1990.

[5] Butterworth, C., et al. Improvement in cervical dysplasia associated with folic acid therapy in users of oral contraceptives. *Am J Clin Nutr*, 35(1):73-82, 1982.

[6] Freudenheim, J., et al. Folate intake and carcinogenesis of the colon and rectum. *Int J Epidemiol*, 20:368-74, 1991.

[7] Block, G., Epidemiologic evidence regarding vitamin C and cancer. *Am J Clin Nutr*, 54:1310S-14S, 1991.

[8] Gey, K.F., et al. Plasma levels of antioxidant vitamins in relation to ischemic heart disease and cancer. *Am J Clin Nutr*, 45(5 Suppl):1368-77, 1987.

[9] Stahelin, H.B., et al. Cancer, vitamins and plasma lipids: Prospective Basal study. *J Natl Cancer Inst*, 73(6):1463-8, 1984.

[10] Prasad, K.N. Modulation of the effects of tumor therapeutic agents by vitamin C. *Life Sci*, 27(4):275-80, 1980.

[11] Gupta, S. Effect of radiotherapy on plasma ascorbic acid concentration in cancer patients. Unpublished thesis—summarized in Hanck, A.B. Vitamin C and Cancer. *Prog Clin Biol Res*, 259:307-20, 1988.

[12] Langer, R., Lee, A. Shark cartilage contains inhibitors of tumor angiogenesis. *Science,* 221:185-87, 1983.

Chapter 7

Headaches

I'm no stranger to headaches. One of my earliest memories is of my mother gently laying cold washcloths on my head and massaging my head and neck as I lay writhing in agony. Although otherwise very healthy and happy, throughout my childhood and well into my adult years, I was often struck by blinding headaches.

As a young physician, I saw patients in five Los Angeles-area hospitals. Arising early in the morning, I always went to the hospitals in a certain order. Before I had left the first hospital, the pain would be crashing through my skull and I would be popping the first of many aspirins and other pain pills.

Then one day, for no particular reason, I went to the hospitals in reverse order, going to the last one first and the first one last. To my great surprise, the headache didn't hit right away. In fact, it didn't appear until I got to the last hospital (which was usually the first one). It took awhile, but I finally realized that my headaches were a response to the stress that I felt at that hospital, which was so burdened with red tape and uncaring administrators that I couldn't get anything done for my patients.

I finally realized that I was not doomed to pain every morning by 10 a.m. My headaches were not inevitable; they were caused by stress. That meant that if I learned to control my stress, the headaches should disappear. I did learn, and they did vanish.

Headache statistics

The numbers are difficult to pin down, but it seems that up to 50 million Americans suffer from chronic headaches. More than $4 billion is spent yearly on aspirin and other over-the-counter remedies, with an additional $300 million being spent on more formal treatments. And the business community loses approximately $5 billion per year due to headache-related absenteeism and other problems.

Types of headaches

There are three types of headaches: 1) muscle contraction ("tension") headaches; 2) vascular headaches caused by the widening or narrowing of blood vessels in the brain or by neurotransmitter abnormalities; and 3) organic headaches caused by various health problems.

Muscle contraction headaches are far and away the most common and most easily treated type of headache. Muscles in the face, neck and scalp tend to tighten up when we're stressed, tired, angry or otherwise upset. Pressure produced by the tensed muscles puts stress on the nerves and blood vessels in the face, neck and head, producing pain and more tension.

The tension pain strikes the forehead, the sides of the head, the back of the neck or all three areas. Many people describe the pain as "a metal band tightening around my head." Muscles in the neck and shoulders may also become knotted. These headaches can last for days, weeks or even months. As if the pain were not enough, recurrent headaches may lead to "secondary" problems such as anxiety, depression, insomnia and nausea. Long-lasting headaches may lead to profound fatigue, chest tightness or chest pain and even thoughts of suicide.

Tension headaches strike both sexes and all ages, although adult females are the most common targets. Stress is usually the culprit, but other factors can pressure the nerves and blood vessels, triggering muscle contraction headaches. Some of these triggers include holding the head or neck in an unusual position, poor posture, a bad pillow, poor or excessive lighting and the grinding of the teeth.

Vascular headaches are caused by the dilation (widening) or constriction (narrowing) of blood vessels in the brain. This widening or narrowing may be caused by alcohol, hangovers, hunger, smoking and certain substances in foods. A sudden rush of blood to the head can also trigger the pain. (Exercising, standing on your head or having sex can trigger vascular headaches in certain people.) Some experts believe that a lack of serotonin, or other chemical imbalances in the brain, may also be to blame.

There are three types of vascular headaches: migraines, cluster headaches and exertion headaches.

Migraines produce terrible, throbbing pain. The pain is usually located on one side of the head, but it may switch sides. "Classic" migraines are heralded by an "aura" (hazy light) or other visual changes, whereas "common" migraines strike with no warning. Migraines may last as long as a few hours or a few days. In addition to the pain, there may also be feelings of confusion, nausea, vomiting, dizziness, weakness and tingling or numbness of the limbs. Vision may be blurry, speech may be impaired and the person may be greatly sensitive to light, odors and sounds. Migraine headaches tend to run in families. Both sexes are struck, but women seem to be the favored target.

Cluster headaches, the second type of vascular headache, occur in groups or clusters. A series of headaches may drag on for weeks or even months. The intense pain strikes with little warning. Usually located over one eye, the pain can cause swelling and tearing of the eye, as well as congestion in the adjacent nostril, and flushing and sweating on the affected side of the face. Clusters typically attack males and may be related to the seasons.

Exertion headaches are the third type of vascular headache. These headaches are triggered by physical activity that causes blood vessels throughout the body, including those in the head, to widen. This causes intense throbbing and pain. Exertion headaches can strike during or just after exercising, and the pain may be severe enough to send the victims to the emergency room. Luckily, these headaches usually disappear with bed rest and are rarely serious.

Organic headaches are symptoms of various underlying medical problems. Anything from inflamed nerves to brain tumors may be to blame for an organic headache, but only 2 percent of all headache sufferers truly have organic problems. Still, the underlying conditions may be serious, so anyone with chronic pain should see a physician to rule out high blood pressure, brain tumors, hemorrhage, sinus disorders, TMJ (temporomandibular joint dysfunction) and other problems.

Signs and symptoms

Symptoms of muscle contraction ("tension") headaches may include a dull, aching pain in the forehead area, on the sides or back of the head and a tightening of the muscles in the scalp, face and neck. With long-lasting or severe headaches there may also be weakness, nausea, fatigue and sensitivity to sound and light.

Symptoms of vascular/migraine headaches may include an "aura" before the headache begins. The aura may produce visual disturbances, such as flashing lights or "halos" around light bulbs. There may also be intense pain on one side of the head, nausea, dizziness, tingling or numbness of the limbs, weakness, vomiting and extreme sensitivity to sound and light.

Symptoms of vascular/cluster headaches may include sudden pain that quickly reaches intense proportions, pain over or behind one eye, swelling and drooping of the affected eye, congestion in the adjacent nostril, flushing and sweating on the affected side of the face, nausea, restlessness and slow heartbeat.

Symptoms of vascular/exertion headaches may include pain during or just after exercising.

Symptoms of organic headaches are many, depending upon the underlying cause. If you have any unexplained, unusual, long-lasting or intense head pain, see your physician immediately, especially if the pain is accompanied by any changes in speech or behavior, any "strange" feelings in the body or any loss of consciousness.

Standard medical treatment

Standard Western medical treatment for headaches consists of:

- Various medications for pain, depression, nasal distress, tense muscles and other symptoms.
- Oxygen therapy.
- Local anesthetics.
- Rest.
- Avoidance of activities or foods that may trigger headaches.

In short, Western medicine's primary focus is on suppressing the symptoms of headaches.

Many people overlook the possibility that their headaches may be caused by various dental or orthodontic problems. Grinding the teeth, holding the jaw in unnatural positions and TMJ (temporomandibular joint) problems are a few of the dental conditions that may cause or contribute to headaches.

An unknown number of headaches may be caused by eyestrain, improper prescriptions for glasses, glare from computer screens and other eye problems. If your headaches seem to be related to eyestrain, rest your eyes regularly and get them checked by an ophthalmologist.

Now let's look at some of the many alternative treatments for headaches. These are not all the possible therapies, because there are too many to investigate in a single chapter. Reading through these alternatives, however, will give you an idea of the many possibilities.

The information on alternative therapies is meant for educational purposes only. I am not endorsing any therapy or suggesting that you see any alternative practitioner. If you have chronic or unusually painful headaches, see your physician.

Acupuncture

Acupuncture points used depend on the cause of the problem. Typically Colon 4 (on the hand), Gallbladder 20 (on the back of the head, just below the skull), Tiyange (in the temples), Yintant (between the eyebrows) and Bladder 1 (near the base of the nail on the little toe) will be used.

In one study, 40 percent of the volunteers reported that their headaches were 50 to 100 percent less frequent and severe.[1] In another study, the frequency of headaches dropped by over 40 percent for six months after five acupuncture treatments.[2]

If stomach upset accompanies the headaches, Stomach 36 (below the knee) will be stimulated, as will local points on the abdomen or stomach. In addition, the acupuncturist may recommend using ice packs, resting, meditation, herbs and rubbing the temples or neck with substances such as Tiger Balm (an over-the-counter preparation that contains camphor and menthol).

Aromatherapy

Aromatherapy uses the aromatic essences of flowers and plants to influence the mind and body. Aromatherapy treatments for headaches vary widely, because there are no standard therapy guidelines for the field. Each aromatherapist approaches headaches as he or she deems best. Essential oils used for headaches include:

- Chamomile (*Matricaria chamomilla*).
- Cardamom (*Elettaria cardamomum*).
- Lavender (*Lavandula officinalis*).
- Marjoram (*Origanum marjorana*).
- Peppermint (*Mentha piperata*).
- Rose (*Rosa spp.*).
- Rosemary (*Rosmarinus officinalis*).

Certain aromas may also be used for the depression that may set in when suffering from chronic headaches. These include:

- Basil (*Ocimum basilicum*).
- Bergamot (*Monarda didyma*).
- Chamomile (*Matricaria chamomilla*).
- Camphor (*Cinnamomum camphora*).
- Geranium (*Pelargonium odorantissimum*).
- Jasmine (*Jasminum officinale*).
- Melissa (*Melissa officinalis*).
- Neroli (*Citrus aurantium*).
- Patchouli (*Pogostemon patchouli*).
- Sandalwood (*Santalum album*).

If the headaches are interfering with sleep, these or other oils may be used:

- Basil (*Ocimum basilicum*).
- Camphor (*Cinnamomum camphora*).
- Lavender (*Lavandula officinalis*).

- Marjoram (*Origanum marjorana*).
- Neroli (*Citrus aurantium*).
- Ylang-ylang (*Cananga odorata*).

The patient may be instructed to inhale the vapors from these oils as they rise from a bowl of water, to mix them in a base oil and use in massage, to wear as a perfume or to mix with the bath water. Treatment length will vary from practitioner to practitioner and according to the patient's condition.

Ayurvedic healing

Like Western medicine, Ayurveda recognizes many potential causes for headaches, including muscle tension and organic problems such as high blood pressure. Ayurveda, however, lists additional causes for headaches, including constipation and stomach distress.

Headaches may manifest themselves in any of the three humors, or primary life forces, in the body.

1. Headaches in the Vata (air) humor are the most common type. Symptoms of Vata-type headaches include severe pain, anxiety, constipation and drying of the skin. Triggers include stress, lack of sleep and mental or physical overstimulation. The Vata-type headache shares characteristics with the muscle contraction "tension" and exertion headaches.

2. Headaches in the Pitta (fire) humor produce a burning pain in the head, anger and light sensitivity. The face and eyes become red and there may be nosebleeds. Like the organic headache, the Pitta-type headache is generally considered to be the result of another disease.

3. Headaches in the Kapha (water) humor produce a dull pain in the head. The patient may also feel nauseated, tired and filled with phlegm. Kapha-type headaches are believed to be caused by problems with the respiratory tract, possibly associated with colds and allergies.

For Kapha-type and Vata-type headaches, herbs that clear out the respiratory system and encourage the coughing up of phlegm are used. These include angelica, basil, bayberry and ginger. Aromatherapy may also be used to help clear out the respiratory system. Because toxins in the bowel may be to blame for the headaches, various herbs and other methods may be used to purge the bowels. Finally, herbs that encourage sleep are used.

Pitta-type headaches call for purgation and general cleansing of the inside of the body, specifically the liver.

Long-term therapy to strengthen the body and emotions may be prescribed.

Chiropractic

"Straight" chiropractors treat headaches by manipulating the spine to correct subluxation and other imbalances. Studies of chiropractic spinal manipulation have shown interesting results on headache pains. In one such study, 150 chronic tension headache sufferers were divided into two groups. One group was given prophylactic spinal manipulation twice a week. The other group took amitriptyline, a prophylactic antidepressant over-the-counter drug used for tension and migraine headaches.

The participants kept track of the frequency and intensity of their pain, and their functional health was measured. At the end of the study period, both the spinal manipulation and medicine groups felt better. Four weeks after treatment ended, however, the medicine group reverted to their prestudy pain. But the spinal manipulation group continued to report less frequent and painful headaches.[3]

The mixed chiropractic treatment for headaches is a combination of manipulation and other therapies, focusing on reducing the tension in the neck muscles.

Mixed chiropractors believe that over 90 percent of all headaches are *primary*, which means that they are not caused by an underlying disease such as a tumor. Although primary headaches can be quite painful, the trouble they cause is limited to the pain and associated symptoms. The remaining 10 percent or less of headaches are, according to this theory, *secondary* headaches brought about by underlying problems such as a brain tumor or meningitis.

When first evaluating a headache patient, the chiropractor will look for "red flags" warning of secondary headaches. These include severe headaches that have begun in the past six months, headaches that are made worse when the patient shifts position, headaches that are progressively more painful and frequent, plus any problems with vision, coordination, memory or awareness. If the mixed chiropractor believes that the headaches are secondary, he or she will refer the patient to a physician.

Mixed chiropractors will most likely treat existing headaches with spinal manipulation, focusing on the neck. They will feel not just the bones, but also the surrounding musculature. Do the muscles on both sides of the spine feel the same? Does one side feel like it has a knot? Are the muscles raised or swollen? Do they feel hot? Sometimes the side-to-side differences are subtle, sometimes they're great.

It is believed that manipulation will help to relieve many headaches in progress because the overwhelming majority of them are related to tension, which yields to manipulation. However, a great number of headache sufferers have ongoing problems with their necks that require two to three manipulations per week for four to six weeks in order to permanently correct the problem. Such therapy will reduce the frequency and/or severity of headaches for many people.

Mixed chiropractors may also call for physical therapy, such as ultrasound or electric muscle stimulation, in addition to the manipulation. Massage or soft-tissue work on the affected muscles may be prescribed. Toward the end of the treatment program the patient might be given exercises to strengthen and balance the muscles.

If there is no improvement within approximately two weeks, the chiropractor will change the therapy. If there is still no improvement after four to six weeks, the patient will most likely be referred out for more diagnostic studies.

In addition, the mixed chiropractor will have conducted a full investigation of the patient's medical and personal history, trying to determine if any foods or other "triggers" are responsible for the headaches. Depending on his or her training and preferences, a chiropractor may also recommend nutritional, homeopathic or other therapies.

The time required to relieve the symptoms and to cure the headaches may vary considerably. When patronizing straight chiropractors, one session may be enough to cure the spinal problems, although continuing treatment for a recurring problem may be required. When patronizing mixed chiropractors, treatment length will depend on what other therapies are used and whether or not your body responds to this kind of therapy.

Color therapy

Red, yellow or *green* may be applied to the abdomen because constipation and other forms of bowel distress are believed to be a common cause of headaches.

- *Red* increases circulation and energy and reduces nervousness. Red is used to treat constipation and malaise. Red should not be used if there is already too much red in the patient (indicated by an overly reddish face, fever, easy excitability or red hair).
- *Yellow* cleanses the bloodstream and the liver while stimulating the nerves. It is good for the anxiety and depression that may accompany chronic headaches.
- *Blue* may be used on the head or directed to the abdomen to treat the liver, which is believed to play a role in some headaches. Blue cools and soothes.

- *Green* is considered a master-healer, good for all conditions, and for helping the body rid itself of toxic substances. Green is also a soothing and cooling color that can help to stabilize the emotions and rebuild the tissues. It is the color of energy, hope and new life.

There are many ways for the color therapist to apply the properly colored light to the patient, including through direct light, gems, jewelry, perfume, clothing and colored glass. Patients can also eat the appropriately colored foods.

- Red foods include radishes, beets, tomatoes, red cabbage, red currants, red plums, watermelon, whole wheat, liver, red wine and grapes. Red metals, chemicals and other substances include barium, cadmium, copper, nitrogen, iron, neon, oxygen, potassium and zinc.
- Yellow foods include bananas, banana squash, eggs, yellow cheese, yellow corn, yellow sweet potatoes, pineapples, lemons, grapefruit and butter. Yellow metals, chemicals and other substances include platinum and magnesium.
- Green foods include green vegetables, peas, beans and lentils. Green metals, chemicals and other substances include barium, chlorophyll, nickel and sodium.
- Blue foods include plums, grapes and blueberries. Blue metals, chemicals and other substances include copper, lead, oxygen and tin.

Folk medicine

Folk remedies for headaches are many and varied. There are absolutely no standard protocols or recipes, but some of the many folk remedies for headaches include:

- Chicken soup is used to help with headaches related to nasal congestion because it helps to unclog nasal passages and sinuses.
- Headbands or scarves soaked with apple cider vinegar may be wrapped around the head for pain relief, or apple cider vinegar may be taken by itself or with honey.
- Slices of apples or raw potatoes are placed on the head to relieve pain.
- A paste can be made of garlic, onions, crushed soda crackers, baking soda, ginger, mint and/or other substances and applied to the head or neck. Or a compress may be saturated with a watery version of the mixture and applied.

Herbal medicine

Herbalists use a wide variety of herbs to treat many headaches. There is no standard herbal protocol for treating disease. Herbs typically used include:

- Feverfew (*Tanacetum parthenium*).
- Jamaican dogwood (*Piscidia erythrina*).
- Lavender (*Lavandula spp.*).
- Lemon (*Citrus limon*).
- Skullcap (*Scutellaria lateriflora*).
- St. John's Wort (*Hypericum perforatum*).
- Vervain (*Verbena officinalis*).
- Wood Betony (*Stachys officinalis*).

Some of the herbs that may be recommended for the tension and fear that may accompany or trigger headaches include:

- Linden (*Tilia europaea*).
- Pasque flower (*Anemone pulsatilla*).
- Vervain (*Verbena officinalis*).

For the depression that may accompany chronic or debilitating headaches, these herbs may be recommended:

- Basil (*Ocimum basilicum*).
- Damiana (*Turnera diffusa*).
- Oats (*Avena sativa*).

Homeopathy

Unlike traditional Western medicine which treats headaches by suppressing their symptoms, homeopathy attempts to cure headaches by helping the body to heal itself. Most of the major homeopathic remedies may be used for headaches, depending upon the patient's symptoms. Some of these remedies include:

- *Belladonna,* which is indicated when the patient seems to be living in a dream world. Symptoms include throbbing pain, which is worse in the front and right side of the head, flushing and sensitivity to light and noise. The pain is better when the patient is lying down and worse with noise, movement and drafts.
- *Bryonia alba,* which is indicated when the patient is irritable and angry and feels cold after a bout of anger. Symptoms include pain that starts in the front of the head and moves back across the top of the head. The pain is made worse by any

movements, warmth or touch and is worse in the morning. Symptoms are better when pressure is applied to the pain, and with rest and cold.

- *Cimicifuga racemosa*, which is indicated when the patient is very talkative and restless and alternately playful and dejected. The headache starts at the back of the head and moves up. Bending over makes the pain worse, warmth makes it better.
- *Glonoinum,* which is indicated when the patient seems confused. The headache produces a throbbing pain, the pulse is full (strong, steady and regular) and the face is flushed red.
- *Lachesis,* which is indicated when the patient is thin and talkative, but moody and suspicious. The head pain extends to the face and shoulders. Open air and warmth relieve the pain, while sleep, pressure and hot drinks make it worse.
- *Nux Vomica*, which is indicated when pain in the back of the head or near either eye is accompanied by nausea and vomiting. Often associated with a hangover.
- *Scutellaria*, which is indicated when the pain is dull and located in the front of the head, when the face if flushed, the eyes hurt and the patient is restless.

Although it is a basic principle of classical homeopathy to use only one remedy at a time, there is a trend among modern homeopaths toward using multiple remedies at once. Using the absolute minimum number of doses necessary is another principle of classical homeopathy. A second dose should not be given until the first has ceased to act, and no more remedies should be given when the body begins to heal. If the right remedy is used, two or three days should be enough to begin many long-term curative processes. If not, another remedy should be selected.

Hypnosis

Hypnosis is often used as an adjunct treatment for headaches. Because it may be difficult to hypnotize someone who already has a headache, the patient may be hypnotized between headaches and given suggestions such as:

"When the pain begins, sit or lie down in a quiet, comfortable place. Take a deep breath, hold it in, then exhale slowly. Concentrate on the top of your head. Feel a cool, relaxed sensation spreading across the top of your head. Concentrate on that pleasant feeling as long as you like. (Pause) Take a deep breath, hold it in, then exhale slowly as you concentrate on your forehead. Feel the cool, relaxed sensation spreading down from the top of your head and across your forehead. (Pause) Take a deep breath, hold it in, then exhale slowly as you concentrate on your face. Feel the cool, relaxed sensation spreading across your face and now around to the back of your head.

"Imagine that you are walking through a snowy field in the winter. You have mittens on your hands, so they're comfortably warm. But you can feel the cold air against your head and face. It's cooling and soothing. You feel relaxed and at peace."

There is no agreed-upon length of time before hypnosis brings results, if any are to be found. Several factors affect the length of treatment: how hypnotizable the client is, the rapport developed between the hypnotist and the client and the severity of the problem. Many people have been helped in just one session. For some, several sessions are required.

Nutritional therapy

It's believed that several common foods and food substances may be responsible for bringing on a good many headaches. There are at least three different ways in which foodstuffs may trigger head pain:

1. By causing blood vessels in the brain to either constrict or dilate.
2. By altering the normal, complex sequence of events necessary to regulate pain in the body.
3. By triggering an allergic response.

Migraine headaches have been linked to many dietary and related factors, including low blood sugar, numerous food sensitivities and the amino acid tyramine.

- *A steady supply of carbohydrates* may help to prevent migraine headaches caused by low blood sugar. Thus, nutritionists may recommend a diet containing plenty of vegetables, fruits and whole grains, eaten as part of many small meals throughout the day, in order to maintain blood glucose levels.
- *Dietary triggers* should be pinpointed and avoided. You may be asked to stop eating many foods, then to reintroduce them to your diet one at a time. This allows you to identify the trigger foods. Common migraine trigger foods include cheese, alcoholic beverages, aspartame (NutraSweet), bananas, chicken livers, coffee, cola and other caffeinated beverages, chocolate, cocoa, cured and/or smoked meats, canned figs, nuts and seeds, onions, citrus fruits, peanut butter, pickled herring and salted

fish, pineapple, sauerkraut, soy sauce, vinegar, yogurt and any foods containing monosodium glutamate (MSG).

- *The amino acid tyramine*, found in peanut butter, chocolate, some cheeses, sauerkraut, alcoholic beverages and other foods, has also been associated with migraines. A tyramine-free diet may help a good number of migraine sufferers.

- *Too much iron* in the body has been linked to increased headaches.

- *A lack of magnesium* may be associated with premenstrual migraine headaches. A study of 3,000 pregnant and nonpregnant women found that magnesium supplements could reduce the severity of their migraine headaches.[4] Good sources of magnesium include spinach, carrots and onions.

- *Omega-3 fatty acids*, found in fish, have helped to reduce the frequency and severity of migraines in 15 patients who were not helped by standard medications.[5]

- *The mineral choline* has been found to be low in people suffering from cluster headaches, both during and between attacks. Choline can be found in lentils, egg yolk and leafy green vegetables.

Supplements

Nutritional experts may recommend a wide variety of vitamins, minerals and other nutrients for headaches, including omega-3 fatty acids, magnesium, choline, copper, vitamins C and E and niacin.

DLPA may also be recommended. DLPA (dl-phenylalanine) is an amino acid with proven painkilling capabilities. Not a painkiller itself, DLPA protects endorphins, which are natural painkillers produced by the body.

Specific foods that aid in treating headaches

A few foods have been found to help sufferers considerably.

- *Seeds, nuts, wheat bran* and other foods containing good amounts of copper should be consumed regularly. Researchers have found that many patients eating low-copper diets need more painkillers than they do when they are on diets with adequate amounts of this mineral. It's believed that copper wards off headache pain by keeping the blood vessels in the brain properly toned.

- *Ginger* has a long history of use for treating headaches, nausea and other problems. Ginger interferes with the production of prostaglandins, substances that play a role in pain. Blocking prostaglandin production helps to relieve pain.

- *Fish*, especially cold-water fish, contain omega-3 fatty acids that can drastically reduce the severity and frequency of migraine pain. Eating salmon, mackerel and other fish high in omega-3 fatty acids several times a week may help to control headaches.

When selecting a nutritional healer, remember that there is no widely-recognized "school" of nutritional therapy and no standards or agreed-upon training for nutritional healers.

Oriental medicine

In Oriental medicine, headaches are believed to be caused by many different factors, such as a blockage in the bladder meridian or coldness or "wind" in the head. One must thoroughly investigate the symptoms (where the pain strikes, how it feels, etc.) in order to determine the cause. Having made a diagnosis, the Oriental medicine physician strives to balance the body's energy with a combination of herbs and spices, diet, acupuncture and other therapies, as necessary.

Herbs and spices

Exactly which herbs and spices and the amount of each will depend upon the patient and his or her condition. Some of the herbs and spices that might be used for headaches are:

- *Peppermint*, a cool and pungent spice that strengthens the lungs and liver.
- *Rosemary*, a warm and pungent spice used for headaches and stomachaches.
- *Spearmint*, a sweet and pungent spice used to quell pain and increase the circulation of energy throughout the body.
- *Sweet basil*, a pungent and warm herb that improves circulation and energy while toning the large intestine, stomach and lungs.

Herbal formulas that might be suggested include *Yan Hu Suo Zhi Tong Pian, Qi Ju Di Huang Wan* and *Er Ming Zuo Ci Wan*.

Diet

Diet plays an important role in Oriental medicine. Foods are selected depending on their flavors, organic actions and other qualities, including energies. There are five food energies: hot, warm, neutral, cool and cold. (The energy has to do with the quality of the food, not its temperature. For example, foods with "hot" energy, such as ginger and black pepper, increase the sensation of heat in the body, even when eaten cold.) In addition to a healthy diet, the Oriental medicine physician may recommend these foods specifically for headaches:

- *Green onion (leaf and head),* warm and pungent vegetables that relieve headaches while strengthening the stomach and lungs.
- *Radish*, a cool and sweet vegetable that detoxifies the body, while strengthening the stomach and lungs.
- *Tea,* a bitter and slightly cold fluid that strengths the heart and lungs, while reviving general health and strength.

Psychoneuroimmunology

Psychoneuroimmunology is a science concerned with the mind/body connection. Mind/body healers attempt to deal with the negative or fearful thoughts that they believe contribute to headaches. There are no standard mind/body healing protocols for headaches, and mind/body healers arise from a variety of health disciplines, so the techniques will vary from healer to healer.

Mind/body healers use positive affirmations to counteract the negative thoughts that may have been contributing to the head pain. Affirmations are typically brief, positive statements that focus on how well one feels and on how the problem is being conquered. The patient might be given several affirmations.

In addition to affirmations for general health, an affirmation to relieve headaches might be worded as follows:

"Like the beautiful mountain air, my head feels light and cool. Like the twinkling stars on a beautiful night, my head feels lively and bright. Like the gentle stream floating forever, I am calm and my good health is endless."

Reflexology

The reflexologist will manipulate the direct reflex areas for the head and brain, which are located in the big toes. The associated reflex areas for the spine, sinuses, eyes and other parts of the body will also be worked on. The spine reflex areas are found on the inner side of both feet. Reflex areas for the sinuses are located on the four small toes of both feet. The reflex area for the eyes is found on both feet where the second and third toes join. Corresponding points on the hands may also be utilized.

To improve general circulation, the intestinal and liver reflex areas may be manipulated. Reflex areas for the stomach and the large and small intestines are found in the arches of both feet. The liver re-flex area is centered on the right foot, in roughly the middle one-third of the foot on the outside. Corresponding points on the hands may also be utilized.

Because reflexology is not a licensed healing art, practitioners may make no claims regarding the treatment of headaches or the length of such treatment.

Advice to headache patients

Although many of my patients have had success with the following program, I only use the general guidelines discussed below after reviewing a patient's personal and medical history, performing a thorough examination and evaluating the laboratory studies to make sure that the program will be beneficial. Please see your own physician before embarking on any treatment program for headaches.

Once I have examined a patient and ruled out any organic causes for head pain, I attempt to identify his or her particular type of head-ache. Correct diagnosis is necessary before effective treatment can begin.

To help give you an idea of what types of headaches you may suffer from, run through the checklists on pages 158 to 159. Check off the items that apply to you. Once you know the kind(s) of headache that you suffer from, you can begin appropriate measures to both treat and prevent them.

Preventing and treating muscle contraction (tension) headaches

Muscle contraction headaches are usually easy to prevent and treat. Simply learning how to deal with stress can eliminate many of the headaches. Here are some techniques for prevention:

- *Reduce the stress in your life.* Look at the pace of your life and see if it is taxing you. Most of us could slow down and avoid making too many changes at once. Do we really need to accomplish all of our goals so quickly? Are we so busy looking ahead that we've lost sight of the good things we already have?
- *Exercise.* At least three times a week, get some exercise. Low-impact exercise, such as walking, swimming or bicycling, will tone the body and release pent-up stress.
- *Relax.* Set aside time every day to relax. A little bit of relaxation can eliminate a lot of stress.
- *Avoid or limit caffeine intake.*
- *Eat a healthful diet.* Make sure to eat a healthful diet based on fresh vegetables and fruits, with plenty of whole grains, small amounts of protein and two to three servings of nonfat dairy

products per day. Reduce or avoid the dangerous "CATS form San Francisco" (caffeine, alcohol, tobacco, sugar, salt). Make sure that you're getting ample amounts of vitamins A, C and E, beta carotene, the B-vitamins and the many minerals.

• *DLPA.* Taking DLPA when you are feeling fine can help to prevent headaches from striking. See the discussion of DLPA earlier in this chapter.

• *Use pain relievers sparingly.* Overusing pain relievers that contain caffeine can lead to tolerance and "rebound headaches."

Should a tension headache strike, I recommend to my patients that they try the following treatments:

• *Massage the scalp, face and full body.* A head and neck massager called Scalpi provides an excellent "hands free" massage.

• *Meditative relaxation.* Try meditative relaxation when stress-induced pain begins to strike in the back of your neck and shoulders. You can do this at home, in the office or in your (parked) car.

Begin by pushing your shoulders up so that they almost touch your ears. Tilt your chin up and your head back, so that the back of your head nearly meets your raised shoulders. Push your neck down and back, into your shoulders, feeling the muscles at the base of your neck contracting. Hold and slowly count to 10. With your mind's eye, see your shoulders and neck relaxing. Feel the tension in the back of your neck and upper shoulders. Slowly relax your neck and lower your shoulders.

Take a slow, deep breath through your nose. Hold it. Let it out slowly through your nose, taking at least five seconds to release it all. Take another slow breath. Fill your lungs. Feel your diaphragm pulling down to open the lungs wide. With your mind's eye, see your diaphragm dropping as your lungs fill. Feel the tension draining out of your head and neck.

Once more, tilt your neck back and lift your shoulders up into your neck. Hold your neck and shoulders tense and slowly count to 10. Now relax your neck and slowly lower your shoulders.

Take a deep breath through your nose. Hold the breath for a moment. Now let it out through your mouth, very slowly, taking at least five seconds to empty your lungs. Take another deep breath, filling up your lungs. Hold it for a moment. Now let it out very slowly. Take five seconds or more to blow it all out. The muscles of your shoulders and the back of your neck should now feel light and tingly.

Repeat this technique as often as you like.

- *Rest with hot or cold compresses to the head.*

- *Drink a caffeinated beverage.* A cup of coffee or other caffeinated beverage may help relieve persistent pain. Caffeine constricts vessels that may have triggered the headache by dilating (widening). Caffeine may also relieve pain by increasing serotonin levels (which helps to relieve pain in general).

- *Over-the-counter and prescription medications.* If none of the other techniques works, you might try an over-the-counter (nonprescription) pain reliever. Should you and your physician feel that it's necessary, prescription antidepressants, tranquilizers, muscle relaxants and other drugs may be used. Bear in mind, however, that all medicines have side effects. But be aware that the stronger the medication, the greater the risk of building up a tolerance and suffering from side effects.

Muscle contraction ("tension") headache checklist

____ The pain feels like a constricting headband or vise, usually across the temples or head.

____ The pain is mild to moderate.

____ The pain may last for days.

____ The pain has no clear beginning or end.

____ The pain usually strikes when I'm stressed, although it may also occur when I'm sleeping.

____ The pain often begins in the morning and gets worse throughout the day.

____ The muscles in my neck and shoulders get knotted.

Migraine headache checklist

____ The pain usually strikes on one side of my head.

____ The pain is moderate to severe.

____ The pain is "throbbing" or "penetrating."

____ The pain usually lasts an average of four to eight hours, but may continue for days.

____ There may be halos, flashing lights or other visual disturbances.

____ I'm sensitive to light and sound during the headache episode.

____ I often feel nauseated and may vomit while having the headache.

____ I may feel dizzy during the headache.

____ I may feel numb in my arm or part of my face during the headache.

____ The headaches may strike during vacations, weekends or other times that I'm *not* feeling stressed.

Cluster headache checklist

____ The pain is excruciating.

____ The pain is "piercing" or "burning."

____ The pain is usually on one side of my face, but it may switch sides.

____ The pain settles behind one of my eyes.

____ My eye tears, swells and droops.

____ I get congestion or a runny nose on the affected side of my face.

____ I have flushing or sweating on the affected side of my face.

____ The pain lasts from 30 minutes to one hour.

____ The headaches strike in clusters of several headaches a day, sometimes for weeks or even months.

____ The headaches seem to start at the same time of the year.

Checking off several items on any one list suggests that you usually get that type of headache. But if you check off several items on more than one list, you are most likely getting tension headaches related to fatigue and stress.

I also advise my patients to keep a log of every single headache that they get. The log helps doctor and patient with diagnosis, treatment and prevention. Make several copies of the headache log on this page and keep careful track of all headache pain.

Headache log

Date _____

Time headache started _____

Time headache ended _____

The pain is located _____

The pain feels like _____

On a scale of 1 to 10, with 10 being worst, the pain rates a ____

Other symptoms _____

Possible triggers * _____

Medication used _____

Other treatment _____

After treatment, on a scale of 1 to 10, the pain rates a _____

* Possible triggers include stress, the let-down period after stress, missing a meal, medication, certain foods, hormonal changes, changes in the weather, lack of sleep, cigarette smoke, withdrawal from caffeine, bright lights, oversleeping, exercise and other factors.

Preventing and treating migraine headaches

- *Avoid migraine triggers.* Certain foods, fatigue, hunger, bright lights, altitude, motion, hormonal factors and changes in the weather can trigger headaches. Staying away from those triggers may relieve the problem significantly. Both becoming overtired or oversleeping can trigger an attack, so make sure that you get enough, but not too much, sleep every night. Hunger, stress, alcohol and bright light can also trigger migraines in susceptible people.
- *Reduce stress.* Although migraines tend to strike *after* a stressful period, they do seem to be related to stress. Reduce your stress as much as possible.
- *Preventive medication.* Discuss the use of preventive medications with your physician if your migraines are lessening the quality of your life.
- *General good health measures.* Healthful eating habits, exercise and other good habits strengthen your overall health, helping you to absorb the stress caused by migraines.

If the migraine has already struck, try the following techniques:

- *Rest in a quiet, dark place with hot and cold compresses.*
- *Vitamin B2.* Discuss using this vitamin, which can reduce pain by over half, with your physician.
- *Scalp and neck massage.*
- *Herbal remedies.* Several herbs are useful, including feverfew, ginkgo biloba, chamomile, coriander, turmeric, bay leaves, skullcap, valerian and willow bark. Be sure to discuss their use with your physician before taking them.
- *Pain medications.* Pain medication is often necessary during a migraine headache. Start with the milder medications such as Midrin before moving on, if necessary, to stronger ones.

Preventing and treating cluster headaches

The dilation of the blood vessels that occurs during a cluster headache can be prevented. In addition to the strategies for preventing tension headaches, you can:

- *Eliminate alcohol, a known headache trigger.*
- *Eliminate dietary triggers.* Avoid any foods and drinks that may trigger your cluster headaches.
- *Avoid cigarette smoke.*
- *Stick to a regular sleeping schedule.*
- *Consider preventive medication.* If your cluster headaches are striking on a daily basis and last for more than 15 minutes, your physician may want to prescribe a preventive medication. I like to use magnesium, a safe and natural calcium channel blocker, as a preventive.

Cluster headaches can be quite severe, so painful that relaxation techniques are not much help once the pain has struck. Deep breathing may help a little to alleviate the fear that accompanies the onset of these attacks. In addition to the techniques for treating tension headaches, you can also try the following:

- *Inhale pure oxygen.* Oxygen can help to lessen the pain of cluster headaches in many people. Discuss this carefully with your physician, especially if you have any pulmonary problems. You'll need a doctor's prescription to get the oxygen from a medical supply house.
- *Pain medication.* For severe headaches that do not respond to other treatments, your physician may prescribe a pain reliever.

Preventing and treating exertion headaches

Exertion headaches can be very painful, but they are rarely serious. Neither are they usually caused by underlying medical problems. Modifying your physical activities should help to lessen the frequency and intensity of your headaches. Take it a little easier. Always warm up before exercising and cool down afterward. Slow down gradually from peak activity. If an exertion headache does strike, lying down in bed, holding cold compresses to your head and massaging your scalp will often quell the pain.

Preventing and treating organic headaches

There are no specific treatment or prevention strategies for organic headaches—it all depends on the underlying cause(s). If you have or suspect that you have organic headaches, see your physician immediately.

When those terrible headaches used to send me to bed crying as a child, I thought I would never be free from them. Now I know that with careful prevention and treatment, most of the pain can be eliminated, often without using strong medications.

[1]   Lenhard, L., Waite, P.M. Acupuncture in the prophylactic treatment of migraine headache: pilot study. *NZ Med J*, 1983, 96, pp. 663-66.

[2]   Laiten, J. Acupuncture for migraine prophylaxis: a perspective clinical study with six months' follow-up. *Am J Chin Med*, 1975, 3, pp. 271-74.

[3]   "Chiropractic Spinal Manipulation Compared to Pharmaceutical Therapy For the Treatment of Headaches," by Patrick D. Boline, D.C., as reported in *AM*, published by the U.S. Department of Health & Human Services, National Institutes of Health, Office of Alternative Medicine, *AM*, November 1993.

[4]   Weaver, K. Magnesium and its role in vascular reactivity and coagulation. *Contemp Nutr*, 12(3), 1987.

[5]   Glueck, C.J., et al. Amelioration of severe migraine with omega-3 fatty acids: A double-blind, placebo-controlled clinical trial. Abstract. *Am J Clin Nutr*, 43:710, 1986.

Chapter 8

Heart disease

Heart disease strikes terror into, well, our hearts. We're frightened, because we know that anything that interferes with our vital pump can abruptly end our lives. There are many types and causes of heart disease, including conditions affecting the heart muscle, the heart valves, the thin sac surrounding the heart and more. There's endocarditis, an inflammation of the inner lining of the heart. Rheumatic heart disease, which may begin innocently as a child's sore throat, may damage heart valves.

Syphilis, a venereal disease, can also attack the heart. And there are heart diseases that result from chronic obstructive lung disease (COLD). You've heard of COLD, although you probably refer to it as emphysema. High blood pressure can cause heart disease. So can blood clots, which may originate in some other part of the body—perhaps the leg—and migrate through the bloodstream to the lungs. There the clot may get stuck in a narrow artery, impeding the exchange of blood between lungs and heart.

The most common form of heart disease, by far, is coronary heart disease (CHD). Commonly called "clogged arteries" or "hardened arteries," CHD comes about when the coronary arteries are clogged by a fatty substance called plaque. When doctors speak of heart disease, we are usually referring to CHD.

Because CHD is so common, the rest of this chapter focuses on this particular type of heart disease. (The high blood pressure that can contribute to heart disease is discussed in Chapter 9.)

Heart disease statistics

Heart disease is the number-one killer in this country today. Every year, more than 1.5 million people suffer heart attacks and more than 500,000 people die of CHD. Sadly, most deaths are preventable.

Signs and symptoms

There are no symptoms in the early stages of CHD. People can function well with 50 percent or more of their coronary arteries blocked.

When symptoms do strike, they may include:

- Angina, chest pain that may radiate to the shoulders and arms, the neck and jaw, the upper abdomen, the shoulders or the back, which is usually related to exertion.
- A "crushing" or "squeezing" feeling in the chest.
- Shortness of breath.
- Heaviness in the chest.
- Fatigue.

What is CHD?

"Coronary" refers to the arteries that supply fresh blood to the heart muscle itself, so CHD is really a problem that begins in these tiny arteries, not in the heart muscle itself or in the heart valves.

Imagine miles of irrigation ditches winding their way through a farm, carrying water to all the crops. Without that water, the crops would die. Suppose that, for some reason, the farmer threw some garbage into the ditches every day. Most of the junk would wash away, but some would remain. Little by little the garbage would build up, although it might take 30 or 40 years. One day, however, one of the ditches would be completely jammed up. No water could get through. All the crops "downstream" of this "junk dam" would quickly die.

CHD is caused by a "dam" made up of cholesterol, fat, blood clots and cellular debris that clog the tiny "irrigation ditches" (coronary arteries) that wind their way through our heart muscles. When a coronary artery becomes blocked and the flow of blood stops, heart muscle "downstream" will die.

Yes, certain genetic factors make us more or less susceptible to CHD, and a very small number of people have genetically determined elevated cholesterol levels. But for most people, CHD is a deadly "junk problem" caused by diet and lifestyle.

CHD risk factors

In medical school, we were taught that most CHD is genetic. If your father had a heart attack, especially in his 50s or younger, your risk of suffering the same was increased. If your mother had a heart attack, the odds were against you. There was nothing that could be done to prevent this genetic predisposition, we were taught. Fortunately, we've learned a great deal about CHD since then and have identified several risk factors associated with heart disease, including:

- Smoking.
- Elevated total cholesterol.

- Elevated LDL ("bad") cholesterol.
- Low HDL ("good") cholesterol.
- High blood pressure (hypertension).
- A family history of heart disease.
- Obesity.
- Stress.
- Diabetes mellitus.
- Lack of exercise.

Being male is also a risk factor. Men have a higher risk of heart disease than do women for most of their lives. After menopause, however, women's risk climbs and the risk begins to equalize.

The cholesterol factor

Cholesterol is a natural substance found inside the cells of humans and animals. Cholesterol is not bad. In fact some hormones, including estrogen and testosterone, are built on a framework of cholesterol. The problem is excess cholesterol.

Babies are born with cholesterol levels of about 80-100 mg/dl (milligrams per deciliter). The average adult's cholesterol level can rise to 220—some even reach 300 or 400. This doesn't have to be the case. In other countries where the diet is low in fat and cholesterol, but high in vegetables and grains, the average adult may have a cholesterol level of 150 or even less.

The average cholesterol level among American adults is somewhere around 220. Unfortunately, the average American with the average cholesterol of 220 may then suffer the average heart attack. Where heart disease is concerned, average is not good.

Three kinds of cholesterol. We usually speak about cholesterol as if it were a single substance. When I check a patient's blood, however, I look his or her total cholesterol, the HDL and LDL. Total cholesterol is what most people are referring to when they speak about cholesterol. I recommend to my patients that they get their cholesterol down to 180 or less. Ideally, it should be 100 plus your age.

HDL (high-density lipoprotein) is the "good" cholesterol. HDL travels through the bloodstream and scavenges cholesterol from the arteries, "pulling" it off the arterial walls and taking it to the liver for disposal. The higher the HDL, the lower the risk of CHD. I like my patients' HDLs to be at 50 or more. (The National Cholesterol Education Plan tells us that a low HDL-cholesterol—35 or less—is an independent risk factor for CHD.)

LDL (low-density lipoprotein) is the "bad" cholesterol that carries cholesterol to the artery walls, where it can stick. The LDL should be 100 or less.

Measuring the risk with CADRIF. CADRIF is a simple ratio that helps you track your risk of heart disease. CADRIF stands for "coronary artery disease risk factor." To figure your CADRIF, simply divide your total cholesterol by your HDL. If your total cholesterol is 280 and your HDL is 30, your CADRIF is 280/30 = 9.3

Your CADRIF should be four or less. The higher the CADRIF, the greater your risk of heart disease.

Another ratio you can use to gauge your risk of heart attacks is the CADRIF 2, which is determined by dividing the LDL by HDL. If your LDL is 150 and your HDL is 50, your CADRIF 2 is three. Your CADRIF 2 should be three or less.

Standard medical treatment

- Medications to lower cholesterol (such as cholestyramine and lovastatin).
- Medications for angina (such as nitroglycerin).
- Medications, such as nitrates, to improve the flow of blood to the heart muscle.
- Medications to strengthen the heart (if it has been weakened by a heart attack), such as digitalis.
- Medications to prevent unwanted blood clots, such as aspirin.
- Medications to dissolve blood clots, such as streptokinase.
- Balloon angioplasty to widen the interiors of the coronary arteries by "squeezing" the blockages against the artery walls.
- Coronary artery bypass surgery.
- Heart transplants for the most severe cases.

As you can see from the list of treatments, standard Western medicine focuses on drugs and medications to either deal with the symptoms or repair the damage that has already occurred.

Now let's take a look at some of the many alternative treatments for heart disease. These are not all the possible therapies, because there are too many to investigate in a single chapter. Reading through these alternatives, however, will give you an idea of the many possibilities.

The information on alternative therapies is meant for educational purposes only. I am not endorsing any therapy or suggesting that you see any alternative practitioner. If you have or suspect that you have heart disease, see your physician.

Acupuncture

Although the treatment varies with the patient's symptoms, four or five acupuncture points are generally used. These include Bladder 14 and 15 (in the upper back between the shoulder blades), the Pericardium point on the lower forearm and Heart 7 (on the wrist crease below the small finger).

If the patient suffers from rapid heart beat (tachycardia), the point known as Pericardium 4 (on the palm side of the lower forearm) may be used. If the heart beat is slow, Heart 5 (on the lower forearm near the wrist) may be used. If the patient has coughed up bloody sputum, indicating a possible blood clot in the lungs, Lung 6 (on the wrist near the base of the thumb) is used. If there is abdominal distention or low back pain, local points in the lower back and Spleen 6 (on the inside of the leg above the inner ankle), called "Sanyinjiao," are stimulated.

Aromatherapy

The goal of aromatherapy is to help relieve symptoms of and strengthen one's resistance to various problems that afflict the heart. There are no standard therapeutic guidelines for using aromatherapy to treat heart disease, so treatment will vary. Essential oils that may be used for clogged, hardened arteries include rosemary (*Rosmarinus officinalis*) and juniper (*Juniperus communis*).

Essential oils that may be used for heart palpitations or heart failure include:

- Camphor (*Cinnamomum camphora*).
- Lavender (*Lavandula officinalis*).
- Melissa (*Melissa officinalis*).
- Neroli (*Citrus aurantium*).
- Peppermint (*Mentha piperata*).
- Rosemary (*Rosmarinus officinalis*).
- Ylang-ylang (*Cananga odorata*).

The patient may be instructed to inhale the vapors from these oils as they rise from a bowl of water, to mix them in a base oil and use in massage, to wear as a perfume or to mix with the bath water. Treatment length will vary from practitioner to practitioner and according to the patient's condition.

Ayurvedic healing

Ayurveda, a 5,000-year-old approach to healing from India, believes that the heart, not the brain, is where the human consciousness lies. Thus, heart disease is related to crises of consciousness, feeling and identity. Emotional problems should always be considered when treating it.

Heart diseases may manifest themselves in any of the three humors, or primary life forces of the body.

- Heart disease in the Vata (air) humor is caused by the drying of body tissue and hardening of the blood vessels. The symptoms of Vata-type heart disease include chest tightness and pain, insomnia, constipation and labored breathing. Fear and restlessness are common.

- Heart disease in the Kapha (water or phlegm) humor has to do with excess: overeating, and too much cholesterol, fat and mucus interfering with the heart. Symptoms of Kapha-type heart disease include coughing, increased salivation, lack of appetite, nausea, fatigue and a heaviness in the chest. Greed and materialism are common.

- Heart disease in the Pitta (fire) humor often manifests as a heart attack. The symptoms of Pitta-type heart disease include a burning sensation in and around the heart, fever, sweating, a feeling of warmth all over the body, dizziness and a yellowish tint to the skin and eyes. Anger and irritability are common.

All heart diseases, regardless of their humors, are treated with mental and physical rest, yoga and meditation. Arjuna is given to stimulate circulation and strengthen the heart. Ashwagandha, guggul and sandalwood may also be given for CHD, angina, hardened arteries and other heart distress. Saffron, hawthorn berries, myrrh, ginger, cinnamon and other herbs may be given as well. Gems and metals may also be prescribed for internal or external use. Gold, ruby and garnet stimulate the heart. Silver, jade, emerald and pearl calm the heart. Yellow sapphire and yellow topaz strengthen the heart.

Treating Vata-type heart disease

An anti-Vata diet is prescribed and the fat-soluble vitamins A, D and E are recommended, as is the "sour" vitamin C.

A ruby or garnet set in gold should be worn on the right ring finger in order to strengthen the heart. Herbs to be used include ashwagandha, arjuna, astragalus, cinnamon, cardamom, comfrey root, garlic, ginseng, guggul, hawthorn berries, licorice, myrrh, rehmannia, sandalwood and zizphus.

The anti-Vata diet includes warm, heavy and moist foods that give one strength. Frequent small meals, mildly spiced and with only a few different types of foods per meal, are recommended. One should not eat when nervous or worried. Your meal should be cooked for you, and you should eat with friends. Many dietary considerations include:

- Wheat, oats, brown rice and couscous are encouraged. Corn grains, buckwheat, millet, rye, barley, granola and dried grains are to be avoided.
- Vegetables, including onions, carrots, beets, parsley, radish, potatoes, tomatoes, fresh corn, fresh peas, turnips, artichokes and okra are helpful. But raw onions, mushrooms, broccoli, cabbage, cauliflower, cucumber, asparagus, spinach, eggplant, lettuce and certain other vegetables are discouraged. The vegetables should be cooked before being eaten.
- Small amounts of fruits are acceptable, but not dried fruit, melons, cranberries or apples.
- Beans, which aggravate Vata, are not allowed, except for mung beans and tofu (which is made from soy beans).
- Fish, chicken and turkey are recommended. Lamb, pork and beef should be avoided.
- Dairy products (except for ice cream) are helpful when warm and spiced. Drink milk by itself. Fermented dairy products, such as yogurt, are better.
- Small amounts of raw or lightly roasted nuts and seeds.
- Oils, which are moist and warm, counteract the elevated Vata. Sesame, almond, olive, avocado, peanut, mustard and coconut oils are helpful. Since they are sometimes hard to digest, the oils can also be applied externally. Margarine, canola, corn, soy and safflower oil are to be avoided.
- Sweeteners such as maple syrup, raw sugar, molasses, honey and fructose (fruit sugar) are helpful, but refined white sugar is not. Most spices are helpful, including garlic, fennel, nutmeg, ginger, basil, cumin, cinnamon, fenugreek, mint, black pepper, cayenne, mustard and horseradish.
- Plenty of fluids help with Vata-type illnesses. Milk, herbal teas and sour fruit juices are helpful. Water is good, but not nourishing enough by itself. Small amounts of alcohol or herbal wines are suggested before or with meals.

Treating Kapha-type heart disease

For Kapha-type heart disease, the treatment includes an anti-Kapha diet that has no dairy products, fatty meats, salt or sugar. Supplements should be kept to a minimum. The B-vitamins are helpful, but the fat-soluble vitamins A, D and E are not recommended.

A ruby or garnet set in gold should be worn on the right ring finger in order to strengthen the heart. Herbs that encourage the breakup of phlegm should be taken. Other herbs include bayberry, cayenne, cinnamon, guggul, motherwort and myrrh. Cinnamon, mustard or camphor may be applied to the chest to ease congestion.

The anti-Kapha diet is light, dry and warm. Cold, oily and heavy foods should be avoided. Three meals a day should be eaten, with lunch being the main meal. Breakfast may be skipped, and weekly fasting is helpful. Most or all of the daily food should be consumed between the hours of 10 a.m. and 6 p.m. Dietary guidelines include:

- Vegetables, which are generally light and dry, are good. Broccoli, cabbage, celery, carrots, peas, mushrooms, asparagus, lettuce, radish, turnips, chard and chilies are good for Kapha types. Sweet potatoes, tomatoes, corn, okra, cucumber and other "wet" foods should be avoided. All vegetables should be steamed and spiced before being eaten.
- Fruit, which is watery, should be avoided. Dried fruit, apples, cranberries and pears are acceptable.
- In general, grains should be avoided. However, some grains, including barley, corn, millet and rye, can be helpful.
- Beans, which are drying and increase air, tend to be good for the watery Kapha diseases. Tofu, mung beans, adzuki beans, kidney beans, soy beans, lima beans, lentils and split peas are good. Chickpeas should be avoided.
- Animal products are harmful and should be avoided. Chicken and turkey are less harmful than beef, pork, lamb and fish.
- Except for goat's milk, soy milk and buttermilk, dairy products should be avoided.
- Nuts and seeds, which tend to be mucous forming, should be avoided. Sunflower and pumpkin seeds may be eaten.
- In general, the heavy and moist oils are bad for Kapha heart disease. Small amounts of corn oil, soy oil, canola, sunflower oil and mustard oil may be used.
- Avoid sweeteners, except for honey, which is drying.
- Spices, such as cayenne, mustard, garlic, ginger, cloves and cardamom, are excellent. Hot spices are especially good.
- Herbal tea, spiced tea and regular tea are good for Kapha-type heart disease. Small amounts of water are acceptable, but it should never be taken cold or as ice.

For Pitta-type heart disease

For Pitta-type heart disease, the treatment includes an anti-Pitta diet that has no red meat, hot spices, greasy foods or alcohol and strictly limits the amount of salt. B-vitamins, vitamin K, calcium and iron are usually recommended.

An emerald set in silver should be worn on the middle finger of the right hand. Herbs to be used include aloe, arjuna, barberry, golden seal, gotu kola, motherwort, myrrh, saffron and shatavari. Sandalwood oil is applied to the chest and to the "third eye" in the middle of the forehead. Meditation reduces pent-up anger, hatred and resentment. Exercise and exposure to the sun are severely limited.

The anti-Pitta diet consists of cool, slightly dry and heavy foods. The foods should be raw and relatively plain-tasting, not cooked in lots of oil or heavily spiced. Three regular meals a day are suggested, with no eating late at night. Guidelines include the following:

- Most vegetables are helpful for Pitta-type heart disease. They should be eaten raw or steamed, but never fried. Cauliflower, celery, broccoli, cabbage, brussels sprouts, mushrooms, asparagus, lettuce, green beans, peas, cucumber, okra, potatoes, parsley and corn are all helpful. Vegetables to avoid include chilies, onions, tomatoes, avocados, carrots, beets, spinach, eggplant, radishes, watercress and seaweed.

- Fruit is helpful, especially apples, pears, pineapple, cranberries, dates, grapes, figs, oranges, raspberries and mangoes. Avoid grapefruit, lemons, limes, bananas, cherries, peaches, strawberries, papaya and apricots.

- Most grains, including whole-grain breads and pastas, are good. Avoid brown rice, corn, rye and buckwheat.

- Beans are good, although they should be eaten with cumin or other spices so as not to upset digestion. Peanuts and lentils should be avoided.

- Meat is generally unhelpful. The white meat of chicken or turkey is acceptable, as is the whites of eggs. Other poultry, meat and fish are not recommended.

- Dairy products are part of the anti-Pitta diet. Milk, cream, unsalted cheeses and cottage cheeses are recommended, but salted cheeses, buttermilk, yogurt, sour cream and ice cream are not.

- Nuts are discouraged because their warm and oily nature can increase the Pitta, which is the opposite of what the anti-Pitta diet is designed to accomplish. Coconut and sunflower seeds may be eaten in small amounts.

- Oils are not helpful in the anti-Pitta diet. Only coconut oil, butter, corn oil and soy oil should be used if oils are absolutely necessary.

- Sweeteners help to cool the fires of Pitta diseases. Sugar (fruit, maple and raw) and honey are helpful. Refined white sugar, molasses and old honey should be avoided.
- Since spices can fuel the heat of Pitta, only selected ones are allowed. These include fennel, cilantro, coriander, mint, parsley and cinnamon.
- Fluids help to cool the fires of Pitta. Black tea, green tea and herb teas are helpful. Avoid spicy teas. Milk and other dairy products are advised, as are fruit and vegetable juices. Alcoholic beverages are forbidden.

Additional treatment for the arteries

Kapha and Pitta types of heart disease are caused by accumulated fats, but the Vata-type is related to the hardening of the arteries. Thus, additional herbs for hardened, clogged arteries may be recommended, including elecampane, garlic, he shou wu, turmeric and salvia.

Color therapy

There are no standard protocols for dealing with heart disease, but color therapists may choose these colors:

Red increases circulation and energy and reduces nervousness. Red is an important color for heart disease because healthy arteries are light red and the heart is dark red. Red should not be used if there is already too much red in the patient (indicated by an overly reddish face, fever, easy excitability or red hair).

Patients can also meditate on the colors or eat appropriately colored foods. Red foods include radishes, beets, tomatoes, red cabbage, red currants, red plums, watermelon, whole wheat, liver, red wine and grapes. Red metals and chemicals include barium, cadmium, copper, nitrogen, iron, neon, oxygen, potassium and zinc.

For angina pain, *magenta* supports the heart action, as do potassium and other minerals that energize the heart. Magenta stimulates the heart and adrenal glands and acts as a diuretic to flush excess fluid from the body. It also helps to calm excited emotions.

There are many ways for the color therapist to apply the proper-color light to the patient, including through direct light, gems, jewelry, perfume, clothing and colored glass.

Herbal medicine

Herbs have been used for many centuries to help relieve the pain, shortness of breath and other symptoms that are associated with heart disease. Herbs typically used to treat the various symptoms of heart disease include garlic (*Allium sativum*), oats (*Avena sativa*) and oolong tea (*Camellia sinensis*).

Herbs that reduce LDL and total cholesterol, both of which are major risk factors for heart disease, include ginkgo (*Ginkgo biloba*), greater periwinkle (*Vinca major*) and mistletoe (*Viscum album*). These herbs help to improve the blood flow in the heart (coronary) and brain (cerebral) arteries, strengthen the walls of the capillaries, reduce capillary inflammation and slow the heartbeat.

Other herbs may be used to strengthen the capillaries and to improve the general circulation. These include:

- Buckwheat (*Fagopyrum esculentum*) to repair the walls of the smaller arteries.
- Cayenne (*Capsicum frutescens*) to warm the body and induce sweating.
- Dandelion leaf to help flush excess fluid from the body.
- Ginger (*Zingiber officinalis*) to stimulate the circulatory system and warm the body.
- *Gui Zhi* (*Cinnamomum cassia*) to warm the body and induce sweating.
- Heartsease (*Viola tricolor*) to strengthen capillary walls.
- Lime blossom (*Tilia europea*) to help flush excess fluid from the body.
- Prickly ash (*Zanthoxylum americanum*) to stimulate the circulation.

For the fear and anxiety that often accompany heart disease:

- Motherwort (*Leonurus cardiaca*).
- Skullcap (*Scutellaria lateriflora*).
- St. John's Wort (*Hypericum perforatum*).

Homeopathy

Traditional Western medicine strives to reduce cholesterol levels, clean out clogged arteries and use medicines to dissolve blood clots. Homeopathy treats heart disease by helping the body to heal itself.

Most of the major homeopathic remedies may be used for heart disease, depending upon the patient's symptoms. Some include:

- *Aconitum napellus*, which is indicated when the patient is very anxious and impatient and can imagine the worst happening. Typically, a very strong pain envelops the heart and left arm. The problem is worse at night and when the patient is warm, and is better with rest and fresh air.

- *Argentum nitricum*, which is indicated when the patient is impulsive and fearful. Chest pain is stronger at night, after eating and with stress. It's better with fresh air and pressure.
- *Aurum metallicum*, which is indicated when the patient is depressed, feels worthless and is very sensitive to pain. Symptoms include depression and night-time chest pain. The patient feels better in the summer and with fresh air.
- *Baryta carbonica*, which is indicated when the patient is very old or very young. Symptoms include hypertension, palpitations and confusion, made worse with exposure to dampness or cold.
- *Cactus grandiflorus,* which is indicated when the patient is sad and in great pain. The pain seems to be "squeezing" the chest, making it difficult to breathe, and is worse around noon and with exertion, but better with fresh air.
- *Glonoine*, which is indicated when the patient is talkative but moody, thin and suspicious. The problem is worse following sleeping and a warm bath, but better with fresh air and a warm compress.
- *Lillium tigrinum*, which is indicated when the patient is depressed and aimless, but hurried. The pain seems to strike on the left side of the body, and is made worse with heat or standing up. Fresh air and activity help relieve the pain.

Should a heart attack occur, homeopaths recommend going to your physician or the emergency room immediately. There are, however, some homeopathic first-aid remedies that may be used to help the patient on the way to the doctor. These include:

- *Aconitum napellus,* which is indicated when the patient has difficulty breathing, is anxious, but feels better sitting up.
- *Cactus grandiflorus,* which is indicated when the attack strikes between approximately noon and midnight, feels as if something is "squeezing" the heart or the pain is severe enough to make the patient cry, shout or whimper.
- *Digitalis,* which is indicated when symptoms include blue skin, numbness and weakness of the left arm, a slow pulse and great fear.

Although it is a basic principle of classical homeopathy to use only one remedy at a time, there is a trend among modern homeopaths toward using multiple remedies at once. Using the absolute minimum number of doses necessary is another principle of classical homeopathy. A second dose should not be given until the first has ceased to act, and no more remedies should be given when the body begins to heal.

If the right remedy is used, two or three days should be enough to begin many long-term curative processes. If not, select another remedy.

Nutritional therapy

Nutritional therapy is an exciting field fueled by a continual stream of new research supporting the idea that what we eat has a tremendous affect on our heart health. Let's look at some of the evidence suggesting that diet and various nutrients can help the heart.

Vitamins and minerals

Beta carotene. Beta carotene, the "plant form" of vitamin A, can be converted into vitamin A by the body. An antioxidant, beta carotene protects against heart disease by inhibiting the conversion of LDL into its more dangerous, oxidized form. The Physicians Health Study found that 50 mg of beta carotene every other day reduced the incidence of major coronary and vascular events.[1] Beta carotene sources include yellow-orange fruits and vegetables (squash, papaya, cantaloupe) and leafy green vegetables (spinach, broccoli and collard greens).

Folic acid. This member of the B-family of vitamins helps to control homocysteine, an amino acid that seems to play a major role in clogging the arteries. In the Physicians Health Study, 271 men who had heart attacks were tested and found to have higher levels of homocysteine than did the healthy men. And when the University of Alabama compared 100 men who had had heart attacks to 100 who had not, the homocysteine was higher in those who had the heart trouble.[2] Good sources of folic acid include green, leafy vegetables, brown rice and carrots. In a test of folic acid's ability to help head off heart problems, 17 elderly patients suffering from arteriosclerosis were given between 5 and 7.5 mg of folic acid daily. As a result, the blood flow through their capillaries improved.[3]

Niacin. Also a member of the B-family of vitamins, niacin has long been known to reduce the total cholesterol and the LDL ("bad") cholesterol, while raising the HDL ("good") cholesterol. In a 12-year study involving close to 4,000 men, those who received niacin supplements were less likely to die of CHD than those who were given placebos. And the higher his cholesterol at the beginning of the study, the more likely a man was to benefit.[4] I may start my patients on 25 to 50 mg, three times a day, gradually increasing up to 2,000 to 5,000 mg per day. I warn my patients about the flushing and tingling sensations that may occur when taking niacin, and I check their liver tests periodically. (Taking one aspirin a day or 500 mg of inositol two to three times a day will reduce or eliminate the flush.)

In another study, patients with high LDL were given various doses of niacin. The vitamin drove the total cholesterol down between

13 percent and 18 percent, and improved the ratio of total cholesterol to HDL (that's the CADRIF ratio).[5] A study with 55 patients found that niacin could push the HDL up by as much as 31 percent.[6] Food sources of niacin include barley, salmon and sesame seeds.

Vitamin B6. Studies involving animals have shown that diets deficient in B6 can lead to hardened, narrowed arteries.[7] This may be because B6 helps to prevent the unnecessary blood clots that can block arteries. B6 is also necessary to control the amino acid homocysteine, which appears to damage artery linings and encourage heart disease. B6 can be found in whole grains, lentils and sweet potatoes.

Vitamin B12. Lack of this vitamin has also been associated with elevated levels of the dangerous homocysteine. Elevated levels of homocysteine, an amino acid produced by the body, can damage the inner surface of arteries. This can be treated and/or prevented with vitamin B12, vitamin B6 and folic acid. Many cardiologists are now using B-vitamins to help prevent coronary artery disease.

Vitamin C. This vitamin helps to protect against CHD in several ways. It plays a role in the conversion of cholesterol into bile acids. If vitamin C is lacking, less cholesterol is converted. Instead, the cholesterol may build up in the arteries, blood and liver.

Vitamin C is also needed for the normal metabolism of blood fats that might otherwise contribute to the "dams" blocking the arteries. It builds the collagen that helps to keep artery walls strong.

Vitamin C is an antioxidant that helps to control the free radicals and other oxidants that can convert LDL into its more dangerous, artery-clogging form.

Vitamin C supplementation can drive down cholesterol in people with high cholesterol and low levels of vitamin C in the blood. Adding pectin, or other agents that bind cholesterol, increases the effect.[8]

The level of vitamin C in the blood has been found to be related to the CHD-related angina pain. The higher the level of vitamin C, the less pain.[9] Good sources of vitamin C include citrus fruits, strawberries and sweet red peppers.

Vitamin E. Vitamin E is an antioxidant that helps to prevent the oxidation-driven conversion of LDL to its more harmful, artery-blocking form. Vitamin E may also "thin" the blood by making the platelets less likely to stick together to form blood clots that can lodge in an already-narrowed artery, thus triggering a heart attack.[10]

The vitamin may play a role in regulating the way that cells lining the arteries proliferate and repair themselves, and may protect them from the damaging oxidants.[11] This helps to prevent the formation of blockages on the artery walls.

Vitamin E supplementation may increase the protective HDL. In a study of 60 patients with elevated cholesterol, 500 IU of vitamin E daily for 90 days increased the HDL and improved the CADRIF ratio.[12]

The amount of vitamin E in the blood may be inversely correlated with death from heart attacks. This means that a greater level of vitamin E in the blood may translate to a lower risk of death.[13] Indeed, a large-scale trial conducted at Harvard Medical School involving over 87,000 female nurses has found that taking vitamin E daily can cut the risk of CHD by over 40 percent.[14] Vitamin E can be found in nuts, peas and green beans.

Calcium. In the proper amounts, the mineral calcium may help to keep cholesterol under control and may prevent dangerous blood clots. Too much calcium may increase the risk of heart disease, especially if there is much too much calcium in relation to magnesium. Sources of calcium include milk, sardines (with bones) and cheese.

Magnesium. A lack of this mineral has been linked to an increased risk of CHD, heart attacks and improper heartbeats (ventricular tachyarrhythmias). For years, I have used magnesium as a first-line treatment for many irregular heart rhythms.

Magnesium supplementation may reduce the total cholesterol, increase the beneficial HDL and prevent unnecessary "clumping" in the blood that can trigger a heart attack.[15] The mineral may also reduce the symptoms of angina or may prevent future attacks.[16]

Magnesium can even help if one is already suffering a heart attack. In a study involving 2,300 people, some patients were given magnesium injections while they were having heart attacks. The injections cut the death rate by 25 percent.[17] Magnesium can be found in almonds, parsley and spinach.

Selenium. The amount of this mineral in the blood and red blood cells may be related to the risk of CHD and heart attacks.[18] The lower the level of selenium, the more the risk. This may be because selenium, like vitamins C and E, is an antioxidant that helps to prevent the conversion of LDL into its more artery-damaging, oxidized form. It may also be because selenium helps to "thin" the blood.[19] When the blood is "thin," there is less chance that unnecessary blood clots will form and trigger a heart attack by lodging in an already-narrowed artery. And among patients who did have heart attacks, those who were then treated with selenium or selenium-rich yeast had fewer second attacks than those who were given a placebo.[20] Good sources of selenium include barley, shrimp and whole grains.

Phytochemicals

Phytochemicals are other substances found in foods that help us to remain healthy. ("Phyto" refers to food.) Neither vitamins nor minerals, the phytochemicals are a remarkably large and diverse group of substances with a variety of duties in the body.

Activated charcoal. This is a special type of capsulated charcoal that is used in hospital emergency rooms as an antidote to many poisons. If warranted, I have my patients start with half a gram and work up to a gram of activated charcoal twice a day, with meals.

One study involved seven patients with elevated cholesterol who had not seen much improvement after 10 years of treatment with cholesterol medicines. When they were given 8 grams of activated charcoal three times a day for four weeks, their total cholesterol fell by 41 percent, and their harmful LDLs by 25 percent. Meanwhile, their beneficial HDLs rose by 8 percent.

Alpha-lipoic acid (Alpha-lipotene). About 50 years ago, scientists discovered a substance in the body that had powerful antioxidant and free-radical quenching effects. This substance, called alpha-lipoic acid, works with other antioxidants to increase their effectiveness against oxidative stress. Nicknamed the "metabolic antioxidant," it helps the body to recycle other antioxidants. Instead of these vitamins being "used up," they're kept available and used again.

Alpha-lipoic acid can also help the body rid itself of toxic heavy metals, such as mercury and cadmium. Furthermore, it prevents glycation, the potentially dangerous combination of sugar and protein in the body. (A common example of glycation is the combination of sugar with proteins in the lenses of the eyes that can result in cataracts.) Alpha-lipoic acid is believed to play a major role in preventing the loss of eye sight that occurs with retinal degeneration.

And as a strong antioxidant, alpha-lipoic acid helps to keep arteries clear by preventing the LDL ("bad") cholesterol from being incorporated into the artery walls. As far as I know, it is the only antioxidant that is both fat and water soluble. This means that it can work inside and outside of the body cells. Alpha-lipoic acid is known by the trade name Alpha Lipotene.

Bioflavonoids. Originally known as "vitamin P," the bioflavonoids are a group of over 200 substances with antioxidant properties. In addition to fighting off the oxidation-driven conversion of LDL to its more dangerous form, the bioflavonoids may "thin" the blood and prevent the formation of potentially deadly blood clots.[21]

Hesperidin, rutin, queretin and catechin are some of the bioflavonoids, which are found in the outer layer, skin and peels of vegetables and fruits, in leafy vegetables, coffee, tea and wine.

Bromelain. An enzyme found in pineapple, bromelain may "thin" the blood and help to clear away debris from artery walls. At least one study has shown that bromelain can relieve the pain of angina, which is associated with CHD.

Lecithin. An antioxidant found in eggs, corn and soybeans, lecithin helps prevent the conversion of LDL into its more dangerous, artery-damaging form. Lecithin may also lower the total cholesterol.

Omega-3 fatty acids. My mother used to tell me to eat fish because it would make me smarter. I don't know if fish is truly a brain food, but exciting evidence suggests that it might be a healthy-heart food.

The omega-3 story began in the 1970s with Danish researchers who noted that Eskimos living in Greenland had very little CHD, despite eating an incredibly high fat diet consisting largely of fatty fish, whale and seal meat. By comparing the diets of the Greenland Eskimos to those Eskimos living in Denmark, who were eating a high-fat, low-fish, Western-style diet, the researchers determined that the omega-3 fatty acids found in fish were heart protectors.

Fatty acids are the building blocks of fat, much as amino acids are used to construct proteins. The typical Western diet contains large amounts of omega-6 fatty acids, while a diet high in fish contains omega-3 fatty acids. Although the omega-3s are found in many types of seafood, deep-sea fish, such as salmon and mackerel, have more than do the "skinny" freshwater fish, such as halibut.

Large-scale studies have shown that eating fish once or twice a week can cut the risk of dying of heart disease in half.[22] In one study, several thousand Swedish men and women were observed from 1969 to 1982. The ones who ate the most fish were least likely to develop CHD or to actually have heart attacks.[23] A longer study, lasting 20 years, tracked 872 men living in the Netherlands. It was found that the more fish they ate, the less likely they were to develop CHD.[24]

Various studies have suggested that the fish oils may:

- Prevent the platelets from unnecessarily sticking together and forming dangerous clots that may lodge in an already-narrowed artery and trigger a heart attack or stroke.
- Reduce the total cholesterol.
- Lower the blood fats (triglycerides).
- Increase the beneficial HDL cholesterol that helps to keep the arteries clean.
- Reduce the pain of angina and make it possible for people with heart disease to exercise longer than normal.
- Reduce the damage to heart tissue, if a heart attack occurs.

Some of these findings have been questioned. And it seems that omega-3 supplements should be taken with vitamin E to prevent oxidation damage to body cells. So the value of omega-3 supplements will continue to be debated. It seems clear, however, that adding fish to the diet is a move toward good health.

Pectin. Pectin is a fiber found in grapefruit, apples and other fruits and vegetables. Eight weeks of pectin supplements pushed the total cholesterol down by 7.6 percent, and the harmful LDL by 10.8 percent.[25] With every one point fall in cholesterol reducing the risk of

CHD by 2 percent, a 7.6 percent drop in cholesterol lowers the risk of heart disease by 15 percent.

The power of grapefruit pectin was studied in pigs, whose cardio-vascular systems are similar to ours. Even when the animals were deliberately fed a high-cholesterol diet, the grapefruit pectin swept away fatty plaque deposits from the artery walls.

Proanthocyanidins. Back in the 1500s, Jacques Cartier explored parts of North America. When his men grew ill from poor nutrition, the Indians helped by showing them how to use tea made from the bark of a certain maritime tree. More than 400 years later, French scientists investigating the bark of a French maritime tree found a class of substances they called *proanthocyanidins.* In the U.S., scientists found what is believed to be an even better source of proanthocyanidins: grape seed extract. Proanthocyanidins are the most powerful antioxidants—more powerful than either vitamin C or vitamin E.

Psyllium seeds. Found in health food stores and in some laxatives, psyllium is a fiber that can help to improve the cholesterol "profile" by lowering the total cholesterol and LDL.

Ubiquinone. Also known as Coenzyme Q10 or CoQ10, ubiquinone is actually a family of related substances known as the ubiquinones. They are so named because they are apparently ubiquitous—found everywhere in the body and in foods such as sardines and mackerel.

Researchers compared healthy people to heart patients and found that the CoQ10 was lower, and both the LDL and total cholesterol were higher in the heart patients.[26] This suggests that CoQ10 may protect against atherosclerosis and CHD. Someday we may use the CoQ10-to-LDL ratio to assess the risk of suffering a heart attack.

CoQ10 has also been used to relieve the symptoms of angina, which are caused by dangerously narrowed coronary arteries and the strain they place on the heart. When men and women with angina were given either CoQ10 or a placebo for four weeks, the ones given the CoQ10 had 53 percent fewer angina episodes and were able to exercise longer on a treadmill.[27] CoQ10 may also help to reduce the risk of heart disease by keeping the blood "thin."[28]

Specific foods that strengthen the heart

Although most studies look at the effects of a single vitamin, mineral or phytochemical, some researchers have studied "whole" foods. Some of the findings are surprising and suggest that there are many tasty ways to keep the heart beating strongly for a long time.

Brewer's yeast. This largely overlooked substance, not found in the typical kitchen, can lower the total cholesterol and LDL while raising the helpful HDL. In one study with normal- and high-cholesterol patients, 11 healthy volunteers were given brewer's yeast. Eight weeks later, 10 of the 11 people with normal cholesterol levels had even lower total cholesterol levels and increased HDL levels. Among the 15 volunteers with high cholesterol, eight enjoyed the same beneficial results.[29]

Garlic. Cholesterol levels tend to rise after a meal, as the body assimilates the cholesterol, fats and other substances in the food. This is especially true after a meal filled with fat and cholesterol. But adding as little as two ounces of garlic juice to a fatty, cholesterol-laden meal can actually lower the cholesterol by up to 7 percent.[30] Another study found that 600 mg of garlic powder a day could push the total cholesterol down by some 10 percent,[31] which translates into a 20 percent decrease in the risk of heart disease. Other research has supported these findings, reporting that garlic can lower both total and LDL cholesterol while raising the HDL ("good") cholesterol.

Garlic's cholesterol-lowering powers also have staying power. A 10-month study found that eating three cloves of garlic (or the equivalent in supplements) a day keeps the cholesterol down for extended periods.[32] And because it contains ajoene and other substances, garlic also helps to keep the blood "thin" and free of potentially deadly blood clots. My favorite garlic supplements are the original AGE (Aged Garlic Extract) capsules, first brought to my attention years ago by Charlie Fox of Wakanaga of America, makers of Kyolic Garlic.

Ginger. Ginger shares heart-helping attributes with its cousin garlic. Ginger interferes with the long sequence of events necessary for blood clots to form. This helps to prevent clots that can lodge in narrowed coronary arteries and set off a heart attack.

Green tea. Popular in Asia for centuries, green tea helps to keep blood pressure under control. The tea contains Epigallocatechin Gallate (EGCG) and other substances that protect the body against the dangers of oxidation, while helping to keep the harmful LDL cholesterol down and the helpful HDL cholesterol up. They also assist in keeping blood pressure under control.

Oat bran. One of my favorite anticholesterol foods, oat bran lowers cholesterol in many people *and* protects against other diseases.

Onions. Onions contain adenosine and other "blood thinners" that help to prevent the possibly fatal blood clots. In addition to "thinning" the blood, onions can help keep the coronary arteries open and clear by increasing the HDL. Eating half a raw onion every day can increase HDL by 20 to 30 percent. Although we can't say for sure that a one-point rise in HDL equals a two-point drop in the risk of CHD, we do know that most people's HDLs are too low and should be increased.

Prunes. Although best known for their beneficial effects on sluggish bowels, prunes also help to protect the heart. In both human and animal studies, prunes had a mild cholesterol-lowering effect.

Soy. Long popular in Asia, soy and soy-based foods, such as tofu, have proven to be heart protectors. If you put people with high cholesterol on a low-fat, low-cholesterol diet, their cholesterol levels usually drop. But if you replace the animal protein in the diet with soy protein, they will drop significantly lower. In fact, one study showed that soy protein could "cancel out" the effect of 500 mg of cholesterol deliberately added to the daily diet. Although soy can lower cholesterol levels in those with normal levels, it works best in people with elevated cholesterol.

Wine. For decades, doctors have been baffled by the "French paradox." We're confused by the fact that the French eat a high-fat diet but have much less heart disease than Americans. The French also smoke more than Americans do and are probably just as stressed. What protects French hearts? It seems that drinking moderate amounts of wine may raise the beneficial HDL while lowering the harmful LDL. Wine also helps to reduce the stress that increases the risk of heart disease and works to keep the blood thin and clot-free. The active heart-boosting ingredients in wine include the phenols. Like vitamins C, E and A/beta carotene, the phenols are antioxidants. (Of course, drinking any kind of alcohol can be dangerous. If you don't drink, don't start now. If you do drink, only drink in moderation.) If you already use alcohol and are not a problem drinker, one glass of wine with dinner will be helpful.

Putting it all together: the healthy diet

The heart-healthy foods mentioned above are just a few of the many that can help to lower the total cholesterol, LDL cholesterol and blood fats, raise the helpful HDL, control oxidation damage, "thin" the blood and otherwise protect the heart.

When people ask me about the best heart foods, I tell them to eat a wide variety of fresh vegetables and fruits, plenty of whole grains and smaller amounts of fish, nonfat dairy products, low-fat meat and occasional nuts and seeds. In other words, a diet rich in the complex carbohydrates found in vegetables and grains, fiber and beneficial phytochemicals. By eating these foods, you're eating less fat and cholesterol.

A great deal of research suggests that this type of diet can lower the cholesterol and blood fats by some 20 percent. Since the risk of heart disease drops 2 percent with every 1 percent drop in total cholesterol, adopting a low-fat, high-fiber, high-complex-carbohydrate diet can reduce the risk of heart disease by up to 40 percent.[33]

Nutritional therapy is a long-term preventive and treatment strategy. It will not, however, stop a heart attack in progress. And in some cases, CHD may have advanced too far and will require other treatments.

When selecting a nutritional healer, remember that there is no widely recognized school of nutritional therapy and no standards or training for nutritional healers. Fortunately, it's hard to go wrong if your diet is based on a variety of fresh vegetables, fruits and whole grains, with smaller amounts of low-fat protein and dairy products.

Oriental medicine

According to Oriental medicine theory, heart attacks or the pain of angina are usually caused by stagnant *chi* (life energy) or blood in the pericardium or heart meridian. This, in turn, may be due to blocked arteries, bacteria or other organisms, poor diet or "invasions" of wind, heat and other factors. Oriental medicine doctors will often work with Western physicians in treating heart disease, striving to strengthen the body with a combination of herbs and spices, diet, acupuncture, "ear acupuncture" and other therapies, as necessary. Treatment will vary according to the type of heart disease and the patient's individual characteristics. The heart disease may be due to an obstruction of the body's energy in the chest, leading to chest pain, palpitations, shortness of breath (often related to cold temperatures) and a greasy white "fur" on the tongue. The problem may also be caused by lack of movement in the heart vessels, leading to shortness of breath, an uneven pulse, a dark purple-looking tongue and a twinge in the chest that radiates to the back and shoulders. Another type of heart disease is related to a lack of both chi and yin. In cases like this, symptoms include shortness of breath, dryness in the mouth, a weak pulse, heart palpitations and vague pain in the chest.

Herbs and spices

Exactly which herbs and spices and the amount of each will depend upon the patient and his or her condition. One of the substances used for heart disease is *licorice,* a sweet substance that "puts the brakes" on acute diseases while strengthening the lungs, stomach and spleen. It also acts as a "command" herb, working with other herbs to improve their effectiveness. There are several herbal formulas for heart disease, including *Su He Xiang Wan, Kuan Hsin Su Ho Wan Styrax* and *Ben Shen Yang Ying Wan.*

Diet

Diet plays an important role in Oriental medicine. Foods are selected depending on their flavors, organic actions and other qualities, including energies. There are five food energies: hot, warm, neutral, cool and cold. (The energy has to do with the quality of the food, not its temperature. For example, foods with "cold" energy, such as bananas and grapefruit, increase the sensation of cold in the body, even if eaten hot.) In addition to a healthy diet, the Oriental medicine physician may recommend these foods specifically for heart disease:

- *Chive root,* a pungent substance that warms the body while promoting energy and keeping the blood from coagulating unnecessarily. It is also used for chest pain.

- *Corn,* which strengthens the stomach and colon, is used for a weak heart.
- *Date,* a warm and sweet fruit that strengthens the spleen while improving energy and blood flow. It is used for heart palpitations.
- *Hawthorn fruit,* a warm, sweet and sour fruit that helps to prevent excessive blood clotting that can lead to heart attacks. It also tones the spleen, liver and stomach.
- *Honey,* a sweet substance that relieves pain while strengthening the lungs, large intestine and spleen. It is used for various forms of heart disease.
- *Logan,* a warm and sweet fruit used for heart palpitations. It strengthens the heart and blood while improving the energy flow.
- *Tea,* a bitter and somewhat cold fluid that helps reduce the swelling sometimes associated with heart disease.

Psychoneuroimmunology

Mind/body healers use positive affirmations to counteract the negative thoughts that have been contributing to the symptoms of heart disease. Affirmations are typically brief, positive statements that focus on how well one feels and on how the disease is being conquered. The patient might be given several affirmations. An affirmation to improve blood flow might be worded as follows:

"My coronary arteries are large, wide tunnels filled with life-giving blood. The blood flows smoothly and easily through my wide-open arteries."

An affirmation to help one stick to his or her diet might be worded as follows:

"I see myself sitting at a beautiful banquet table filled with delicious and healthful foods. I happily reach for the healthful foods that strengthen my heart, delighting in their delicious taste."

An affirmation for heart and general health may be worded as follows:

"My heart beats like a perfect clock, never missing a beat. I am peaceful and serene, content and confident."

The patient will be instructed to repeat these and other affirmations several times a day.

Reflexology

For circulatory problems and angina (chest pain), the heart reflex area on the foot will be manipulated. This is located in the center of the ball of the left foot. Corresponding points on the hands may also be used.

Associated reflex areas used for angina are the solar plexus and adrenal glands. The solar plexus reflex areas are below the balls of the feet, in the midline. The reflex areas for the adrenal glands are found at approximately the middle of the feet, slightly to the inside. Corresponding points on the hands may also be utilized.

To improve general circulation, intestinal and liver reflex areas may be manipulated. Reflex areas for the stomach and the large and small intestines are found between the balls and heels of both feet. The liver reflex area is located on the right foot, in roughly the middle one-third of the foot, on the outside. If the pain radiates to the left arm and shoulder, the shoulder and arm areas will be manipulated as well. Corresponding points on the hands may also be used.

Other exciting approaches

Chelation therapy

Many physicians use chelation to reverse the narrowing of the arteries called *atherosclerosis*. The idea is simple: Inject EDTA (ethylenediaminetetraacetic acid) into the body, where it will "chelate" (bind) with calcium plaques blocking the flow of blood in the patient's arteries. The calcium, bound to the EDTA, comes off the artery walls, allowing blood to flow more freely. The EDTA/calcium mix later flows out of the body with the urine. EDTA also removes heavy metals, such as lead, and cuts down on inflammation brought about by free radicals. The chelating solution is administered via an intravenous (IV) drip, and the typical chelation session takes between two and four hours. Vitamins and minerals may be added to the chelating solution. About 20 to 30 sessions may be required. Physicians who perform chelation generally put their patients on healthful diets and recommend antioxidants and good health habits.

Many studies have reported good results with chelation therapy, claiming that blood flow improves in up to 80 percent of the patients treated. Angina, the chest pain associated with CHD, is also reported to abate with chelation. However, some other studies have not borne out the early promise. The proponents of chelation therapy are sponsoring additional studies, so we'll know more in the future.

Advice to heart patients

Although many of my patients have had success with the following program, I only use the general guidelines discussed on the next page after reviewing a patient's personal and medical history, performing a thorough examination and evaluating the laboratory studies to make sure that the program will be beneficial. Please see your own physician before embarking on any treatment program for heart disease.

Smoking, high fat or high cholesterol diets, high blood pressure, stress, obesity and lack of exercise are major risk factors for CHD. Fortunately, it is possible to reduce or eliminate many of these risk factors. And because they are also risk factors for many other diseases, including some forms of cancer, when you take steps to protect yourself from CHD, you protect yourself from other diseases as well. Here are the "Seven Steps to Heart Health" I explain to my patients:

1. If you smoke, stop. Immediately.
2. Switch to a diet rich in the complex carbohydrates (with moderate amounts of protein), and low in fat, cholesterol and sodium. Make fresh vegetables, fruits and whole grains the mainstay of your diet.
3. Take antioxidants, such as the 4 ACES (vitamin A as beta carotene, vitamins C and E and the mineral selenium), alpha-lipoic acid (Alpha Lipotene), green tea, proanthocyanidins and coenzyme Q10.
4. Keep your cholesterol levels under control. Your total cholesterol should be less than 180. Ideally, it should be 100 plus your age. Your HDL ("good") cholesterol should be 50 or above. Your LDL ("bad") cholesterol should be 100 or less. Your CADRIF (total cholesterol divided by HDL) should be four or less.
5. Have your blood pressure checked regularly or learn to check it yourself at home. If it's high, have it treated immediately. Ask your doctor if it is feasible and safe to treat your high blood pressure with dietary and lifestyle changes alone. Try to avoid drugs, unless they are necessary. (See Chapter 9 for more on elevated blood pressure.)
6. Exercise regularly. This strengthens the heart muscle and reduces stress. Exercisers tend to live longer and to have less CHD than nonexercisers. Remember that exercise alone is not enough. If you exercise but eat a high-fat diet, you're still at risk of a heart attack.

What kind of exercise is best for preventing heart disease? Any exercise that keeps your heart beating at 70 to 85 percent of its maximal rate for 20 to 30 minutes, three times a week. Brisk walking is an excellent exercise. Jogging, bicycling, aerobics and swimming are also fine exercises. (Be sure to check with your doctor before beginning or changing your exercise program.)

Use your heart as a guide when exercising. If it's continually beating at 70 to 85 percent of your maximal heart rate during exercise, you're exercising well. (The following chart shows the 70 to 85 percent range by age.)

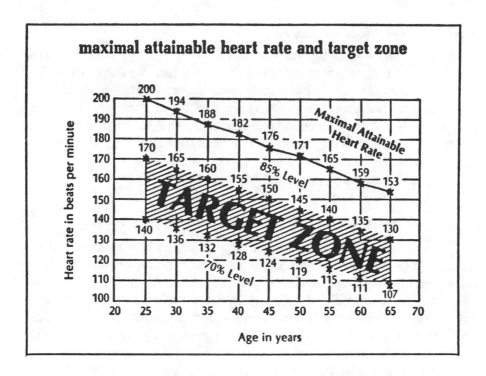

maximal attainable heart rate and target zone

7. Learn how to recognize and avoid stress. Some stress is necessary and beneficial, such as the stress of falling in love or the stress that keeps you going so you can finish a job on time. Most of the stress we face, however, is absolutely unnecessary and very unhealthy.

One of my friends, Smitty, discovered the hard way how stress can harm the heart. A 53-year-old executive, Smitty was in his usual harried mood one morning. There was a big meeting at work, but he had overslept and traffic was horrendous. He snapped out some instructions as he rushed past his secretary and shouted at the copy clerk because his reorganization report wasn't colored in the exact shade of blue he had ordered.

Sitting in the executive board room, Smitty felt his heart slamming against his chest wall as the CEO and president raked him and his plan over the coals. Humiliated and convinced that he would be fired, he could felt tightening in his chest and neck as he shuffled back to his office. He sat at his desk, unable to work, trying to convince himself that his chest pain was caused by stomach acid. He reviewed the meeting over and over again in his head, wondering what he could have done or said. He kept his wife up late that night, going over what had happened. Smitty never did find out if the company intended to fire him, because he died of a heart attack early the next morning.

Stress raises blood pressure

Make a fist with your left hand, thumb on top. Put your fist up to your breastbone, slightly to the left of center. Squeeze your fist, strongly, rhythmically. That's how your heart beats some 100,000 times a day, pushing four or so quarts of blood through your body every minute. When you're stressed or exercising, even more blood is pumped. It all seems very mechanical, yet it is possible for thoughts to harm the heart by pushing up the blood pressure, as well as the cholesterol, and by causing the heart to beat abnormally.

Back in medical school I learned a simple formula:

Blood pressure = cardiac output x arterial resistance

This means that blood pressure depends upon how much blood the heart pumps per unit of time (cardiac output) and how difficult it is for the blood to move through the "pipes" (arterial resistance).

Blood pressure goes up if your heart pumps faster or harder, if your arteries narrow or if there's more fluid to pump. Blood pressure drops if your heart beats slower or more gently, if your arteries widen or if there's less fluid to pump (if you lose blood, for example).

Stress can make the heart beat harder and faster. When we're frightened, worried, angry or otherwise stressed, the brain stimulates the sympathetic nervous system. This then prompts the adrenal medulla (the inside part of the adrenal glands) to pump out adrenaline-like substances. These, in turn, increase the heart rate and the strength of the heartbeats. Blood pressure goes up.

That's not all. When the hypothalamus, the "pilot" of the brain, "reads" all of your negative thoughts and other signs of stress, it tells the pituitary to release ACTH. This ACTH goes down to the adrenal glands (on top of the kidneys). There the ACTH directs the outer part of the adrenal glands to put out hormones, including aldosterone and 40-some varieties of cortisone. Among other things, these hormones cause your body to retain sodium and water. Extra water and sodium means that there's more fluid in the bloodstream that has to be pumped throughout the body. This elevates the blood pressure.

And there's more. With chronic stress, the blood vessels constrict or "tighten up." When these "pipes" get smaller, it's harder for the blood to flow through, which means blood pressure goes up. Plus, with chronic stress, the chemistry of the blood changes, making it more likely to clot. This means there's a greater chance that a clot will form and trigger a heart attack by getting stuck in a partially narrowed artery in the heart.

It's a simple formula: Negative thoughts equal stress, and stress equals elevated blood pressure. And remember, most of the time stress is not what happens to us, it's our perception of what's happening. "They" are not responsible for our being stressed. Most of the time "we" are, thanks to our angry, unhappy thoughts.

Stress increases cholesterol

Put your fist back up to your chest, let it stand in for your heart again. Look down at that fist, at the back of it. See the veins just under the skin? Imagine that these are some of your coronary arteries, those arteries that supply fresh, oxygen-rich blood to the heart muscle itself. I remember, from the days when I used to do autopsies, that some of these vital arteries are only as wide as the tip of a pencil.

Suppose that you've been eating the high-fat, cholesterol-rich Standard American Diet (SAD) and that some of your coronary arteries have become narrowed, but not fatally. Let's say that you have a 50-percent blockage in one artery and a 60- or 75-percent narrowing in another. You can do reasonably well with these kinds of blockages, unless...

You begin to think "negative thoughts." You're angry, frustrated, depressed, humiliated. These negative thoughts can cause cholesterol levels in the body to rise. Many studies have shown this relationship between stress and elevated cholesterol. If you stress people by throwing them into ice cold water, for example, their cholesterol will rise. If you threaten them, if you tell them they're going be fired or they are going to have to take difficult tests, their cholesterol levels will also go up.

Years ago, studies of doctors, lawyers and accountants showed that all three of these groups had elevated cholesterols because of bad diets. However, even though they did not change their diets, the accountants' cholesterol levels went up further during tax season (as compared to the doctors and attorneys). The accountants were eating the same food, but they were under increased stress, which caused this rise in cholesterol. So even if you're on a healthy diet, you may find that stress is keeping your cholesterol high. And that puts you at increased risk of heart disease and stroke.

Again, notice how important our perception is. It was the accountants' feeling of being rushed and under the gun that lead to the rise in cholesterol. It was their thoughts that caused the problem. Many studies have shown that stressful conditions can cause cholesterol to soar by as much as 30 percent.

Stress and elevated cholesterol are intimately related. Anger, fear, "hurry-itis," feeling that you are a failure and other negative thoughts increase blood pressure and cholesterol. These thoughts are killers.

Stress and sudden death

Can stress kill, suddenly, right on the spot? I believe it can and does happen. Suddenly flooding the body with high-voltage chemicals such as adrenaline, noradrenalin and ACTH can cause the coronary arteries to constrict, impeding the flow of blood to the heart muscle. It can also overwork the heart muscles, raise blood pressure by constricting the peripheral arteries and make the heart beat abnormally.

A 60-year-old man brought his wife to the emergency room. She was pronounced dead on arrival, and he immediately collapsed. The doctors slapped an EKG (electrocardiogram) onto his chest and found that he was suffering from ventricular fibrillation (the heart could not pump blood through the body). This grieving man, who had no symptoms of a heart problem before, suddenly had a heart attack and died. This is not an unusual case. A study in a highly respected medical journal described how the stress of public speaking can cause the heart to beat in irregular and potentially dangerous ways.

Anger, fear, frustration, rage, "unforgiveness" and other negative, stressful thoughts are like germs—they're germs of the mind that can raise blood pressure, elevate cholesterol and disrupt the heart's normal rhythm. Negative thinking is a disease. The cure is to give yourself a daily "prescription" of positive thoughts. As a physician with more than 40 years of experience in the "front lines" of crisis medicine, I believe that positive thoughts are a very powerful medicine, a medicine that can help many of us live young and healthy to a very old age.

There is a homeopathic remedy called L.72 Anti-Anxiety that seems to be almost as powerful as valium. Available from Enzymatic Therapies, it is a complex mixture of many remedies, including Cicuta virosa 4x, Ignatia 4x, Staphsagria 4x and Asfoetida 3x. I have found this to be an effective anxiolytic for people whose elevated blood pressure was due to nervousness or anxiety. I also use an herb called Kava kava *(piper methysticum)* to relieve anxiety.

A brief review

1. Quit smoking.
2. Switch to a diet based on fresh vegetables, fruits and whole grains, with small amounts of nonfat dairy and animal products.
3. Protect your heart with antioxidants.
4. Keep your cholesterol under control.
5. Have your blood pressure checked regularly, and have it treated if it is high.
6. Exercise regularly.
7. Learn how to recognize and avoid as much stress as possible.

These are seven steps that we can all adopt to reduce the risk of CHD and many other diseases as well.

[1]   Gaziano, J.M., cardiology fellow, Harvard U. Presented at the Am Heart Association Scientific Session, Dallas, Texas. Reported in *Medical World News*, Jan. 1991.

[2]   Mason, M. The vitamin B breakthrough. *Hippocrates*, Sept 1995, p.57.

[3]   Kopjas, T.L. Effect of folic acid on collateral circulation in diffuse chronic arteriosclerosis. *J Am Geriatr Soc*, 14(11):1187-1966.

[4]   Berge, K., Canner, P. Coronary Drug Project: Experience with niacin. *Eur J Clin Pharmacol*, 40:49-51, 1991.

[5]   Keenan, J., et al. Niacin revisited: A randomized, controlled trial of wax-matrix sustained-release niacin in hypercholesterolemia. *Arch Intern Med*, 151:1424-32, 1991.

[6]   Luria, M.H. Effect of low-dose niacin on high-density lipoprotein cholesterol and total cholesterol/high density lipoprotein cholesterol ratio. *Arch Intern Med*, 148:2493-95, 1988.

[7]   Rinehard, J.F., Greenberg, L.D. Vitamin B6 deficiency in the Rhesus monkey. *Am J Clin Nutr*, 4:318-25, 1956. Rinehard, J.F., Greenberg, L.D. Arteriosclerotic lesions in pyridoxine deficient monkeys. *Am J Pathol*, 25:481-96, 1949.

[8]   Ginter, E., et al. Vitamin C in the control of hypercholesterolemia in man. *Int J Vitam Nutr Res Suppl*, 23:137-52, 1982.

[9]   Riemersma, R.A., et al. Risk of angina pectoris and plasma concentrations of vitamins A, C and E and carotene. *Lancet*, 337:1-5, 1991.

[10]   Steiner, M. Influence of vitamin E on platelet function in humans. *J Am Coll Nutr*, 10(5):466-73, 1991. Creter, D., et al. Effect of vitamin E on platelet aggregation in diabetic retinopathy. *Acta Hematol*, 62:74, 1979.

[11]   Boscobionik, D., Szewczyk, A., Azzi, A. Alpha-tocopherol (vitamin E) regulates vascular smooth muscle cell proliferation and protein kinase C activity. *Arch Biochem*, 286:264-70, 1991. Hennig, B., et al. Protective effects of vitamin E in age-related endothelial cell injury. *Int J Vitam Nutr Res*, 59:273-79, 1989.

[12]   Cloarec, M.F., et al. Alpha-tocopherol: Effect on plasma lipoproteins in hypercholesterolemic patients. *Isr J Med Sci*, 23(8):886-92, 1987.

[13]   Gey, K.F., et al. Inverse correlation between plasma vitamin E and mortality from ischemic heart disease in cross-cultural epidemiology. *Am J Clin Nutr*, 53:326S-34S, 1991.

[14]   Stampfer, M.J., et al. Vitamin E consumption and the risk of coronary heart disease in women. *New Eng J Med*, 328(20):1444-49.

[15]   Davis, W.H., et al. Monotherapy with magnesium increases abnormally low high-density lipoprotein cholesterol: A clinical essay. *Curr Ther Res*, 36:341, 1984.

[16]   Cohen, L., Kitzes, R. Magnesium sulfate in the treatment of variant angina. *Magnesium*, 3:46-49, 1984.

[17]   *The Lancet*, Jun. 27, 1992.

[18]   Kok, F.J., et al. Decreased selenium levels in acute myocardial infarction. *JAMA,* 261(8):1161-4, 1989. Virtamo, J., et al. Serum selenium and the risk of coronary heart disease and stroke. *Am J Epidemiol*, 122:276, 1985.

[19]   Stead, N.W., et al. Selenium (Se) balance in the dependent elderly. *Am J Clin Nutr,* 39:677, 1984. Schiavon, R., et al. Selenium enhances prostacyclin production by cultured epithelial cells: Possible explanation for increased bleeding times in volunteers taking selenium as a dietary supplement. *Thrombosis Res*, 34:389, 1984.

[20]   Korpela, H., et al. Effect of selenium supplementation after acute myocardial infarction. *Res Commun Chem Pathol Pharmacol,* 65:249-52, 1989.

[21]   Robbins, R.C. Flavones in citrus exhibit antiadhesive action on platelets. *Int J Vitam Nutr Res*, 58:418-21, 1988. Puliero, G., et al. Ex civo study of the inhibitory effects of Vaccinium myrillus (Bilberry) anthrocyanosides on human platelet aggregation. *Fitoterapia*, 60(1):69-75, 1989.

[22]   Dromhout, D. n-3 fatty acids and coronary heart disease. *BNF Nutr Bull,* 15:93-102, 1990.

[23]   *Br Med J*, 293:426, 1986.

[24]   Dromhout, D., et al. The inverse relation between fish consumption and 20-year mortality from coronary heart disease. *N Engl J Med,* 312:1205-9, 1985.

[25]   Cerda, J.C., et al. The effect of grapefruit pectin on patients at risk for coronary heart disease without altering diet or lifestyle. *Clin Cardiol*, 11(9):589-94, 1988.

[26]   Janaki, Y., Sugiyama, S., Ozawa, T. Ratio of low-density lipoprotein cholesterol to ubiquinone as a coronary risk factor. Letter. *N Engl J Med*, 324(11):814-15, 1991.

[27]   Kamikawa, T., et al. Effects of coenzyme Q_{10} on exercise tolerance in chronic stable angina pectoris. *Am J Cardiol*, 56:247, 1985.

[28]   Kato, T., et al. Reduction of blood viscosity by treatment with coenzyme Q_{10} in patients with ischemic heart disease. *Int J Clin Pharmacol Ther Toxicol*, 28(3):123-6, 1990.

[29]   Elwood, J.C., et al. Effect of high-chromium brewer's yeast on human serum lipids. *J Am Coll Nutr,* 1:263, 1982.

[30]   *The Natural Healing and Nutrition Annual, 1992.* Bricklin, M., ed. Emmaus, PA: Rodale Press, 1992, p.143.

[31]   Ernst, E., et al. Garlic and blood lipids. *Br Med J*, 291:139, 1985.

[32]   Ibid.

[33]   Anderson, J.W., Gustafson, N.J. High-carbohydrate, high-fiber diet: Is it practical and effective in treating hyperlipidemia? *Postgrad Med*, 82(4):40-55, 1987.

Chapter 9

Hypertension

Hypertension is elevated blood pressure, the "silent killer" responsible for a great deal of heart disease and other serious health problems. "Hyper" means "high" and "tension" refers to blood pressure.

A long-time patient named Sarah once came to my office for her regular checkup. Her husband, John, came along with her. We got to talking, and soon John was describing how his supervisors were giving him trouble at work, how he was putting in extra hours and how the company was trying to cut their pay. He became very agitated, his face grew flushed and his voice harsh as he pounded one hand into the other for emphasis.

This got me worried, because I knew that simply talking about unhappy events can elevate the blood pressure. I had John lie down while I measured the blood pressure in both of his arms. As I feared, it was high: 180/120. I believed John's high blood pressure was related to the stress of telling us how difficult work was, so I kept him lying down for 45 minutes, then rechecked his blood pressure. It was now only moderately elevated at 140/95 in both arms.

"But I didn't feel anything, Dr. Fox," he protested. "I felt fine."

Patients often tell me that they feel fine, even if their blood pressure is sky high. It's important to remember that hypertension is the "silent killer." In most cases, you don't know anything is wrong until quite a bit of damage has already occurred.

What is blood pressure?

Blood pressure is a measure of the relationship between cardiac output and arterial resistance: how much blood the heart pumps per second or minute (output) and how easily it flows (resistance).

The heart of the average person beats 60 to 100 times a minute, each time pumping out three to five ounces of blood. This is the cardiac (heart) output. As for resistance, ideally, our arteries and arterioles (smaller arteries) should be wide-open, flexible highways carrying blood throughout the body. As the blood surges through, the arteries should be able to stretch and relax, to give and take with the flow. Unfortunately, the high-fat standard American diet, emotional state, lack of exercise and other factors can combine to make the arteries narrow and inflexible. It is harder for the blood to flow through the body as the resistance increases.

If the heart beats faster and/or harder, or the arteries become narrower and less flexible, blood pressure goes up. (Other factors may be involved, including instructions from the nervous system to the muscles surrounding arterioles to squeeze down, making the arterioles smaller and increasing the resistance.)

What do the two numbers mean?

Blood pressure is given as two numbers (such as 120/80). The first number represents the systolic pressure, the pressure when the heart is contracting. The second number is the diastolic pressure, the pressure when the heart is resting.

There is no "perfect" blood pressure number. Blood pressure of 120/80 is considered average and healthy, but there is room for variation. Some people have much lower pressures, but it's perfectly normal and healthy for them.

Hypertension is generally defined as blood pressure of 160/95 or more. I believe blood pressure should be lower; certainly under 140/90. The lower it is, the smaller your chances of having a cardiovascular catastrophe.

Hypertension statistics

It is estimated that one in every four Americans has hypertension, whether they know it or not. That comes to about 60 million Americans at risk for big trouble. Although adults are most commonly afflicted, high blood pressure can develop at any age.

How does hypertension harm us?

With hypertension, the heart must work harder to pump the blood throughout the body. Eventually the heart muscle enlarges as the heart grows in a desperate attempt to keep the blood flowing. Unless the pressure is brought down, the heart may eventually fail.

Ironically, hypertension also causes the blood vessels to become thicker, increasing the resistance and pushing the blood pressure even higher. This process, which is called reactive arteriosclerosis, jeopardizes the entire cardiovascular system, increasing the risk of heart disease, stroke, kidney failure, blindness and gangrene.

Signs and symptoms

A "silent killer," hypertension gives no warnings in its early stages. In advanced cases there may be:

- Headaches.
- Nosebleeds.
- Dizziness.
- Confusion.

Possible causes

There is no single cause of hypertension. Likely triggers include:

- Smoking.
- Stress.
- Chronic alcoholism.
- High-sodium diet.
- Lack of potassium or calcium in the diet.
- Lack of exercise.
- A family history of hypertension, heart disease, stroke or kidney failure.
- Certain medications, including birth control pills.

Possible complications and long-term effects

If untreated, hypertension may cause heart problems (enlargement of the heart, heart attack, heart failure), stroke, kidney failure, pulmonary edema, visual disturbances (hypertensive retinopathy) and other problems.

Standard medical treatment

Standard Western medical treatment for hypertension consists of:

- Four main types of medications to lower blood pressure: 1) beta blockers, such as Tenoramin, 2) calcium channel blockers, such as Cardizem, 3) Angiotensin-I-converting enzyme inhibitors, such as Zestrin and 4) the very newest, Antiotension-II receptor blockers such as Cozaar.
- Diuretics, such as Dyazide and hydrochlorothiazide to flush excess fluid out of the body. 8
- Recommendation to stop taking certain other prescription and over-the-counter drugs that can elevate blood pressure.
- Recommendation to consume less sodium.
- Recommendation to lose weight.
- Recommendation to reduce stress.

- Regular monitoring of blood pressure at the doctor's office.
- Exercise.

In brief, Western medicine's primary thrust is to lower the pressure with medication. Less attention is paid to altering the patient's lifestyle.

Now let's look at some of the many alternative treatments for hypertension. These are not all the possible therapies, because there are too many to investigate in a single chapter. Reading through these alternatives, however, will give you an idea of the many possibilities.

The information on alternative therapies is meant for educational purposes only. I am not endorsing any therapy or suggesting that you see any alternative practitioner. If you have or suspect that you have high blood pressure, see your physician.

Acupuncture

Three points are commonly used for hypertension: Kidney 3 (between the inside ankle and the Achilles tendon), Bladder 23 (in the lower back) and Liver 2 (in the web between the large and first toe).

If the patient is dizzy or has a headache, Gall Bladder 20 (at the base of the skull) may be used. If there are stomach problems as well, Conception Vessel 12 (midway between the navel and the breast bone) may be used. And if the patient is troubled by sputum or mucus, Stomach 30 (on the lower leg) will be stimulated.

To help with general weakness, Stomach 36 (below the knee) may be needled and an herb called moxa applied to the skin and burned. Spleen 6 (on the inside of the lower leg about three finger breadth up from the inside ankle) may be used as well.

Hypertensive patients often receive one treatment per day, lasting 15 to 30 minutes each time. As they improve, the number of weekly treatments drops. The points should be well stimulated; the person should feel the chi, the electrical sensation, with each treatment.

Aromatherapy

Aromatherapy treatments for hypertension vary widely because there are no standard therapy guidelines in the field. Essential oils that may be used to reduce blood pressure include:

- Clary (*Salvia sclarea*).
- Hyssop (*Hyssopus officinalis*).
- Lavender (*Lavandula officinalis*).
- Marjoram (*Origanum marjorana*).
- Melissa (*Melissa officinalis*).
- Ylang-ylang (*Cananga odorata*).

The patient may be instructed to inhale the vapors from these oils as they rise from a bowl of water, to mix them in a base oil and use in massage, to wear as a perfume or to mix with the bath water. Treatment length will vary from practitioner to practitioner and according to the patient's condition.

Ayurvedic healing

Because, according to Ayurvedic theory, the heart is believed to be the seat of human consciousness, elevated blood pressure indicates that the patient may be undergoing a crisis of consciousness, feeling and identity.

Hypertension may manifest itself in any of the three humors (primary life forces) in the body.

- When manifested in the Vata (air) humor, the blood pressure may suddenly jump up or down. Likc thc blood pressure, the pulse will be erratic. Emotional states involving worry, nervousness, insomnia or work fatigue may be involved.

   The treatment for Vata hypertension is similar to that for Vata-type heart disease. (See Chapter 8.) Garlic and nutmeg may be especially helpful.

- When manifested in the Kapha (water) humor, hypertension makes one tired, obese and swollen with fluids. The blood pressure tends to remain consistently high.

   The treatment is similar to the treatment for Kapha-type heart disease. (See Chapter 8.) Cayenne, garlic, motherwort and myrrh may be especially helpful herbs.

- When manifested in the Pitta humor, the fire of Pitta is reflected in a red face and eyes, as well as headaches, anger, nosebleeds and photosensitivity (sensitivity to light).

   The same treatment for Pitta-type heart disease is used for Pitta-type hypertension. (See Chapter 8.) Aloe gel and barberry may be helpful. Aloe and rhubarb may be used as purges.

Color therapy

There are no standard protocols for dealing with hypertension, and the time it takes to see results is not known with any certainty.

Color therapists often choose *green,* a soothing, calming color which stabilizes the emotions, relieves tension, opens the capillaries and lowers blood pressure. It is the color of growth, new life and energy. In addition to hypertension, green is used to treat nervous disorders, shell shock, overstimulation, irritation and exhaustion. Since green and blue are often interchangeable, *light blue* may be used.

Green foods include green vegetables, peas, avocados and kiwi-fruit. Green metals and chemicals include aluminum, carbon, chlorophyll, chlorine, cobalt, nickel, nitrogen, platinum and sodium.

Herbal medicine

Herbalists use a wide variety of herbs to treat many diseases and symptoms. There is no standard herbal protocol for treating hypertension. Much depends upon the herbalist's background. Herbs typically used include:

- Guelder rose (*Viburnum opulus*).
- Hawthorn (*Crataegus spp.*).
- Ju hua (*Chrysanthemum morifolium*).
- Kava root (*Piper methysticum*).
- Linden (*Tilia europaea*).
- Wood betony (*Stachys officinalis*).
- Yarrow (*Achillea millefolium*).

These herbs help to reduce blood pressure by dilating (opening) the arteries. They also strengthen the heart muscles, "calm" the heart and provide an overall sense of relaxation.

Homeopathy

Homeopathy attempts to cure hypertension by helping the body to heal itself. Most of the major homeopathic remedies may be used, depending upon the symptoms. Some of these remedies include:

- *Aurum metallicum*, which is indicated when the patient is depressed and lacks self-esteem. Symptoms include depression and nighttime chest pain. The problem tends to be worse at night and with cold, damp weather. It's better during the summer and with fresh air.
- *Baryta carbonica*, which is indicated when the patient is very young or very old, and shy. The blood pressure may be very high, the pulse feels hard and full and there are palpitations.
- *Belladonna,* which is indicated when the disease seems to strike suddenly.
- *Coffea cruda*, which is indicated when the patient is creative but anguished, alternatively laughing and weeping. The headaches make sleeping difficult, and there are strong palpitations. Emotional or intellectual stimulation, noise, cold, alcohol and coffee make the pain worse. The pain is better when the patient is lying down or is warm.

- *Iodum*, which is indicated when the patient is sensitive, irritable and dark-haired. Symptoms include depression and anxiety, nasal congestion and palpitations brought on by little or no exertion.
- *Lachesis*, which is indicated when the patient is talkative and moody, thin and suspicious. The symptoms include a very rapid heart beat, chest pain, headaches, nosebleeds and a weak pulse. Fresh air and warm compresses help with the problem. Hot drinks and pressure make it worse.

A homeopathic remedy called L.72 Anti-Anxiety is also useful for those whose hypertension is related to stress. Although it is a basic principle of classical homeopathy to use only one remedy at a time, there is a trend among modern homeopaths toward using multiple remedies at once. Using the absolute minimum number of doses necessary is another principle of classical homeopathy. A second dose should not be given until the first has ceased to act, and no more remedies should be given when the body begins to heal. With the right remedy, two or three days should be enough to begin many long-term curative processes. If not, another remedy should be selected.

Hypnosis

Hypnosis has been used as an adjunct treatment for hypertension. Although it is not a cure for elevated blood pressure, it can help people learn to control the stress that has been associated with hypertension. Hypnosis and post-hypnotic suggestions can help one remain calm in situations that would ordinarily trigger stress reactions.

The hypnotist's primary goal is to help the patient learn to remain calm when faced with stressful situations that might elevate the blood pressure. Patients may be taught relaxation techniques and then hypnotized. While hypnotized, they can be given post-hypnotic suggestions telling them that when they feel themselves becoming angry or stressed, they will automatically enter into the relaxed but alert states they achieved while practicing the relaxation techniques. This helps to keep the body from setting off the "fight or flight response" that can worsen hypertension. A typical suggestion might be:

"Imagine that you are caught in traffic. Cars are everywhere and it's impossible to move ahead. The side streets are jammed, there's no where else you can go. You're late for work. How do you feel? [The patient will respond by describing negative feelings.] Imagine that you're still in the car. You're hot with anger. [Pause] Take a deep breath. [Pause] Let it out. [Pause] Feel your body cooling off as you blow out your anger. See yourself sitting calmly in your car, listening to your favorite music, cool and calm. [Pause] You know that there's nothing you can do but wait. You know that the best thing to do is enjoy your music. You feel cool and calm as you ride out the traffic jam. [Pause] When you get caught in traffic, take a deep breath, hold it for a moment, then let it out. Do that a few times, feeling yourself cooling off as you do. Remember that all you can do is wait, so you might as well enjoy the wait and keep your pressure low."

Some hypnotists will attempt to influence their patient's physiology. They may suggest, for example, that resistance to the blood flow in the hypnotized patient's arteries is being reduced. They may use images to suggest falling blood pressure, making hypnotic suggestions such as:

"Imagine that you are in the most beautiful, peaceful place you can think of. It might be the beach, a mountain stream or your own bedroom. Imagine that you can hear a steady hum. This hum represents your blood pressure. The higher your blood pressure, the louder the hum. Listen to the humming of high blood pressure. [Pause] Now take a deep breath. Hold it. Let it out. As you do so, feel your entire body relaxing and the hum fading away.

Feel a wonderful sense of peace and relaxation washing over your entire body as the hum fades into the background and your blood pressure drops to safe levels. Again, take a deep breath. [Pause]. Hold it. Let it out, feeling your body relax and the hum fade away as your blood pressure drops to safe levels. Several times during the day, and whenever you feel yourself getting stressed, take a deep breath. As you let it out, feel your body relaxing and your blood pressure dropping down to normal."

There is no agreed-upon length of time before hypnosis brings results, if any are to be found. Several factors affect the length of treatment: how hypnotizable the client is, the rapport developed between the hypnotist and the client and the severity of the problem. Many people have been helped in just one session. For some, several sessions are required.

Nutritional therapy

The grocery store and the supplement shelves are filled with wonderful tools that can help to reduce elevated blood pressure. For many of my patients, changing the diet is a major step toward reducing the blood pressure and weaning them away from their potentially dangerous medications.

Vitamins, minerals and other substances

A wide variety of vitamins and minerals have proven their mettle in scientific studies conducted at major research centers across the country. The following are some of the findings:

Vitamin C. The amount of vitamin C in the blood appears to be related to the risk of developing hypertension. In a study of 170 healthy men and women ranging in age from 19 to 70, the higher the blood pressure, the lower the levels of vitamin C in the blood.[1]

Another study involved 20 adults, eight of whom had normal blood pressure. The remaining 12 had borderline hypertension. All 20 were given 1 gram of vitamin C or a placebo daily in random order for six weeks each. (In other words, some were given the vitamin C for six weeks and then the placebo, while the others received the placebo first, then the vitamin.)

Blood pressure dropped in both the hypertensive and the normal groups when they were on vitamin C. The systolic pressure (the first number) fell by an average of 6.3 "points," while the diastolic pressure (the second number) dropped by an average of 6.9 "points."[2] Good sources of vitamin C include citrus fruits, kale and parsley.

Calcium. A great deal of research has linked low calcium levels to elevated blood pressure.[3] When 7,000 men of Japanese descent were examined, researchers found a strong link between blood pressure and calcium (as well as potassium).[4]

In the large-scale First National Health and Nutritional Examination Survey (NHANES 1), people with elevated blood pressure were found to be taking in 18 percent less calcium than those with normal pressure. The study's results suggested that getting enough calcium might be more important for avoiding hypertension than watching sodium intake.[5]

Those who have hypertension may consider eating more calcium-containing foods or even taking calcium supplements because several studies have found that calcium supplementation can lower blood pressure modestly in those with normal and elevated pressures.[6] Good sources of calcium include milk and milk products such as cheese and yogurt.

Magnesium. This important mineral helps to relax the involuntary muscles surrounding the blood vessels, which reduces the resistance to the flow of blood and lowers pressure. (Remember, pressure equals cardiac output times resistance. Lowering the resistance automatically reduces the pressure.) Magnesium's action is similar to that of the much more expensive drugs called calcium channel blockers.

People with lower magnesium levels tend to be taking more blood pressure medicines than people with normal magnesium levels.[7] And when researchers investigated over 60 different factors in the diets of

615 men of Japanese ancestry, they found that magnesium intake was the factor most strongly linked to normal blood pressure.[8] Magnesium can be found in apples, broccoli and tomatoes.

Potassium. Frequently low in the elderly, potassium is another important mineral that helps to keep blood pressure at healthy levels. When 233 children, ranging in age from 5 to 17, were followed for an average of seven years, researchers found that those eating the larger amounts of potassium had lower systolic pressures (the first number).[9]

In a study testing whether or not potassium could lower elevated blood pressure, 37 patients with mild hypertension were given either potassium or a placebo every day. About 15 weeks later, blood pressures in the potassium group had dropped significantly compared to the placebo group.[10]

Vegetarians, who tend to get more potassium in their diets than nonvegetarians, also tend to have much less hypertension. Good sources of potassium include orange juice, bananas and apricots.

Coenzyme Q10. Also known as ubiquinone, coenzyme Q10 is often found to be deficient in hypertension patients.[11] When 18 people with hypertension were tested with coenzyme Q10 and a placebo, the coenzyme Q10 pushed systolic pressure down by 10.6 "points" and diastolic pressure down by 7.7 "points."[12] Coenzyme Q10 is manufactured by the body but can also be found in certain foods, such as sardines and mackerel.

L-tryptophan. This essential amino acid may reduce blood pressure in people with essential hypertension.

Omega-3 fatty acids. When Danish scientists studied the Eskimos in Greenland who seemed to have some extra protection against heart attacks, they found that the omega-3 fatty acids in the fish they ate could also guard against hypertension. The omega-3s don't seem to reduce pressure in people with normal blood pressures. But when the pressure is at least mildly elevated, omega-3 supplementation can significantly drive down both the systolic (first number) and diastolic (second number) pressures. Omega-3 fatty acids are found primarily in cold water fish, such as salmon and mackerel.

Taurine. Taurine is an amino acid that apparently plays a role in regulating blood pressure. When 19 people with borderline high blood pressure were given either taurine or a placebo for seven days, both the systolic and diastolic pressures fell significantly in the taurine group. The placebo group did not enjoy the same results.[13] Some significant sources of taurine include beef, fish, veal, lamb and milk.

Foods that aid in the treatment of hypertension

A great many foods have been found to be of value in treating hypertension. These include bananas, garlic, milk, potatoes, pumpkins, tropical fruits and yogurt.

Bananas. Bananas are high in the mineral potassium, which has been shown to reduce blood pressure.

Garlic. Large amounts of this aromatic vegetable have been shown to reduce blood pressure. In one study, blood pressure dropped by an average of 20 "points" in three months.[14] Garlic may lower blood pressure by helping the smooth muscles surrounding the blood vessels to relax. This reduces the resistance to blood flow and allows the pressure to fall.

Milk. Milk contains good amounts of calcium, an essential mineral with a proven ability to help keep blood pressure in the desirable range.

Other calcium, magnesium or potassium-rich foods that can help to keep blood pressure under control include broccoli, dandelion greens, cheese, okra, sardines with bones, tofu, wheat bran, wheat germ, dried beans, pumpkin, watermelon, whole-wheat flour, nuts, raisins, prunes, figs and avocados.

Putting it all together: the healthy diet

I've had a great deal of success in treating my hypertensive patients with diet, exercise and lifestyle changes. As a result, in many cases my patients are able to slowly cut back on their medications. Some patients are even able to completely stop their medications.

The general approach is to use nutritional means to help patients to lose weight, increase the amount of fiber and fresh, raw vegetables in their diets and to cut back on dietary fat, salt, sugar, alcohol and caffeine. Rather than tell my patients to eat so many ounces of broccoli or rice, I point out that the more fresh vegetables, fruits and grains one eats, the better. Following this simple dietary guideline is a great start: Have four to five servings of vegetables, two to three servings of fruit and two servings of grains daily, with no added salt.

When selecting a nutritional healer, remember that there is no widely recognized school of nutritional therapy and no standards or agreed-upon training for nutritional healers.

Oriental medicine

Oriental medicine has a multifaceted approach to treating hypertension. The Oriental physician's first step is to determine the reason for the elevation, which may be due to problems such as a disturbance in the balance and flow of energy in the gall bladder or heart meridians. The doctor then strives to relieve the symptoms and strengthen the body with a combination of herbs and spices, diet, acupuncture and other therapies, as necessary.

Herbs and spices

Exactly which herbs and spices and the amount of each will depend upon the patient and his or her condition. Herbal formulas that may be used include *Chiang Ya Wan* and *Yun Nan Te Chan Tian Qi Pan.*

Diet

Diet plays an important role in Oriental medicine. Foods are selected depending on their flavors, organic actions and other qualities, including energies. There are five food energies: hot, warm, neutral, cool and cold. (The energy has to do with the quality of the food, not its temperature.) The Oriental medical physician may recommend foods that lower blood pressure and "soften" the arteries, such as:

- *Banana,* a cold and sweet fruit that "greases" the intestines and detoxifies the body while lowering the blood pressure.
- *Celery,* a sweet and bitter vegetable that helps to lower blood pressure.
- *Corn silk,* a sweet food that tones the liver and gall bladder and reduces the nasal inflammation seen with some allergies.
- *Kelp,* a cold and salty food that helps to "soften" the arteries.
- *Mung bean sprouts,* which help to "soften" the arteries.
- *Persimmon,* a sweet and cold food that strengthens the heart, lungs and large intestine while lowering the blood pressure.
- *Tomato,* a somewhat cold fruit that lowers the blood pressure.

Psychoneuroimmunology

Mounting scientific evidence backs the argument that stress can raise blood pressure. Mind/body healers attempt to deal with the stressful thoughts that they feel contribute to hypertension using positive affirmations to counteract them. Affirmations are typically brief, positive statements that focus on how well one feels and on how the disease is being conquered. The patient might be given several affirmations.

An affirmation to reduce blood pressure might be worded as follows:

"With my arteries open wide, my heart beating smoothly and calmly, my blood flows gently through my body. Like a gentle stream on a cool spring day, it flows easily."

An affirmation for reduced stress might be worded as follows:

"Always calm and cool, I find it easy to handle all my tasks and to interact with everyone. Challenges are chances to be creative; deadlines are opportunities to excel."

Reflexology

The direct reflex area used for hypertension is the heart area, which is near the center of the ball of the left foot. Corresponding points on the hands may also be utilized. Associated areas to be manipulated include the solar plexus, adrenal glands, kidneys and big toe areas. The solar plexus reflex areas are below the balls of the feet, in the midline. The adrenal reflex areas are at approximately the middle of the foot, slightly to the inside. The kidney reflex areas are about midway down the feet, slightly to the inside of the midline. Corresponding points on the hands may also be utilized.

Water therapy

Water therapy has been used as an adjunct to other therapies for hypertension, but is not offered as a cure.

- Drinking distilled water immediately upon awakening in the morning to stimulate the kidneys, reduce the amount of water in the body and reduce blood pressure.
- Various massages to stimulate and help the body dispose of "toxins" that may be pushing the blood pressure up. Rubbing the body with a dry, rough cloth and cold water friction massages are among the massage techniques used.

There are no widely accepted protocols for water therapy, so practices may vary from practitioner to practitioner.

Advice to hypertension patients

Although many of my patients have had success with the following program, I only use the general guidelines discussed below after reviewing a patient's personal and medical history, performing a thorough examination and evaluating the laboratory studies to make sure that the program will be beneficial. Please see your own physician before embarking on any treatment program for hypertension.

More advanced cases of high blood pressure may require medication, but I've found that changing a person's diet and lifestyle is often all it takes to bring the pressure back to normal. Here's the eight-step program I often use with my hypertension patients:

1. If the blood pressure is dangerously elevated, get it down as quickly and safely as possible, using medications when necessary. Some medicines work well with relatively mild side effects. I tell my

patients that we must quickly lower the blood pressure to prevent a "brain attack" (stroke). As soon as the lifestyle and other changes begin taking effect, however, we can often reduce and eventually eliminate the medications altogether.

2. Change your lifestyle and eliminate as much stress as possible. In the case of emotional stress, the problem is not what happens to us, but, rather, how we respond to it. "Thought disease" can cause hypertension, but we can help to protect ourselves by learning to look upon challenges as NICE (new, interesting, challenging experiences), rather than to view them with FUD (fear, uncertainty and doubt).

"Thought disease," the major scourge of our time, is caused by germs of the mind such as anger, fear, frustration, loneliness, alienation, unforgiveness and others. But we unknowingly bring "Thought disease" on ourselves. Other people do not make us think harmful, negative thoughts. We, and only we, decide what we will think.

3. Learn meditation and relaxation techniques to help keep stress at bay.

4. Maintain normal body weight. Shedding excess fat is very important and can help bring high blood pressure back down to normal.

5. Adopt a high complex-carbohydrate diet based on fresh vegetables, whole grains and fruit, with smaller amounts of low fat protein and dairy products. Avoid the dangerous "CATS from San Francisco" (caffeine, alcohol, tobacco, sugar, salt and fat).

6. Take carefully calculated doses of magnesium, calcium, potassium and other supplements.

7. For unremitting anxiety, I recommend a homeopathic remedy put out by Enzymatic Therapies called L.72 Anti-Anxiety. It is a complex mixture of many remedies, including *Cicuta virosa 4x, Ignatia 4x, Staphsagria 4x* and *Asfoetida 3x*. I have found this to be an effective anxiolytic that I've used to help people whose elevated blood pressure was due to nervousness or anxiety. I also use an herb called Kava kava *(piper methysticum)* to relieve anxiety.

8. In many cases, it may be helpful to undergo a 24-hour Ambulatory Blood Pressure Monitoring (ABPM) to detect "hidden" hypertension. ABPM can also show what drives your pressure up—work, traffic, tense family situations, etc. Later, ABPM is a valuable tool for following the course of improvement during treatment.

Blood pressure goes up and down during the day, as we commute, work, eat lunch, meet with friends, relax, play softball, go shopping, laugh, converse and get angry. If your blood pressure is checked only once during a medical visit, it won't reveal the entire picture.

It's a good idea to have your blood pressure checked by a doctor. You should also check it regularly at home, as well. One reading, especially in a doctor's office where the patient may be nervous, is not enough to establish a diagnosis of high blood pressure. However, the blood pressure reading must be taken correctly if it is to be of any value. (A surprising number of health care professionals do not measure patients' blood pressures properly.)

The ABPM blood pressure monitor consists of a blood pressure cuff worn around the upper arm and a small box-like device that can be worn like a purse or attached to the belt. The patient wears the device for 24 hours. The patient also keeps a diary of everything done during the day. The readings are computer-analyzed and compared to the diary to find out exactly how the patients' blood pressure responds to everyday events and stresses.

Using the ABPM, I've found many "hidden" hypertensives, as well as situations where blood pressure is usually normal, but rises dangerously when the patient is in stressful situations (such as arguing with a spouse or being harassed at work).

How should blood pressure be taken?

Simply talking about certain subjects can raise the blood pressure, so you should be silent, seated, relaxed and calm. Eating may falsely elevate the reading, so some time should have passed since your last meal. Your arm should be relaxed and at the level of the heart—not higher up or hanging down. Your fist should be relaxed. (Clenching your fist can raise your pressure.) You should not be pushing against anything with either arm. You shouldn't be chewing gum, and should not have recently had coffee, smoked a cigarette or taken over-the-counter drugs containing caffeine or phenylpropanolamine (a medicine used to suppress appetite). And you should be silent.

The blood pressure cuff should fit snugly around the upper arm, just above the elbow. It should be at the level of your heart, and not hanging down low. The first time, the doctor should take your pulse at the wrist. With one hand on your pulse, the other pumping up the blood pressure cuff, he or she should keep pumping until the pressure has obliterated the pulse. Now above the systolic pressure, he or she can let pressure out of the cuff, listening for the first sound with the stethoscope.

When I find elevated blood pressure, I usually ask the patient to lie down and relax. Then I repeat the reading after he or she has rested for 20 minutes, often finding that the pressure has fallen to acceptable levels.

Your blood pressure should always be measured in both arms. With certain diseases, the pressure will be different, and finding significantly different pressure from right arm to left can be an important diagnostic clue. On the first visit, if your blood pressure is elevated in both arms, it should be measured in your legs as well. If it is low in the legs, a diagnosis of coarctation (a localized narrowing of the aorta) may be made.

Getting the right blood pressure reading is an important first step in combating hypertension. Although hypertension is a potentially serious problem, it can often be controlled.

[1]   Moran, J., et al. Dietary antioxidants and blood pressure—extended study. *Clin Res*, 39:A41, 1991.
[2]   Osilesi, O., et al. Blood pressure and plasma lipids during ascorbic acid supplementation in borderline hypertensive and normotensive adults. *Nutr Res*, 11:405-12, 1991.
[3]   McCarron, D.A., Morris, C.D. Metabolic considerations and cellular mechanisms related to calcium's antihypertensive effects. *Fed Proc*, 45:2734-38, 1986.
[4]   Criqui, M.H., et al. Dietary alcohol, calcium and potassium. Independent and combined effects on blood pressure. *Circulation*, 80(3):609-14, 1989.
[5]   Harlan, W.K., et al. Blood pressure and nutrition in adults. The National Health and Nutrition Examination Survey. *Am J Epidemiol*, 120:17-27, 1984. McCarron, D.A., et al. Blood pressure and nutrient intake in the United States. *Science*, 224(4656):1392-98, 1984.
[6]   Moore, T.J., The role of dietary electrolytes in hypertension. *J Am Coll Nutr*, 8 Suppl S: 68S-80S, 1989.
[7]   Wester, P.O., Dyckner, T. Magnesium and hypertension. *J Am Coll Nutr*, 6(4):321-28, 1987.
[8]   Joffres, M.R., et al. Relationship of magnesium intake and other dietary factors to blood pressure; the Honolulu heart study. *Am J Clin Nutr*, 45(2):469-75, 1987.
[9]   Gelijnse, J.M., et al. Sodium and potassium intake and blood pressure change in childhood. *Br Med J*, 300:899-902, 1990.
[10]   Sinai, A., et al. Controlled trial of long term oral potassium supplements in patients with mild hypertension. *Br Med J*, 294:1453-56, 1987.
[11]   Yamagami, T., et al. Bioenergetics in clinical medicine. Studies on coenzyme Q10 and essential hypertension. *Res Commun Chem Pathol Pharmacol*, 11:273, 1975.
[12]   Digiesi, V., et al. Effect of coenzyme Q10 on essential arterial hypertension. *Curr Ther Res*, 47:481-5, 1990.
[13]   Fujita, T., et al. Effects of increased adrenomedullary activity and taurine in young patients with borderline hypertension. *Circulation*, 75:525, 1987.
[14]   *Food—Your Miracle Medicine*. Jean Carper. New York, HarperPerennial, 1993, pp. 85-6.

Chapter 10

Menopause

"Even though I hated having my period every month for 35 years," one of my patients explained, "I was a little disappointed when it stopped. I just didn't feel like a woman any more."

The "change of life" is a perfectly normal but often frightening and confusing time for women. Sometime during her 40s or 50s, a woman's production of the hormone *estrogen* falls to the point where she no longer ovulates or menstruates. This does not occur suddenly during a well-defined period of time. Instead, it creeps up on a woman as she goes through a long process called the *climacteric*, a 10-to-15-year period during which the body undergoes significant changes. The climacteric usually starts during the mid-30s or early 40s when hormonal production begins to drop. Hormones continue to fall throughout the climacteric.

The early part of the climacteric is called the *perimenopause* when some women notice that their periods are becoming irregular (they may remain regular for other women). Perimenopause may last for several years before sliding into menopause, which officially begins when a woman has completed her last menstrual cycle. Of course, she doesn't know that it is her final cycle until some time has passed. Menopause mostly occurs sometime between the late 40s and mid-50s.

Menstrual periods may become heavier or lighter, longer or shorter, more or less frequent, or even absent for months before returning. Although menopause is usually defined as a single event (the last menstrual period), the loss of menstruation is just the most visible of the many changes that women undergo. These may include:

- Hot flashes.
- Nervousness.
- Dizziness.
- Depression.
- Mood swings.
- Thinning of the bones.
- Weight gain.
- A difference in breast size.

- An irregular or rapid heart beat.
- Difficulty holding the urine (stress incontinence).
- Vaginal dryness, itching or other discomfort.
- More or less interest in sex.
- Skin changes such as dryness and increased moles.

Some women have an "easy" menopause: irregular periods, then finally no periods at all. Others are annoyed by mild to moderate but tolerable symptoms, such as hot flashes. A smaller number of women suffer severely enough to seek medical help. If a year has passed since a woman's last period, she is usually considered to be *post menopausal*. Her symptoms may continue, however, for many years.

Osteoporosis

Perhaps the most serious common "side effect" of menopause is the thinning of the bones known as *osteoporosis*. With the drop in estrogen, the bones lose density and strength, leading to an increased risk of fractures. Although men and women both lose bone mass as they age, women are at greater risk of fractures because they tend to have thinner bones to begin with, may have been on nutrient-poor weight-loss diets at some point and may have lost calcium during pregnancy. The low estrogen levels and lack of physical activity that come with advancing age also contribute to the "thinning" of the bones.

Osteoporosis often sneaks up silently. For many, the first obvious symptom is a broken hip. X-rays can detect thinning bones but are not routinely performed. Some possible symptoms to watch for include backaches, a cracking sound in the back associated with sudden back pain, spinal deformity, loss of height, loosening of the teeth due to degeneration of the jaw bone and bones that break "too easily." Some women develop a "dowagers hump," which doctors call a *kyphosia*, at the juncture of the neck and upper back.

The risk of osteoporosis increases with age, smoking, heavy alcohol use, a family history of osteoporosis, long-term use of certain drugs (such as cortisone), surgical removal of the ovaries, radiation therapy for cancer of the ovaries, poor nutrition and other factors. Fine-boned women should pay special attention to preserving their bone mass, because they can't afford to lose *any* of it.

There is no way to cure osteoporosis. Once the bone material is lost, it won't come back. However, eating plenty of calcium-rich foods (such as milk and cheese), taking calcium supplements, eating a well-balanced diet rich in nutrients and participating in regular weight-bearing exercise (such as walking) can help prevent further bone loss. It also helps to avoid any activities that jar the bones or increase the risk of falling.

Standard medical treatment

- Vaginal creams.
- Antidepressants or medications to treat specific symptoms.
- Calcium supplements, vitamin D and osteoporosis medication.
- Estrogen replacement therapy (also called hormone replacement therapy).

When to seek help

Most women pass through menopause with relatively few problems, but you should have a regular checkup when signs of menopause begin to show. Make sure that these signs are due to "the change" and not other problems, such as a tumor. To verify that you are going through menopause, the doctor will mostly likely do blood tests, including two pituitary tests called FSH (follicle stimulating hormone) and LH (leutinizing hormone), and will check your blood estrogen.

In addition, if you have excessive bleeding, bleeding between periods, unusually difficult or painful periods, bleeding six months or longer after your last period or other unexplained symptoms, it's a good idea to be examined, just to rule out other diseases.

The information on alternative therapies is meant for educational purposes only. I am not endorsing any therapy or suggesting that you see any alternative practitioner. If you have or suspect that you are having any difficulties related to menopause, see your physician.

Acupuncture

Acupuncture points that might be used to maintain good health are similar to those used for infertility. These include points in the lower abdomen (between navel and pubic bones), Spleen 6, Kidney 3 (behind the ankle), lower back points and Colon 4 (on the hands).

Aromatherapy

Aromatherapy treatments for problems related to menopause vary widely, but essential oils that may be used include: chamomile (*Matricaria chamomilla*), cypress (*Cupressus sempervirens*), fennel (*Foeniculum vulgare*). For irregular, scanty or difficult periods, these essential oils may be recommended:

- Basil (*Ocimum basilicum).*
- Clary (Salvia sclarea).
- Jasmine (*Jasminum officinale).*
- Juniper (*Juniperus communis).*
- Lavender (*Lavandula officinalis).*

- Melissa (*Melissa officinalis*).
- Peppermint (*Mentha piperata*).
- Rose (*Rosa spp.*).

For depression that some women suffer during menopause, these or other essential oils may be selected:

- Basil (*Ocimum basilicum*).
- Bergamot (*Monarda didyma*).
- Camphor (*Cinnamomum camphora*).
- Geranium (*Pelargonium odorantissimum*).
- Jasmine (*Jasminum officinale*).
- Lavender (*Lavandula officinalis*).
- Neroli (*Citrus aurantium*).
- Ylang-ylang (*Cananga odorata*).

These or other oils may be prescribed for skin problems associated with menopause:

- Benzoin (*Styrax benzoin*).
- Chamomile (*Matricaria chamomilla*).
- Geranium (*Pelargonium odorantissimum*).
- Hyssop (*Hyssopus officinalis*).
- Myrrh (*Commiphora myrrha*).
- Neroli (*Citrus aurantium*).
- Sandalwood (*Santalum album*).

For anxiety or nervous tension, the aromatherapist may suggest:

- Bergamot (*Monarda didyma*).
- Camphor (*Cinnamomum camphora*).
- Cypress (*Cupressus sempervirens*).
- Jasmine (*Jasminum officinale*).
- Lavender (*Lavandula officinalis*).
- Melissa (*Melissa officinalis*).
- Patchouli (*Pogostemon patchouli*).

And for insomnia, these and other oils may be suggested:

- Basil (*Ocimum basilicum*).
- Marjoram (*Origanum marjorana*).
- Rose (*Rosa spp.*).
- Sandalwood (*Santalum album*).

The patient may be instructed to inhale the vapors from these oils as they rise from a bowl of water, to mix them in a base oil and use in massage, to wear as perfume or to mix in bath water. Treatment length will vary, depending upon the practitioner and the patient's condition.

Ayurvedic healing

Ayurveda associates menopause with aging, which is a Vata (air) stage of life. Thus, the symptoms of menopause experienced by some women are similar to the symptoms seen when the Vata humor "rises" and upsets the normal balance of the body. Vata-type menopausal symptoms tend to include depression, anxiety and insomnia. Menopause may also manifest itself in the other two humors. Women with Pitta-type symptoms are often angry and suffer hot flashes. Kapha-type symptoms include listlessness, weight gain and feelings of mental and physical heaviness. The type of treatment depends upon the humor in which the woman's menopausal symptoms are manifesting.

Treatment for Vata-type menopause

Since menopausal symptoms are generally associated with an excess of Vata (air), a common approach is to "reduce" the Vata to proper levels utilizing oils, incense, herbs and a special diet.

Sesame, almond and olive oil are among the oils that may be used in massage or placed on specific parts of the body, such as the mouth and ears. Herbs may be mixed with the oils. The vapors from essential oils, such as wintergreen, cinnamon or sandalwood, may be inhaled. Incenses, such as myrrh, frankincense and musk, may also be inhaled.

Anti-Vata herbs include ashwagandha, arjuna, astragalus, cinnamon, cardamom, comfrey root, garlic, ginseng, guggul, hawthorn berries, licorice, myrrh, rehmannia, sandalwood and zizphus. Also helpful are herbs that help to strengthen the female reproductive system, such as aloe, saffron, kapikacchu, lycium and white peony.

The anti-Vata diet includes warm, heavy and moist foods that give one strength. Frequent small meals, mildly spiced and with only a few different types of foods per meal are recommended. One should not eat when nervous or worried. Your meal should be cooked for you and you should eat with friends. (For a more complete description of the anti-Vata diet, see Chapter 8.)

Treatment for Pitta-type menopause

Women who display anger and suffer from frequent and severe hot flashes may be suffering from menopausal symptoms associated with excess Pitta (fire). For them, treatment would aim to "reduce" the Pitta to proper levels. Anti-Pitta treatment for menopause may utilize oils, incense, herbs and a special diet.

Oils use to combat Pitta-type symptoms include coconut and sesame. The Ayurvedic doctor may recommend taking clarified butter, called *ghee*, internally or using it for massage. In addition, inhaling the vapors from essential oils made from gardenia, honeysuckle, lotus and iris may be recommended, as well as incense made from saffron, jasmine or geraniums.

Herbs to be used include aloe, arjuna, barberry, golden seal, gotu kola, motherwort, myrrh, saffron and shatavari. Sandalwood oil is applied to the chest and to the "third eye" in the middle of the forehead. Meditation and other techniques are used to reduce the pent-up anger, hatred and resentment. Exercise and exposure to the sun are limited.

The anti-Pitta diet consists of cool, slightly dry and heavy foods. The foods should be raw and relatively plain-tasting, not cooked in lots of oil or heavily spiced. Three regular meals a day are suggested, with no eating late at night. (For a more complete description of the anti-Pitta diet, see Chapter 8.)

Treatment for Kapha-type menopause

If the menopause is manifesting in the Kapha (water) humor, the woman may feel unmotivated, tired and bloated. Her treatment would be an anti-Kapha regimen.

Mustard oil is often recommended as is linseed oil. If the woman is suffering from a great excess of Kapha, however, the doctor may recommend avoiding all massage and cooking oils. Inhaling the vapors from essential oils made from cedar, pine and sage, as well as incense made from basil, frankincense and cedar, may be suggested. Herbs to break up phlegm and ease chest congestion include bayberry, cayenne, cinnamon, guggul, motherwort and myrrh. Cinnamon, mustard or camphor may be applied to the chest to ease congestion.

The anti-Kapha diet is light, dry and warm. Cold, oily and heavy foods should be avoided. Three meals a day should be eaten, with lunch being the main meal. Breakfast may be skipped, and weekly fasting is helpful. Most or all of the daily food should be consumed between the hours of 10 a.m. and 6 p.m. (For a more complete description of the anti-Kapha diet, see Chapter 8.)

Color therapy

Although there are no standard protocols for dealing with menopause, color therapists often choose the following colors: Blue is a cooling, soothing color used to increase vitality and energy. It helps relieve menstrual difficulties and nervous irritability. Yellow, the color of joy, helps to soothe the emotions and relieve depression. It is used for mental fatigue and for stimulating activity. Green is the color of energy and youth. It stimulates the nervous system and soothes the emotions. It is used to treat exhaustion, irritability, sleeplessness and nervous disorders.

There are many ways for the color therapist to apply the properly colored light to the patient, including through direct light, gems, jewelry, perfume, clothing and colored glass. Patients may also meditate on colors and eat the appropriately colored foods.

- Blue foods include plums, grapes and blueberries. Blue metals and chemicals include copper, lead, oxygen and tin.
- Yellow foods include bananas, banana squash, eggs, yellow cheese, yellow corn, yellow sweet potatoes, pineapples, lemons, grapefruit and butter. Yellow metal and chemicals include platinum and magnesium.
- Green foods include green vegetables, peas, beans and lentils. Green metal and chemicals include barium, chlorophyll, nickel and sodium.

Herbal medicine

Herbs typically used to treat menstrual irregularity, hot flashes and vaginal discomfort include:

- Blue cohosh (*Caulophyllum thalictroides*).
- Chaste tree (*Vitex agnus-castus*).
- Damask rose (*Rosa damascena*).
- Golden seal (*Hydrastis canadenis*).
- Ladies mantle (*Alchemilla vulgaris*).
- Motherwort (*Leonurus cardiaca*).
- Sage (*Salvia officinalis*).
- Vervain (*Verbena officinalis*).

These herbs may be recommended for insomnia:

- Hops (*Humulus lupulus*).
- Jamaican dogwood (*Piscidia erythrina*).
- Limeflower (*Tilia europaea*).
- Passion flower (*Passiflora incarnata*).
- Wild lettuce (*Lactuca virosa*).

Herbs typically used for depression include:

- Basil (*Ocimum basilicum*).
- Borage (*Borago officinalis*).
- Damiana (*Turnera aphrodisiaca*).
- Gentian (*Gentiana lutea*).
- Mugwort (*Artemisia vulgaris*).
- Oats (*Avena sativa*).
- Rosemary (*Rosemarinus officinalis*).
- Rue (*Ruta graveolens*).
- St. John's Wort (*Hypericum perforatum*).

- Vervain (*Valeriana officinalis*).
- Wormwood (*Artemisia absinthum*).

For anxiety, these or other herbs may be suggested:

- Linden (*Tilia europaea*).
- Skullcap (*Scutellaria lateriflora*).
- Vervain (*Valeriana officinalis*).
- Wood betony (*Stachys officinalis*).

Homeopathy

Homeopathy attempts to relieve some of the "symptoms" of menopause by strengthening the body. The "remedies" (medicines) selected by the homeopath will depend upon the patient's symptoms, plus her physical, mental and emotional state. Most of the major homeopathic remedies may be used for the symptoms of menopause:

- *Bellis perennis,* which is indicated when the woman is frequently tired and has a constant backache.
- *Cimicifuga racemosa,* which is indicated when the woman is very talkative and restless. Her emotions may swing from troubled to happy, and she may be fearful of disease or death. She often has headaches and a feeling of doom centered in her stomach.
- *Sanguinaria,* which is indicated when the right side of the body is more troubled than the left. The woman suffers from itching all over her body, heavy vaginal discharge, sore breasts and headaches on the right side of her head.
- *Sepia,* which is indicated when the woman is worn out and weak. She is likely to be sad and to display indifference to her job or family. She feels cold, despite flushing often. She shies away from intercourse because it is difficult or painful for her.

For the painful intercourse that may accompany menopause, the homeopath may suggest several remedies, including:

- *Apis mellifica,* which is indicated when the woman is restless, tearful and apathetic. She may feel sluggish and feverish, especially in the afternoon. Her pelvis feels sore and her vagina "tight."
- *Belladonna,* which is indicated when the woman is a "dreamer" whose symptoms are made worse by noise or being touched. Her vagina feels sore and "burning," and she may bleed after engaging in intercourse.

For depression, several remedies may be suggested, including:

- *Aconitum napellus,* which is indicated when the woman is anxious and fearful. She feels better after resting or being outside, but worse at night or when lying on her left side.
- *Lachesis*, which is indicated when the woman is talkative, suspicious, thin and moody. She prefers to be by herself and may be especially depressed in the morning.

Anxiety may be treated with these or other remedies:

- *Arsenicum album,* which is indicated when the woman is cool, restless and has fears of great disease or death. She is fault-finding and demanding. Even minimal activity tires her out. Symptoms are worse when she is cold, during wet weather and late at night. Heat makes her feel better.
- *Borax*, which is indicated when the woman is nervous and annoyed by sudden noises or activity. She may become nauseated by excessive anxiety, and hot flashes may keep her awake at night. Noise, warm weather and downward motion increase her symptoms, while pressure and cold water decrease them.

These or other remedies may be recommended for insomnia:

- *Arsenicum album*, which is indicated when the woman is chilly and frightened of dying. She tends to wake up in the middle of the night and restlessly walks around the house.
- *Coffea cruda*, which is indicated when the woman is filled with thoughts and ideas, her emotions swinging. She is sensitive to noise and can't stop thinking about things.
- *Lycopodium clavatum*, which is indicated when the woman is physically weak but has a sharp mind. Although lacking in self-confidence, she tends to "rise to the occasion." She tends to wake up in the very early morning and can't stop thinking about things long enough to get back to sleep.
- *Sulphur*, which is indicated when the woman is depressed, weak and lazy. She tends to argue and grumble a lot and suffer from recurring symptoms. She is a very light sleeper, often awakened by small noises.

Other homeopathic preparations may be used for vaginal dryness, fatigue, flushes and other problems as the practitioner sees fit.

Although it is a basic principle of classical homeopathy to use only one remedy at a time, there is a trend among modern homeopaths toward using multiple remedies at once. Using the absolute minimum number of doses necessary is another principle of classical homeopathy.

A second dose should not be given until the first has ceased to act, and no more remedies should be given once the body begins to heal. If the right remedy is used, two or three days should be enough to begin many long-term curative processes.

Nutritional therapy

Although good nutrition in general is important for menopausal women, some vitamins and phytochemicals seem to be especially helpful. Phytochemicals are health-giving substances found in foods. ("Phyto" refers to "food.") Neither vitamins nor minerals, the phytochemicals are a remarkably large and diverse group of substances with a variety of duties in the body. Let's look at some of the nutrients and phytochemicals that may be recommended to help a woman deal with the symptoms of menopause.

Vitamin E. We've known for decades that the antioxidant vitamin E can be helpful for menopausal women. In 1949, the effect of vitamin E on menopausal symptoms was studied on 66 women with "vasomotor" difficulties (a dilating or "widening" of the blood vessels). They were given between 20 and 100 mg of vitamin E in the form of alpha tocopherol for an average of 31 days each. As a result, 31 of the 66 reported "excellent" relief, with another 16 enjoying "fair" benefits. When the women stopped taking the vitamin, their symptoms reappeared.[1]

Even more effective than vitamin E alone is a combination of vitamins E and C, plus calcium. Food sources of vitamin E include broccoli, nuts and tomatoes.

Boron. Although most people are not aware that boron is found in food, this overlooked mineral can help to soften menopausal symptoms. Boron appears to work by increasing the levels of certain forms of estrogen. Some studies suggest that eating boron-rich foods or taking boron supplements may raise estrogen levels as high as those found in women taking estrogen-replacement therapy. Three or four apples a day or three to four ounces of peanuts may supply boron-deficient women with all they need. Boron is also found in pears, raisins, peaches, almonds, honey, peas, beans and lentils.

Phytoestrogens. Phytoestrogens are estrogen-like compounds found in certain foods, such as soybeans and flaxseed. These phytoestrogens act like mild estrogens within the body, helping to relieve many of the symptoms of menopause. In a 1990 study, 25 post-menopausal women ranging in age from 51 to 70 had soy flour, red clover sprouts and linseed added to their diets for two weeks each. At the end of the six-week period, laboratory examination of vaginal cells from the women showed an increase in estrogenic activity. The benefits quickly disappeared once the women went back to eating their regular diets.[2]

Bioflavonoids. Sometimes called "vitamin P," the bioflavonoids give citrus fruits their orange and yellow colors. But they do more than that: It seems that some of them bear a structural resemblance to estradiol, a form of estrogen.

The combined effects of bioflavonoids and vitamin C were tested on 94 women complaining of hot flashes. The bioflavonoid/vitamin C combination relieved the troublesome hot flashes in 53 percent of the women and lessened them in another 34 percent. There was, however, a mildly unpleasant perspiration odor.[3] In another study, bioflavonoids combined with vitamin C successfully relieved nighttime leg cramps, bruises and spontaneous nose bleeding in menopausal women.[4] Bioflavonoids can be found in oranges, grapefruit and tangerines.

L-tryptophan. This amino acid is a precursor to the neurotransmitter *serotonin*, which helps to prevent depression. Although more study is needed, it appears that low levels of tryptophan in the blood are related to estrogen and to the depression some women face during menopause. If this theory is proven by further research, L-tryptophan may be used as a natural antidepressant and mood modulator for menopausal women. Food sources of L-tryptophan include beef, pork, lamb, veal and cheese.

Melatonin. A natural hormone produced by a part of the brain called the *pineal gland*, melatonin helps us to sleep at night. In fact, the pineal gland releases melatonin only when it's dark and no light is striking the retinas of the eyes. Its secretion is turned off by light.

Many adults frequently endure nights of little sleep, and insomnia is a common symptom associated with menopause. According to Ray Sahelian, M.D., author of *Melatonin: Nature's Sleeping Pill,*[5] as little as 1 mg of melatonin, taken two hours before going to bed, may help to ease sleeping problems. (The average dose is 3 mg.)

Other nutrients. Although they do not specifically relieve menopausal symptoms, several vitamins and minerals are very helpful in keeping a woman as strong and healthy as possible during what can be a difficult time of life. Chief among these are the 4 ACES: vitamin A in the form of beta carotene, vitamins C and E and the mineral selenium. (Beta carotene is the "plant" form of vitamin A, found especially in carrots and other yellow, orange and green vegetables.)

Oriental medicine

Oriental medicine looks upon menopause as a normal function of the female body, and not as a disease or disorder that must be fought with medicines and hormones. Instead of telling women that they must take hormones to avoid the hot flashes and other symptoms of menopause, the Oriental medicine physician will use diet, herbs, exercise, acupuncture and other means to maintain the woman's good health and to relieve any symptoms that do occur. Oriental medicine is very clear about this: Filling a menopausal woman's body with hormones is an unnatural state; the body wishes to have lower levels of certain hormones at this point in life.

To help relieve symptoms of menopause and to strengthen the body, the Oriental medical doctor may recommend a combination of herbs and spices, diet, acupuncture or "ear acupuncture" as necessary.

Herbs and spices

- *Sweet basil,* a warm and pungent substance that improves energy and circulation while regulating menstruation.
- *Cinnamon twig,* a warm and pungent substance that tones the heart and lungs.
- *Ginseng,* a warm, sweet and slightly bitter herb that improves energy and works against vaginal difficulties.

Herbal formulas that may be recommended include *Da Bu Yin Wan* and *He Che Da Zao Wan.*

Diet

Foods are selected depending on their flavors, organic actions and other qualities, including energies. There are five food energies: hot, warm, neutral, cool and cold. (The energy has to do with the quality of the food, not its temperature.)

Advice to menopause patients

Although many of my patients have had success with the following program, I only use the general guidelines discussed below after reviewing a patient's personal and medical history, performing a thorough examination and evaluating the laboratory studies to make sure that the program will be beneficial. Please see your own physician before embarking on any treatment program for menopausal symptoms.

There is no single remedy for the many ailments that *may* trouble menopausal women, but there are a number of things one can do. There are general measures to improve overall health and specific measures for individual symptoms:

- Eat a highly nutritious diet to ensure that you are getting all the nutrients you need without burdening your body with excess fat, salt, sugar, alcohol and caffeine.
- Take supplements of the 4 ACES (vitamin A/beta carotene, vitamins C and E and the mineral selenium). These antioxidant nutrients help the body to resist the ravages of aging while strengthening the immune system.
- Try body creams containing Mexican yam root, a strong, natural, nontoxic progesterone-like compound.

- Take supplements of the bioflavonoids naturally found in citrus fruit. For many of my patients, 500 mg, two to three times per day, has worked quite well.
- Learn how to recognize and reduce stress. Stress does not cause menopause, but it can certainly make any symptoms that you have seem worse. Try meditation, exercise, yoga and other stress-reducing measures.

For hot flashes:

- Take vitamin E supplements, which have been used for 50 years to treat hot flashes. I often begin my patients on 400 IU of vitamin E a day, working up to 800 IU daily.
- Consider taking GLA (gamma linolenic acid), naturally found in borage, black currants and evening primrose oil.
- Try Dong Quai, which has been called the "female ginseng." This "smooths out" the mood and bringing on relaxation.
- Consider other herbs such as Hawthorn berry, yam root, black cohash and blue cohash.

For sexual difficulties and vaginal dryness:

- Have regular sex. It's a remedy for many sexual difficulties.
- Use vitamin E creams made from marigold flower, aloe vera and/or the Mexican yam for vaginal dryness.
- Avoid alcohol, caffeine and the antihistamines found in many cold remedies. All three can dry the mucus membranes.

For sleeplessness:

- Consider melatonin, often called "nature's sleeping pill."
- Try herbs such as passion flower, hops, skull cap and valerian.

For osteoporosis:

- Engage in regular weight-bearing exercise. The more you force your bones to support your weight, the more likely they are to remain strong. Walking, jogging, aerobics and dancing are good exercises for the lower body. Light weight lifting will help to keep the bones of the upper body strong.
- Eat plenty of calcium-containing foods (such as dairy products) and take calcium supplements, if necessary. Menopausal women should be getting at least 1,500 mg of calcium per day (roughly the amount in a quart of milk).
- Eat foods high in boron, a mineral that helps the body "hang on" to its calcium. Boron is found in apples, pears, grapes and other fruit, as well as in legumes, nuts and honey.

- Make sure that you are getting enough of the trace mineral manganese. You'll find manganese in pineapples, nuts, spinach, beans and whole wheat.
- Vitamin D is necessary for the absorption of calcium, so include plenty of vitamin D foods in your diet (such as vitamin D-enhanced milk). Your skin can also make vitamin D when exposed to the sun. Supplements are helpful, but too much vitamin D is dangerous.

For Restless Leg Syndrome:

- A common cause of menopausal sleep problems, Restless Leg Syndrome (Ekhom Syndrome) can cause itching, pain and "creeping" and "crawling" feelings in the legs and thighs. Restless Leg sufferers move their legs or walk in an attempt to relieve the problem. Although usually harmless, Restless Leg may be a prelude to nerve problems related to kidney failure. It may be helped taking by calcium, magnesium, potassium and vitamin E before going to bed.

Practical tips

For hot flashes: Layer your clothing, putting one lightweight item over another. If you become hot, remove your jacket or sweater. Wear clothing made of absorbent material, such as cotton. Don't wear silk blouses or other clothes that show perspiration stains. Air out stuffy rooms in your house. Purchase a small fan that you can set on your night table or desk. When a flash hits, direct the cool air right to you.

For vaginal dryness or irritation: Use a simple, nonirritating, non-drying soap. Temporarily set aside any soaps, lotions or bath preparations that are even the least bit irritating or drying. When you're at home in the evenings, wear a nightgown, long T-shirt or other clothing that allows air to circulate by your genitals. Having intercourse often will help to keep the vaginal walls strong. Generous amounts of foreplay will help overcome dryness before intercourse.

To help you sleep: Don't drink coffee, cola or any other drinks that contain caffeine for several hours before bedtime. Instead, have a glass of warm milk or take a warm bath. Try not to nap during the day, or you may not be tired enough to go to sleep at bed time. Meditation or relaxation techniques before bedtime will also help to prepare you for sleep by releasing tension and clearing the mind.

Try not to argue with your spouse or discuss distressing situations right before bed. In fact, it may help to give your mind time to "wind down" from a busy day. And if you find yourself watching the clock at night, put the clock where you can't see it or get rid of it altogether.

Experiment with different pillows and room temperatures to create the most comfortable environment possible. If noise bothers you, try wearing ear plugs. A slightly noisy fan that makes a steady hum can help to mask the sounds of a television playing in an other room, cars driving by and dogs barking. You can also purchase "sound machines" that make "white noise." Get blackout shades, hang up heavier curtains or wear eye shades to eliminate any offending light.

Avoid sleeping pills. Although they may work at first, you'll eventually build up a tolerance to their effects.

Finally, some women report that nightly sex or simple caressing helps them to sleep.

For varicose veins: Exercise often to increase leg circulation. Don't stand, sit in one position or cross your legs for long periods of time. Avoid tight-fitting garters, knee-high nylons or anything else that might impede circulation. Wear support hose. If you already have varicose veins, sit with your feet elevated as often as you can.

These are just a few of the many simple ways you can deal with menopausal annoyances. In addition, maintain your ideal weight, stay mentally and physically active, reduce your stress as much as possible and make sure that you take time to enjoy life.

A final note: before you take estrogen

Should women routinely begin estrogen replacement therapy at menopause? Many doctors think so and are prescribing the hormone treatment to increasingly large numbers of women. Some 10 million American women are on hormone therapy, at a cost of billions of dollars per year. Estrogen prescriptions doubled between 1982 and 1992.

The doctors who prescribe the hormones insist that they are safe and effective. Yet, according to a report in the June 15, 1995 issue of the *New England Journal of Medicine*, there is a "substantial increase in the risk of breast cancer among older women who take these hormones." As for estrogen's effectiveness, half of the women who begin estrogen therapy stop within a year. Estrogen replacement therapy has its place, but it is not as safe as women have been led to believe, it is not as effective as has been advertised and it is not the only choice for dealing with the symptoms of menopause and aging. Still, women regularly come to my office carrying estrogen pills or prescriptions that were given to them by a gynecologist at the first mention of any menopausal symptoms. Are the possible benefits of hormone replacement therapy worth the real possibility of serious side effects? Most of the women I see aren't sure about this because their doctors never explain the therapy's down side.

There are some reasons for taking estrogen, including relief from menopausal symptoms, a lowered risk of heart disease and protection against thinning bones. However, there are other safe, simple and effective ways of achieving the same goals without using estrogen and *without* the side effects of estrogen therapy, which are considerable.

They include cancer of the breast and uterus, potentially lethal blood clots, gallstones, nausea, vomiting, chest pain, severe headaches, dizziness, abnormal bleeding from the uterus, skin problems, plus swelling and tenderness of the abdomen.

Doctors tell women that the risk of osteoporosis (thin bones) rises at menopause. They explain that estrogen therapy keeps the bones strong. *But they rarely mention that exercise, calcium and vitamin D can do the same thing, without the side effects of estrogen therapy.*

Doctors tell women that the risk of heart disease rises dramatically after menopause. They urge women to take estrogen to protect the heart, *neglecting to add that a healthful diet, exercise, stress management and antioxidant vitamins protect the heart just as well, without estrogen's side effects.*

Vitamins, minerals, herbs, creams, simple dietary changes, exercise and, yes, even regular sex can reduce or eliminate most of the symptoms of menopause. At the same time, these simple measures also protect a woman's heart, strengthen her bones, increase her energy level and energize her immune system

The medical establishment treats menopause like a disease. Before you agree to take estrogen, remember that there are safe and effective, natural approaches to reducing the symptoms of menopause and slowing the aging process. Estrogen replacement therapy certainly has its place, but it is not for everyone.

If it is right for you, ask your doctor about natural progesterone rather than the synthetic progesterone called "protestins." The natural progesterones are not easy to find, so your doctor may have to find a pharmacy able to prepare the natural hormone. (Women's International Pharmacy can. The number is 1-800-279-5708.)

Throughout the world, the majority of women go through menopause without taking many medicines or requiring treatment. A subset of women need care and should see their doctors. Most women, however, will do quite well with the natural remedies I've discussed.

[1]   Finkler, R.S. The effect of vitamin E in the menopause. *J Clin Endocrinol Metab*, 9:89-94, 1949.

[2]   Wilcox, G., et al. Oestrogenic effects of plant foods in postmenopausal women. *Br Med J,* 301:905-6, 1990.

[3]   Smith, C.J. Non-hormonal control of vaso-motor flushing in menopausal patients. *Chic Med*, 67(5):193-5, 1964.

[4]   Horoschak, A. Nocturnal leg cramps, easy bruisability and epistaxis in menopausal patients: Treated with Hesperidin and ascorbic acid. *Del State Med J*, Jan 1959, pp. 19-22.

[5]   Sahelian, Ray. *Melatonin: Nature's Sleeping Pill.* Marina Del Rey, Calif: Be Happier Press, 1995.

Chapter 11

Pain

Pain is that hammer banging on your head, the vise squeezing your back, the knife ripping through your finger joints, the constant dull ache in your knees, the needle flashing through your belly. And pain is more than a physical sensation. It is a constant reminder of our fragility and a nagging fear that someday things may be worse.

We suffer greatly from back pain, arthritis, headaches and cancer pain. Back pain is a major problem; the incidence is staggering. About 80 percent of the population will, at some time, have back pain serious enough to interfere with regular activities or require a trip to the doctor.[1]

No one knows exactly how many Americans suffer from pain. Perhaps some 70 million of us go to our doctors looking for pain relief every year. At one point or another, an estimated one in every three Americans will be in serious pain. For some of us, the pain is manageable and fleeting, signifying nothing more than a temporary, correctable problem. For others, the pain may be chronic, despite the best efforts of traditional and alternative healers.

Possible causes

- Physical injury.
- Problems with digestion.
- Degenerative diseases, such as arthritis.
- Cancer.
- Stress.
- Congenital defects (birth defects).
- Nerve disorders.
- Autoimmune diseases, such as Sjogren's Syndrome.
- Circulatory problems leading to various problems, such as angina pectoris.
- Muscle strains.
- Inflamed tendons.
- Infections.

- Hormonal changes, causing problems such as sore breasts in women.
- Poor posture.

In many cases, however, we don't know why someone hurts.

Types of pain

Although there are many ways of looking at pain, for the purposes of this chapter I'm going to divide it into two "types": *acute* and *chronic*.

Acute pain is usually a sudden pain that "hits" hard when you smash your thumb with a hammer or stub your toe. Acute pain is a messenger, telling you that something is wrong, that body tissue is being damaged. Acute pain is "designed" to get your immediate attention and to make you stop the harmful behavior. Therefore, it serves a useful purpose.

Chronic pain, however, serves no such purpose. In many cases, it appears for no obvious reason at all and refuses to leave, lingering for days, months or even years. Whereas acute pain is the bearer of bad news, chronic pain is, itself, the bad news. Hit by a pain that has no rhyme or reason, unable to get relief, frequently depressed and unable to sleep, chronic pain patients may lose hope. Acute pain is "good" for us because it is a warning, but chronic pain can ruin us.

Standard medical treatment

- Pain medications such as aspirin, Tylenol, Fiorinal, Percocet and Demerol.
- Sedatives, such as Valium and Xanax.
- Antidepressants, such as Elavil.
- Muscle relaxants, such as Paraflex and Robaxin.
- Anticonvulsants, such as Tegretol.
- Nerve blocks.
- Surgery (especially with back pain).
- Physical therapy (including massage, heat and cold and electrical stimulation).
- Psychological counseling.

Now let's take a look at some of the many alternative treatments for pain. These are not all the possible therapies, because there are too many to investigate in a single chapter. Reading through these alternatives, however, will give you an idea of the many possibilities.

The information on alternative therapies is meant for educational purposes only. I am not endorsing any therapy or suggesting that you see any alternative practitioner. If you have any serious, suspicious, unexpected or unusual pain, see your physician.

Acupuncture

The exact treatment for pain depends upon where the pain is located. Needles will be inserted into the appropriate local areas (near the pain), as well as in overall points such as Colon 4. If the pain is caused by cold and dampness, an herb called *moxa* will be placed on appropriate points on the skin and then burned. According to reports published in *Acupuncture* and elsewhere, acupuncture produces significant relief in cases of backache, low back pain, headaches, migraines, shoulder pain, tennis elbow, knee pain and other types of pain.

Color therapy

Color therapists have no standard methods for dealing with pain, which will vary with the type of pain one has and the practitioner's preferences. For example, back pain may be treated with *green*, a soothing and cooling color that works on both the mind and body. The color of energy and hope, green is considered a master-healer, good for all conditions and for helping the body rid itself of toxic substances.

Green foods include green vegetables, peas, beans and lentils. Green metal and chemicals include barium, chlorophyll, nickel and sodium.

Homeopathy

While many traditional Western therapies are geared toward simply relieving the pain, homeopathy attempts to cure pain by helping the body heal itself. As with other healing arts, the remedies that might be used for pain depend upon the type of pain from which one is suffering. Backache remedies, for example, might include:

- *Aesculus hippocastanum*, which is indicated when the patient is irritable and despondent. Symptoms include a continuous dull ache in the lower back that is worse when the patient is walking or bending over. The pain is worse in cool temperatures, better in the summer and open air.

- *Ledum palustre,* which is indicted when the patient feels cold, suffers from various symptoms and the pain seems to move diagonally across the body (such as from the left leg up and across the body toward the right shoulder). The pain is worse with heat and at night, better with cold.

- *Ruta graveolens*, which is indicated when the patient is weak, restless, filled with despair and feeling as if the pain has spread all over the body. It's worse when lying down or with cold weather, better when moving.

Other homeopathic preparations may be used as the practitioner sees fit. (See, for example, the homeopathic headache remedies discussed in Chapter 7.)

Although it is a basic principle of classical homeopathy to use only one remedy at a time, there is a trend among modern homeopaths toward using multiple remedies at once. Using the absolute minimum number of doses necessary is another principle of classical homeopathy. A second dose should not be given until the first has ceased to act, and no more remedies should be given once the body begins to heal. If the right remedy is used, two or three days should be enough to begin many long-term curative processes. If not, another remedy should be selected and given a chance to work.

Hypnosis

Although hypnosis does not "cure" underlying organic problems, it does allow one to handle the physical and often emotional effects of the pain more easily. Generally speaking, hypnosis can be used to help the patient relax, reduce anxiety and gain "control" over the pain.

After hypnotizing the patient and inducing a very relaxed state, the hypnotist may use suggestions such as these to help the patient control and diminish the pain:

"Concentrate your focus on your [pained body part]. Notice the pain in your [body part]. With your mind's eye, see the pain as a redness over the area. Completely relax all the muscles around your [body part]. Feel all the tension flowing out of those muscles as the entire area completely relaxes. And as the muscles relax, your [body part] begins to cool down. As the wonderful cooling sensation spreads through your [body part], notice how the redness fades away. With your mind's eye, see the hot redness turning to a blue coolness as the wonderful cooling sensation spreads through your [body part]. Your [body part] muscles are completely relaxed. The entire area is completely relaxed and pleasantly cool, the formerly red pain turning into a soft blue mist over your [body part].

"Concentrate on the pleasant, cool blue mist over your [body part]. Notice how relaxed and healthy your [body part] feels when covered by the mist. With your mind's eye, see that blue mist growing thicker and richer, becoming a beautiful, cool, relaxing blanket that covers your [body part]. With that cool blue blanket in place, you feel comfortable and calm."

The hypnotist would then give suggestions, saying that whenever the patient liked, he or she could sit or lie down in a comfortable, quite place and put him- or herself in a self-induced hypnotic trance. In that trance, the patient would relax completely, visualize the pain as a redness, then replace it with the cool, calming blue blanket.

Of course, this is not the only approach that might be used, but it illustrates the general technique. Hypnosis is also used prior to surgery to help ease tension and speed the patient's recovery.

There is no agreed-upon length of time necessary before a patient can feel the benefits of using hypnosis to treat pain. Several factors may affect the length of treatment: how hypnotizable the client is, the rapport developed between the hypnotist and the client and the severity of the pain. Many people have been helped in just one session. For others, several sessions are required.

Nutritional therapy

Several vitamins and other substances have been shown to be of value in treating pain. They include:

Vitamin B1 (Thiamin). Back in the 1960s, European researchers found that large doses (10 to 30 grams) of B1, given intravenously, reduced certain types of pain.[2] More recently, 133 headache, backache and "nerve pain" patients, whose pain had persisted despite medications and physical therapy, were given 1 to 2 grams of thiamin twice daily. As a result, 78 percent of the headache patients reported improvement, as did 71 percent of those with back pain and 62 percent of the "nerve pain" volunteers. (Slightly over 10 percent of the headache patients complained of nausea.)[3] Good sources of B1 include almonds, split peas and whole grains.

Vitamin B12. Some interesting studies have shown that B12 is also useful in treating pain. Injections of B12 have been used for many years to treat tic doloreaux, a painful twitch. When 400 people with spine pain and sensory disturbances were given injections of 5,000 micrograms (mcg) of B12 daily, 50 percent of them reported "very good" or "good" relief from pain within six to 16 days. The others reported "satisfactory" relief, except for 10 who did not respond at all.[4]

In another study, two weeks of treatment with 10,000 mcg of B12 daily produced marked pain relief in people with degenerative neuropathy. When cancer patients were given the same doses, 27 percent reported complete relief within two weeks, while 33 percent enjoyed some improvement.5 Food sources of B12 include fish, eggs and cheese.

Vitamin C. Like B12, vitamin C's anti-pain properties have been tested in cancer patients. In severely ill victims, 10 grams a day produced significant relief.[6] The vitamin has also been used to treat volunteers suffering from gum sensitivity and muscle pain following medical procedures (such as bronchoscopy, in which a tube is pushed into the "wind pipes"). Intravenous injections of the vitamin have been used to help resolve the pain of pancreatic cancer. Vitamin C can be found in citrus fruits, lima beans and kale.

Vitamin E and copper. Although more study is needed, it appears that vitamin E and the mineral copper may help to relieve pain by stimulating endorphins, the body's built-in pain killers.[7] Good sources of vitamin E include wheat germ and whole grains. Copper can be found in beans, lentils and oysters.

Selenium. A low intake of this mineral may be linked to muscle pain.[8] A 1985 Swedish study reported that middle-aged women with long-term back and shoulder pain had lower levels of selenium in the blood than did healthy controls. The study also found that giving selenium plus vitamin E to the women often improved their response to standard physiotherapy.[9] Good sources of selenium include turkey, radishes and mushrooms.

Capsaicin. This "hot stuff," which is found in chili peppers, is being investigated as a promising painkiller. Capsaicin doesn't "cure" pain, rather it appears to block the transmission of pain signals along the nervous system. Capsaicin-based medicines and capsaicin injections have been used to treat arthritis, "nerve pain," headaches, post-herpes zoster neuritis and other painful conditions.

DLPA. In 1972, Drs. Candace Pert and Solomon Snyder showed that morphine (a powerful painkilling drug) fits into certain nerve cell structures in the brain like a key fits its lock. In other words, morphine can "unlock" previously unknown powers of the brain. But this was a puzzling discovery. Why do human brain cells have specific structures that interact with morphine? Were we humans supposed to be taking morphine all of our lives?

These two scientists, along with others, proposed a simple yet revolutionary explanation: The human brain must produce its own form of morphine. That would explain why morphine could "turn on" certain brain cells. Studies at major universities around the world showed that the brain does, in fact, produce many hormone-like chemicals that resemble morphine. These chemicals were named the *endorphins*, because they are endogenous (produced by the body) and similar to morphine. Unfortunately, the same body that produces endorphins also destroys them.

The scientists quickly reasoned that some people may be in chronic pain because their bodies do not produce enough endorphins or because they overproduce the "endorphin-killers." In either case, these people have low endorphin levels, allowing pain that would normally be filtered out to "get through" to the brain. Somehow the body's natural balance is upset, and the result is chronic pain that serves no purpose, other than to make its victims miserable.

Dr. Seymour Ehrenpreis of the Chicago Medical School found that the amino acid DLPA (dl-phenylalanine) naturally protects the endorphins.

Studies have shown that DLPA allows the patient's natural levels of endorphins to rise, reducing or eliminating long-standing chronic pain.

In the first study of DPA (a form of DLPA) on humans, 10 chronic pain patients were given the amino acid. These people were suffering from back pain, arthritis, headaches and other forms of long-standing pain that had not been helped by standard therapies. The result was "good to excellent" pain relief for all 10.[10] Later studies confirmed that DLPA or DPA could reduce or eliminate pain in many long-term sufferers, without significant side effects or costs.

Although DLPA does work against pain, it's not like aspirin or other medications in that it does not work right away. Instead, it may take from two days to six weeks for DLPA's "endorphin-guarding" activities to allow the body's endorphin levels to rise enough to block pain. DLPA also strengthens the pain-killing effects of aspirin.

DLPA is available in health food stores. (See the section, "Advice To Pain Patients" for more information on DLPA.)

Note: I recommend against taking DLPA during pregnancy or lactation. Pregnant or lactating women should not expose the fetus or newborn to anything except their normal diet. Anyone suffering from the genetic disease phenylketonuria (PKU) or on a phenylalanine-restricted diet should not take DLPA. I do not recommend the use of DLPA for children under the age of 14. For more information on DLPA, see our book DLPA To End Chronic Pain and Depression.

To combat the anxiety that often accompanies pain and makes it worse, I often recommend two nutritional substances. The first is a homeopathic remedy that seems to be almost as powerful as valium for reducing anxiety. Called L.72 Anti-Anxiety, it's a blend of many remedies, including *Cicuta virosa 4x, Ignatia 4x, Staphsagria 4x* and *Asfoetida 3x*. I also use an herb called Kava kava *(Piper methysticum)*. Both these substances have helped many of my patients break the cycle of pain/anxiety/more pain. They are available from Enzymatic Therapies.

In addition, a number of foods may help to quell pain, including chili peppers (which contain capsaicin), onions, garlic and peppermint.

When selecting a nutritional healer, remember there is no widely recognized school of nutritional therapy and no standards or agreed-upon training for nutritional healers. The exception is the Registered Dietitians, who tend to be conservative in their recommendations.

Oriental medicine

Pain is often caused by stagnant energy that has built up in one or more areas of the body. If that is the case, part of the treatment is to use acupuncture to disperse this excess energy, allowing the body to return to balance. Pain is treated with a combination of herbs and spices, diet, acupuncture and other therapies, as necessary.

Herbs and spices

Exactly which herbs and spices and the amount of each will depend upon the patient and his or her condition. Many herbs and spices may be recommended for pain, depending upon the type and location of the problem. These include:

- Star anise (*Illicium verum*).
- Fennel (*Foeniculum vulgare*).
- Cinnamon bark (*Cinnamomum zeylanicum*).
- Garlic (*Allium sativum*).
- Clove (*Eugenia aromatica*).
- Dried ginger (*Zinbiger officinale*).
- Nutmeg (*Myristica fragrans*).
- Black and white pepper.
- Caraway seed (*Carum carvi*).
- Spearmint (*Mentha spicata*).
- Licorice (*Glycyrrhiza glabra*).

Many herbal formulas are available for pain, including:

- For abdominal pain, *Ren Dan* and *Ping Wei Pian*.
- For back pain, *Yao Tong Pian* and *Die Da Zhi Tong Gao* (which is applied as a plaster to the afflicted area).
- For pain due to an injury, *Tieh Ta Yao Gin* and *Shang Shi Bao Zhen Gao* (which is applied as a plaster to the skin).
- For rheumatic pain, *She Xiang Zhui Feng Gao* and *Shang Sui Zhi Tong Gao*, both of which are applied as plasters to the skin.
- For rheumatic joint pain, *Chin Kao Tien Shang Wan* and *Du Huo Tisheng Wan*.

Diet

Diet plays an important role in Oriental medicine. Foods are selected depending upon their flavors, organic actions and other qualities, including energies. There are five food energies: hot, warm, neutral, cool and cold. (The energy has to do with the quality of the food, not its temperature. For example, foods with "hot" energy, such as red pepper and cinnamon bark, increase the sensation of heat in the body, even when eaten cold.)

Psychoneuroimmunology

Mind/body healers use positive affirmations to counteract the negative thoughts that have been contributing to the intensity of the pain. Affirmations are typically brief, positive statements that focus on how well one feels and on how the disease is being conquered.

An affirmation to counter pain might be worded as follows:

"My muscles and joints move easily and smoothly. Nothing can hold me back today!"

An affirmation to help resist the depression and despair that often accompany chronic pain may sound like this:

"Things get better every day as I move forward, accomplishing my goals one by one. With each triumph, I look for more new, interesting and exciting challenges."

Relaxation/visualization

The way one responds to pain can either increase it or decrease it. "Telling" yourself that you are relaxed can help to reduce stress and pain in many cases. Here's a two-part technique that has helped many chronic pain patients reduce their stressful reactions to pain, physically relax, sleep better and actually reduce the amount of pain.

Set aside 10 to 15 minutes at least twice a day to focus on physical relaxation. Turn off the lights and the phone, loosen tight clothing and sit in a comfortable chair with a high back. Lay your hands on your knees and rest your feet comfortably on the floor.

Begin by relaxing your muscles

Close your eyes tightly. Close them even tighter and hold them closed as you count very slowly to 10.

Slowly relax your eye muscles, but keep your eyes closed. Take a slow, deep breath in through your nose, and hold it. Now let it slowly out through your mouth. Relax and open your eyes. Take another slow, deep breath and hold it. Let it slowly out through your mouth.

Now grimace and "show your teeth" to tighten the muscles of your mouth. Tilt your chin up and, teeth still bared, open your lips as wide as possible. Then contract your cheek and neck muscles. Hold that pose tightly as you slowly count to 10. Relax. Take a slow, deep breath in through your nose and hold it. Let it out slowly.

Firmly but gently contract the muscles in the back of your neck by pressing your head against the back of your chair. Keep pushing as you slowly count to 10. Let your head fall slowly forward a little as you relax. Take a slow, deep breath in through your nose and hold it. Now let it slowly out through your mouth.

Lift your shoulders as high as you can. Tilt your head back until you can almost touch your shoulders with the back of your head. Push your neck back and down into your shoulders, feeling the muscles at the base of your neck tightening. Hold that position as you slowly count to 10. Relax. Take a slow, deep breath in through your nose and hold it. Let it slowly out through your mouth. Repeat the same pattern as you complete the following movements. (Relax and take a slow, deep breath between each movement.)

Raise both arms in front of you, about shoulder level, with the palms toward the floor. Squeeze both hands into tight fists. Bending your wrists down but keeping your arms up, push your fists down toward the floor, as hard as possible. Hold as you count slowly to 10.

Once again, raise your arms out in front of you, at shoulder level. This time, however, your palms should be facing up. Squeeze your hands closed into tight fists. Bend your arms at the elbow until your clenched fists are near your ears. Hold that pose, arm and hand muscles tight, as you slowly count to 10.

Straighten your legs out in front of you. Raise your feet off the floor, your legs straight. Lift them to the level of the seat of your chair, toes pointing forward, and hold them there as you slowly count to 10.

Now "remove" your pain

You're still sitting in the chair with your feet on the floor and your eyes closed. With your mind's eye, focus on the part of your body that hurts. Identify the exact location of the pain, its center point and its outermost boundaries. With your mind's eye, draw a circle around your pain. Imagine that your "circle of pain" is rising out of your body, up into the air. Slowly feel it moving up and out, taking as much time as you need to let that pain move up and out of your body.

Feel your pain becoming smaller as it moves out of your body. Smaller and smaller, it keeps moving up and out of your body.

When it has left your body, use your mind's eye to watch the circle of pain drift away and vanish. Notice how good you feel.

Reflexology

Reflexology, the application of pressure to the feet, helps to relieve tension, improve the circulation, stimulate the nerves and normalize the functioning of the organs and glands through a series of pressures, stretches and general movements of the feet.

The treatment for pain will depend upon which part of the body hurts. If, for example, chronic back pain is the problem, the reflexologist will manipulate the direct reflex areas corresponding to the spine, as well as the associated reflex areas for the adrenals and solar plexus. The spine reflex areas are found on the inner sides of both feet. The adrenal gland reflex areas are at approximately the middle of the arch, slightly to the inside. The solar plexus reflex areas are below the balls of the feet, in the midline.

Advice to pain patients

Although many of my patients have had success with the following program, I only use the general guidelines discussed below after reviewing a patient's personal and medical history, performing a thorough examination and evaluating the laboratory studies to make sure that the program will be beneficial. Please see your own physician before embarking on any treatment program for pain.

I began seeing patients during my second year as a medical student in the 1950s. Chronic pain patients were constantly in and out of the hospitals—patients that we could not help. We doctors treated pain patients by ourselves back then, without the help of a psychologist to handle emotional upsets, without the assistance of a skilled social worker to identify and rectify certain home problems, without dentists, chiropractors, physical therapists and others at our sides.

This began to change toward the end of the 1960s as allied health professionals fought to have their voices heard. By the 1970s, many new treatments were used for chronic pain: biofeedback, meditation, acupuncture, nutrition, hypnosis, electrotherapy, group therapy and other modalities that proved their value. The power also began to shift from the physician back to the patient, where it belonged. And we learned that pain must be treated as a multifaceted problem, strongly influenced by the things that make a person who and what he or she is. We started to view the patient as part of a family, a circle of friends and various social, cultural and religious groups—a person who works, plays and lives in his or her own individual manner.

Here are eight important points that I use as a basis for building individualized anti-pain programs for many of my chronic pain patients. They are designed to strengthen the patient mentally and physically so the body has the best possible chance to heal.

1. Take control of your health.
2. Assemble a multidisciplined team to assist you.
3. If you're overweight, slim down.
4. Working with your physician, eliminate as many of your medications as you safely can.
5. Use the appropriate nutrients to strengthen natural defenses.
6. Use DLPA, as necessary, to relieve pain and lift your mood.
7. Exercise as much as possible. You can always do *some* exercise, even while sitting in a chair.
8. Believe that you are going to get better.

Now, let's take a closer look at the eight points.

1. *Take control of your health.* We doctors have been telling people to passively wait for us to "fix" them. We were wrong. Healing is quickest

and most sure when the patient takes control of his or her own health, playing an active role in the decision-making and the treatment.

2. *Assemble a multidisciplined team to assist you.* The chronic pain equation is complex and too difficult for a single healer to solve. There are many factors contributing to pain: the patient, the patient's feelings and fears, the doctor's attitude, the "germs," the medicines and treatments, the family and more. There is rarely a single cause for chronic pain. It often takes a team of experts, including perhaps a neurologist, orthopedist, chiropractor, physical medicine specialist, physical therapist and psychologist, to solve complex pain problems. The team should be led by your personal physician, the one who knows you best and whom you trust.

3. *If you're overweight, slim down.* I have seen many patients whose pain was worsened by their obesity, and many who felt much better when they shed their excess pounds. Not only that, but eating a low-fat, low-cholesterol diet based on fresh vegetables, fruits and whole grains and small amounts of lean meat and nonfat dairy products means that you'll have fewer other diseases to complicate your pain.

Vegetables are sources for many vitamins, minerals and enzymes, as well as dietary fiber. A diet including plenty of vegetables also lowers blood fats. If you cook your vegetables, do so for as short a time as possible—just until they are tender and crisp. Eat more raw than cooked vegetables, as cooking destroys many vitamins and minerals.

Fruits are packed with vitamins, minerals and fiber and are appetizingly sweet. Eat them whole and fresh, rather than cooked, canned, frozen or dried. Two to four fruits per day are recommended.

Whole grains are rich sources of B vitamins, minerals, fiber, low-fat protein and complex carbohydrates. Use whole grains as cereal or in breads and pasta. The number-one ingredient in breads, cereals or pasta should be a *whole* grain.

Legumes are dried beans and peas, such as black beans, garbanzos, Great Northern beans, kidney beans, lentils, lima beans, red beans, small white beans and split peas. Legumes are high in vitamins B1, B6 and others. They're high in minerals such as iron and copper, high in fiber, low in fat and contain up to 20 percent protein.

Protein provides the building blocks of the body's structures—muscles, organs, tissues, even fluids. It also helps to stabilize the blood sugar. Eat two to three small servings of low-fat protein daily, such as vegetable proteins, fish and white meat of chicken or turkey.

Dairy products are the most concentrated and easily absorbable source of calcium. Drink nonfat milk or buttermilk, eat plain nonfat yogurt or low-fat cheese. Two to three servings per day are recommended to help prevent the thinning of the bones (osteoporosis).

Nuts and seeds are delicious, but are also high in fat. Use them sparingly, just to add flavor or crunch to your foods. Avoid salted, roasted or coated nuts and seeds.

Water is a terrific weight loss aid, as it actually helps to reduce water retention. And we need lots of water to ensure proper functioning of the kidneys as well as replenishment of fluid to all of the body's cells. Drink eight or more 8-ounce glasses of water daily.

4. *Working with your physician, eliminate as many of your medications as you safely can.* Many patients have come to my office with grocery bags filled with the 20 to 30 medications they've been given. The inevitable side effects of drugs complicate matters, often making patients feel worse. Simply stopping the unnecessary medications has helped many patients.

5. *Use the appropriate nutrients to strengthen your natural defenses.* The following is the basic supplementation plan I use for pain, modifying it to each patient's needs.

- *Beta carotene.* 25,000 IU (15 mg) of beta carotene, twice a day. Get as much beta carotene from food as possible. Dark green leafy vegetables and yellow orange fruits and vegetables tend to be high in the plant form of vitamin A, which is called beta carotene. Eat two to three whole carrots a day because carrots have 8,000 to 10,000 IU of beta carotene. Three and one-half ounces of broccoli contain 2,500 IU of beta carotene.

- *B vitamins.* A B-complex vitamin containing 50 mg of the major B vitamins, taken twice a day.

- *Vitamin C.* Start with 1,000 mg of vitamin C, twice a day.

- *Vitamin E.* About 200 to 400 IU of vitamin E in the form of D-alpha-tocopherol, taken twice a day.

- *Minerals.* I tell my patients to take 50 mg of zinc, 100 mcg of selenium, 100 to 200 mcg of chromium and 350 mg of magnesium, all twice a day, and others as necessary.

6. *Use DLPA as necessary to relieve your pain and lift your mood.* When appropriate, I start my chronic pain patients on 375 mg of DLPA, three times a day taken right after breakfast, lunch and dinner. If there is no improvement, I increase the dose to 750 mg, three times a day. It takes about a week to begin to feel the improvement.

7. *Exercise as much as possible.* Exercise helps to keep the muscles strong, "lubricate" the joints, burn off calories and help you feel good about yourself. Whenever possible, and without hurting yourself, get out there and exercise. Even if you can only walk around the block, keep active. Almost everyone can do some form of exercise.

8. *Believe that you are going to get better.* Several years ago, doctors at the University of Tennessee Center For Health Science measured

the endorphin levels in 32 patients who were suffering from chronic pain. Then they gave the patients a placebo, a "sugar pill" that had no medicinal effect, although they told the volunteers that this was a medicine that would help relieve their pain.

Sometime later, 14 of the 32 reported feeling better. That's not unusual, because the "placebo effect" works 30 to 40 percent of the time. What was unusual, however, was that when the doctors retested those 14, they found that their endorphin levels had gone up. It was the endorphins, not the placebos, that relieved the patients' pain. But what made the endorphins rise? Not the placebo, but the patients' *belief*. Just by thinking they would get better, they changed their biochemistry (increased their endorphins) and healed themselves.

This study, and others like it, prove that what we believe plays an important role in our health. That's why it's important to believe that you can and will get better. Strong belief is a very powerful medicine.

[1]   Nachemson, A.L. "The Lumbar Spine: An Orthopaedic Challenge." *Spine*, 1:59-71, 1976.

[2]   See, for example: Lenot, G. Note sur l'aneurine, anesthesique general. *Ann Anesthesiol Franc,* 7(suppl 1):173-75, 1966. Mazzoni, P., Valenti, F. Un nuovo anestetico generale per via endovenosa—la tiamina. *Acta Anesth* (Padova), 15:815-28, 1964.

[3]   Quirin, H. Pain and vitamin B1 therapy. *Bibl Nutr Dieta,* (38):110-1, 1986.

[4]   Hieber, H. Die behandlung vertebragener schmerzen und sensibilitatsstorungen mit hochdosiertem hydroxocobalamin. *Med Monatsschr*, 28:545-48, 1974.

[5]   Dettori, A.G., Ponari, O. Efetto antalgico della cobamamide in corse di neuropatie periferiche di diversa etiopatogenese. *Minerva Med*, 64:1077-82, 1973.

[6]   Creagan, E.T., et al. Failure of high-dose vitamin C (ascorbic acid) therapy to benefit patients with advanced cancer. *N Engl J Med*, 301:687-90, 1979.

[7]   Kryzhanovskii, G.N., et al. [Endogenous opiod system in the realization of the analgesic effect of alpha-tocopherol.] *Biull Eksp Biol Med,* 105(2):148-50, 1988. Bhathema, S., et al. Decreased plasma enkephalins in copper deficiency in man. *Am J Clin Nutr*, 43:42-46, 1986.

[8]   van Rij, A.M., et al. Selenium deficiency in total parenteral nutrition. *Am J Clin Nutr*, 32:2076-85, 1979.

[9]   Jameson, S., et al. Effekter av selenvitamin E-behandling till kvinnor med lang variga arbetsrelaterade nack-och skuldersmartor. En dubbelblindstudie. *Lakaresallskapets Riksstamma*, 1985.

[10]   *Advances in Pain Research and Therapy*, Vol. 3. Bonica, J., et al., eds. New York: Raven Press, 1978, p. 479.

Chapter 12

Ulcers

I can't remember how many times I was called upon to pass a thin, flexible tube called a gastroscope down a patient's throat in order to look into his or her stomach. As I maneuvered the tip of the scope around the patient's stomach, I'd see the protective mucosal lining looking glossy and red. Too many times, however, I also saw a yellowish/whitish sore eating into the mucosal lining, proof that the patient had an ulcer.

Ulcers are erosions or "sores" in the lining of the gastrointestinal (GI) tract. Essentially a long hollow tube over 20 feet long, the GI tract fills with acids and other substances that digest food. These acids would also digest the walls of the stomach itself if not for the protective mucosal layer that lines its interior. But if something happens to that lining, acid and enzymes can begin to eat away at the walls of the GI tract, possibly "burning" right through them.

Ulcer statistics

As many as 10 percent of all Americans will suffer from an ulcer at some point in their lives. Some of those will not realize that they have an ulcer because the symptoms will be mild and the problem will eventually take care of itself.

Signs and symptoms

The signs and symptoms of an ulcer, which might be gentle or strong, may include:

- A burning or gnawing pain in the upper abdomen or below the breast bone. The pain is often relieved by eating.
- Pain that strikes right after eating, or not until hours later.
- Pain that is present off and on for several days, disappears for a while, then returns.
- Pain at night that awakens one from sleep.
- Loss of appetite.
- Weight loss.

- Weight gain (due to eating to relieve ulcer pain).
- Bloody stools (hematochezia).
- Black stools (melena).
- Nausea.
- Vomiting.
- Vomiting blood (hematemesis).
- Antacids usually relieve, but may sometimes cause the pain.

Types of ulcers

Ulcers can arise in many parts of the gastrointestinal tract, from the esophagus all the way down to the rectum. In this chapter, we're primarily talking about ulcers of the stomach and duodenum (the first 12 inches of the small intestine).

The most common are called *peptic ulcers* or *PUD (peptic ulcers disease)*. Of these, *gastric ulcers* are ulcers that arise in the stomach, while *duodenal ulcers* usually strike in the first part of the duodenum. When viewed through a gastroscope (a long tube pushed through the mouth into the stomach and small intestine), peptic ulcers have a "hole" in the middle and are surrounded by a raised area of inflamed mucosal tissue.

Possible causes

Many factors can play a role in peptic ulcer disease. Sometimes there is a single cause, such as the use of cortisone.[1] Sometimes there are multiple causes, such as smoking and alcohol abuse. Recently, we have identified a new cause: a bacteria called *Helicobacter pylori*. Other factors that might contribute to ulcers include:

- Certain medicines, such as aspirin and other nonsteroidal anti-inflammatory drugs.
- Reserpine, a drug sometimes still used to lower elevated blood pressure and relieve anxiety.
- Liver disease and other chronic ailments.
- Emotional stress.
- Cancer.
- Hot and spicy foods and other dietary factors (in certain susceptible people).

Even though the latest medical information blames the germ *Helicobacter pylori*, I believe that most ulcers arise because of stress, alcohol, tobacco, drugs and other factors that disrupt the flow of oxygen to a small area of the mucosa (lining) of the stomach or duodenum. This results in inflammation and a loss of the mucosal barrier that normally protects the lining of the stomach or duodenal wall. Now the acid and pepsin (a stomach enzyme that starts digesting protein in the stomach) start penetrating the lining and "burn" their way deeper into the stomach or duodenal wall.

I believe that another major, overlooked cause of ulcers is physical stress. Stress ulcers usually arise quickly following severe traumatic injuries, massive burns and sepsis ("blood poisoning"). About 90 percent of all patients with major burns or massive injuries will develop stress ulcers, often multiple ulcers. I recall looking into the stomach of one patient who had 13 discrete stress ulcers, all of them bleeding.

Shock can also cause stress ulcers. "Shock" is a medical term used to describe a condition in which the blood pressure suddenly drops due to a problem with the circulatory system.

Possible complications and long-term effects

Untreated or poorly treated, ulcers can produce a variety of problems. They include perforation, penetration into other organs, hemorrhage, pain and obstruction.

Perforation. Ulcers can perforate—or eat a hole—all the way through the lining of the stomach or duodenum, allowing acid, pepsin and anything that happens to be there to flow into the abdominal cavity. This causes an inflammation of the lining of the abdominal cavity called peritonitis, which can leave you sick for a very long time or even kill you.

Penetration into other organs. The ulcer, whether it is gastric or duodenal, can penetrate into other organs. If, for example, the ulcer eats through the stomach into the pancreas, pancreatic enzymes may be dumped into the abdominal cavity, "digesting" everything in their path. This condition, called acute pancreatitis, may be fatal or it could leave you in chronic pain for the rest of your life.

Hemorrhage. If the ulcer penetrates a blood vessel, the patient may bleed internally (hemorrhage). If the bleeding is slow, the victim will suffer from anemia and all its various consequences, including weakness and increased susceptibility to infections. The patient may vomit blood, have black tarry stools or even have reddish-colored, loose stools. More serious cases of bleeding can cause a severe, possibly fatal drop in blood pressure.

Pain. Chronic pain is another possible complication of ulcers. One can be incapacitated for years by the pain, becoming depressed and anxious and suffering from a diminished quality of life.

Obstruction. When ulcers heal, scar tissue forms. If it forms in a narrow area, such as in the exit from the stomach (pylorus), the scar can cause a blockage that must be surgically removed.

Standard medical treatment

- Antacids to "neutralize" stomach acid.
- Medications called "H$_2$ blockers," such as Tagamet and Zantac, that reduce stomach acid. Also a newer class of acid reducers called Proton Pump Inhibitors, such as Prilosec.
- Carafate or other drugs that "coat" the ulcers, acting like an "internal Band-Aid."
- Antibiotics, in case of infection.
- Diet.
- Stress reduction.

Although the standard medications usually relieve the ulcer, it is not uncommon for the problem to return.

The latest treatment is "triple therapy" aimed at the *Helicobacter pylori*. This consists of two antibiotics called metronidazole (Flagyl) and tetracycline, plus bismuth subsalicylate (Pepto-Bismol). Early studies suggest that the "triple therapy" can eliminate the problem once and for all in up to 90 percent of all patients. Unfortunately, the two-week course of medication includes taking a lot of pills that produce unpleasant side effects. Many patients "drop out" of the therapy too soon, stopping their medications as soon as the pain begins to disappear. But some bacteria may remain in the GI tract and sooner or later the symptoms can start up again.

Now let's take a look at some of the many alternative treatments for ulcers. These are not all the possible therapies, because there are too many to investigate in a single chapter. Reading through these alternatives, however, will give you an idea of the many possibilities.

The information on alternative therapies is meant for educational purposes only. I am not endorsing any therapy or suggesting that you see any alternative practitioner. If you have or suspect that you have an ulcer, see your physician.

Acupuncture

Acupuncture can be used to help ulcers by returning the body's energy flow to normal. Some of the points that might be used include Conception Vessel 12 (between the navel and breastbone), Stomach 36 (on the lower leg), Spleen 6 (on the lower leg), Liver 3 (on the foot) and Spleen 4 (on the inside of the foot, about where the arch starts). Various points on the back may also be used.

Aromatherapy

Essential oils used for peptic ulcers may include:

- Chamomile (*Matricaria chamomilla*).

• Geranium (*Pelargonium odorantissimum*).

These or other essences may be used for nausea:

• Basil (*Ocimum basilicum*).

• Cardamom (*Elettaria cardamomum*).

• Fennel (*Foeniculum vulgare*).

• Lavender (*Lavandula officinalis*).

• Melissa (*Melissa officinalis*).

• Rose (*Rosa spp.*).

• Sandalwood (*Santalum album*).

The patient may be instructed to inhale the vapors from these oils as they rise from a bowl of water, to mix them in a base oil and use in massage, to wear as a perfume or to mix with the bath water. Treatment length will vary from practitioner to practitioner and according to the patient's condition.

Ayurvedic healing

According to Ayurvedic theory, ulcers are mainly due to stress and anxiety, although sour or spicy foods can be contributing factors. The acid that burns the lining of the stomach or small intestines indicates that ulcers are largely a Pitta (fire) disorder. Kapha (water) ulcers are caused by problems with the protective mucus lining of the stomach, in which case the proper amounts of acid normally present become dangerous. Vata (air) ulcers are related to nervousness and mental fatigue.

The treatment for all three types of ulcers includes a bland diet including herbs to help the body heal itself. These herbs include aloe, licorice, slippery elm and comfrey root. Additional treatment depends upon the humor in which the ulcer has manifested.

• When ulcers manifest in the Pitta (fire) humor, pain and burning are problems. Additional herbs, such as barberry, coptis, gentian and golden seal, are used.

• When ulcers manifest in the Vata (air) humor, pain, anxiety and a feeling of coldness are the major problems. Applying heat to the stomach can be helpful.

• Ulcers rarely manifest in the Kapha (water) humor because Kapha types are less likely to be anxious or worried. Ulcers that do manifest in the Kapha humor tend to produce nausea, a feeling of heaviness and dull pain. Cayenne, black pepper and other spices that encourage digestion are often indicated.

Color therapy

For duodenal ulcers, blue light will be directed to the abdomen and head. For gastric ulcers, yellow light will be directed to the abdomen and blue light to the head.

Blue has antibacterial properties, helping to fight the *Helicobacter pylori* bacteria that is believed to play a major role in ulcers. A cooling color, blue reduces nervousness. Blue foods include plums, grapes and blueberries. Blue metals and chemicals include lead, oxygen and tin.

Yellow assists with cleansing the digestive system and stimulating both the digestive and nervous systems. It also purifies the blood and helps to relieve depression. Yellow foods include bananas, banana squash, eggs, yellow cheese, yellow corn, yellow sweet potatoes, pineapples, lemons, grapefruit and butter. Yellow metals and chemicals include platinum and magnesium.

There are no standard protocols for dealing with ulcers, so treatment may vary from practitioner to practitioner. The time it takes to see results is not known with any certainty.

Folk medicine

Folk remedies for ulcers are many and varied. There are absolutely no standard protocols or recipes. Some of the folk medicines for ulcers and ulcer-related symptoms include:

- Drinking milk.
- Drinking cabbage juice.
- Eating raw or cooked plantains (relatives of the banana).

Herbal medicine

Herbalists use a wide variety of herbs to treat many diseases and symptoms. There is no standard herbal protocol for treating ulcers. Much depends upon the herbalist's individual background. Herbs typically used include:

- Chamomile (*Matricaria chamomilla*).
- Cloves (*Syzygium aromaticum*).
- Comfrey root (*Symphytum officinale*).
- Fennel (*Foeniculum officinale*).
- Ginger (*Zingiber officinalis*).
- Licorice (*Glycyrrhiza glabra*).
- Meadowsweet (*Filipendula ulmaria*).
- Passion flower (*Passiflora incarnata*).
- Peppermint (*Mentha piperita*).

- Slippery Elm *(Ulmus fulva)*.
- St. John's Wort (*Hypericum perforatum*).
- Sweet flag (*Acorus calamus*).
- Valerian (*Valeriana officinalis*).

Homeopathy

Most of the major homeopathic remedies may be used for ulcers, depending upon the patient's symptoms. Some remedies include:

- *Argentum nitricum*, which is indicated when the patient is fearful, impulsive and intolerant to heat. The stomach is distended with gas. Pain in the stomach is relieved by belching, cold, pressure and cold temperatures. The pain is made worse by warmth and stress.
- *Arsenicum album,* which is indicated when the patient is cold in temperature and fears death. His or her stomach pain may be burning but, oddly enough, it feels better when heat is applied. Symptoms are generally worse at night. The patient is very thirsty, although nauseated. The pain is worse late at night and if the patient is cold.
- *Lycopodium clavatum,* which is indicated when the patient is physically weak, irritable and lacking in self-confidence. The patient eats little and craves sweets. Gas and abdominal distention are present.
- *Nux vomica,* which is indicated when the patient is thin, irritable, cool in temperature and highly sensitive to light, noise, odor and the presence of people. The stomach often feels heavy and nausea is common. The pain feels better in the evening, after sleeping and with pressure. It is worse in the morning, after eating and in dry or cold weather.
- *Sepia,* which is indicated when the patient is worn out and thin, depressed, weepy and has a cold temperature. The patient suffers from diarrhea, vomiting, nausea, belching and bloating. The pain is better with heat and exercise. It is made worse by cold temperatures.

Although it is a basic principle of classical homeopathy to use only one remedy at a time, there is a trend among modern homeopaths toward using multiple remedies at once. Using the absolute minimum number of doses necessary is another principle of classical homeopathy. A second dose should not be given until the first has ceased to act, and no more remedies should be given when the body begins to heal. If the right remedy is used, two or three days should be enough to begin many long-term curative processes. If not, another remedy should be selected.

Nutritional therapy

Nutritional therapy uses foods and food components (such as vitamins and minerals) to prevent and treat a variety of illnesses. One of the main principles underlying nutritional therapy is that the body is able to heal itself in many cases, given the right "tools." The tools are, of course, all of the various vitamins, minerals, amino acids and other substances found in foods.

Nutritional healers may recommend a wide variety of vitamins, minerals and other nutrients for ulcers, including vitamins A, C and E and the mineral zinc.

Vitamin A. This "anti-infection" vitamin has helped people suffering from gastric ulcers. In a study conducted in the early 1980s, one group of chronic ulcer patients was given antacids only and a second group received antacids plus vitamin A. Four weeks later, 38 percent of the antacids-plus-vitamin-A group had completely recovered, compared to only 18 percent of the antacids-only group. This suggests the possibility that vitamin A more than doubles the effectiveness of antacids. (A third group in this study took antacids, vitamin A and medicine. The 36 percent recovery rate in this group was about the same as in the antacids-plus-vitamin-A group, suggesting that the addition of the ulcer medication was of no value.)[2]

Vitamin A may also help prevent the development of ulcers often seen with physical stress, such as burns or major injuries. Stress patients were divided into groups, one of which received vitamin A daily. Only 18 percent of those given the vitamin showed signs of developing stress ulcers, compared to over 60 percent of those who did not get the vitamin.[3] Vitamin A can be found in beef and chicken livers, milk and cheese.

Vitamin C. As far back as 1944, researchers noted that people suffering from chronic peptic ulcers tended to consume inadequate amounts of vitamin C.[4] Other studies have shown that low levels of vitamin C in the blood may be related to an increased risk of bleeding from peptic ulcers.[5] Good sources of Vitamin C include citrus fruits, cantaloupe and cabbage.

Vitamin E. A lack of vitamin E has been associated with ulcers. As far back as 1958, we've known that volunteers deliberately given a low-E diet tended to develop gastric ulcers.[6] Russian studies have shown that giving supplemental vitamin E helps to heal peptic ulcers. Vitamin E is found in wheat germ and nuts.

Zinc. The mineral zinc may protect against ulcers by preventing the damage to the tiny vessels of the circulatory system that has been associated with damage to the protective mucosal barrier of the stomach. When gastric ulcer patients were given either zinc sulfate or a placebo, the ulcers in the zinc group shrunk three times as much as did the ulcers in the placebo group.[7] Good sources of zinc include oysters, green peas and whole grains.

Eliminating harmful foods

A great many common foods and foodstuffs, including alcohol, caffeine, tea, decaffeinated coffee and sugar, have been associated with ulcers. Although these substances may not cause ulcers, they appear to increase the symptoms in some people. Thus, the nutritional healer will suggest that you stop consuming these and possibly other foods, then add them back to your diet one by one to see what happens.

Specific foods that aid in treating ulcers

Finally, the nutritional healer may suggest foods that have helped many ulcer patients. For many years, physicians have believed that a bland, low-fiber diet was best for ulcer patients. New research, however, suggests that the old dietary regimen was actually harmful and that a high-fiber diet is better.[8]

Studies and anecdotal evidence suggest that ulcers may be prevented or healed by bananas, cabbage, cinnamon, figs, ginger, licorice, seaweed and tea. Surprisingly, hot peppers may also help.

In a test of the effectiveness of cabbage against ulcers, 26 patients were given a milk diet plus concentrated cabbage juice; 19 patients were given the milk diet plus a placebo drink with no cabbage juice. Three weeks later, X-rays showed ulcers healing in 92 percent of the cabbage juice group, but only 32 percent of the placebo group.[9]

When selecting a nutritional healer, remember that there is no widely recognized school of nutritional therapy and no standards or agreed-upon training for nutritional healers.

Oriental medicine

Oriental medicine does not have a single approach to treating ulcers. Instead, the Oriental medicine doctor looks for the cause of the ailment and treats accordingly. With duodenal ulcers, for example, the underlying problem may have to do with excesses or deficiencies of energy in the stomach or spleen meridians. (Many ulcers are "cold" ulcers arising out of a lack of energy, whereas excess energy leads to "hot" ulcers.) In addition, the doctor will take a careful history and perform a thorough examination to make sure that the patient really has an ulcer, and not gall stones or problems with the pancreas or lungs. Once the problem has been correctly identified, the Oriental medicine physician will work to relieve the symptoms and strengthen the body with a combination of herbs and spices, diet, acupuncture, "ear acupuncture" and other therapies, as necessary.

Herbs and spices

Exactly which herbs and spices and the amount of each will depend upon the patient and his or her condition. For bleeding ulcers, herbal formulas such as *Yei Yao* and *Yunnan Piayao* may be recommended. For nonbleeding ulcers, *Sai Mei An* may be suggested.

Diet

Diet plays an important role in Oriental medicine. Foods are selected depending on their flavors, organic actions and other qualities, including energies. There are five food energies: hot, warm, neutral, cool and cold. (The energy has to do with the quality of the food, not its temperature. For example, foods with "cold" energy, such as lettuce and watermelon, increase the sensation of cold in the body, even when eaten hot.) In addition to a healthy diet, the Oriental medicine physician may recommend these foods specifically for ulcers:

- *Chinese cabbage,* a sweet vegetable that strengthens the stomach and large intestine.
- *Soybean oil,* used specifically for duodenal ulcers to lubricate the intestine.
- *Sesame oil,* a cool and sweet oil that detoxifies and lubricates the body.

Psychoneuroimmunology

Mind/body healers use positive affirmations to counteract the negative thoughts that have been contributing to the symptoms of ulcers. Affirmations are typically brief, positive statements that focus on how well one feels and on how the illness is being conquered. An affirmation to reduce ulcer pain might be worded as follows:

"My stomach is like a calm stream, its pleasant, cool waters flowing gently through."

Although ulcers may not be caused by stress, there does appear to be an association between angry thoughts and ulcer pain. Thus, the mind/body healer might use affirmations to help promote happiness:

"Like a child at play, I am delighted by everything I see, touch or do. Every day is an opportunity to find new wonders and do new things."

Reflexology

To treat ulcers, areas on the feet corresponding to the stomach and small intestines are manipulated. The stomach reflex areas are found in about the middle third of the bottom of the feet, on the inside. The small intestines reflex areas are found on the bottom of both feet, slightly beyond the heels (toward the toes), but not all the way to the middle.

Associated reflex areas will also be manipulated. These include the areas corresponding to the solar plexus, diaphragm and adrenal glands. The solar plexus reflex areas are below the balls of the feet, in the midline. The diaphragm reflex areas are across the bottom of the balls of the feet. The adrenal gland reflex areas are at approximately the middle of both feet, slightly to the inside.

Advice to ulcer patients

Although many of my patients have had success with the following program, I only use the general guidelines discussed below after reviewing a patient's personal and medical history, performing a thorough examination and evaluating the laboratory studies to make sure that the program will be beneficial. Please see your own physician before embarking on any treatment program for ulcers.

The first step in treating ulcers is to make the right diagnosis. With a careful review of the patient's personal and medical history, physical examination and appropriate studies, we can learn:

- Whether this is a new (acute) ulcer that has appeared or an older (recurrent) ulcer that has been reactivated.
- Whether or not scar tissue left by an ulcer has deformed the stomach or duodenum.
- If the ulcer is penetrating or "eating" its way through the stomach or intestinal lining.
- How big the ulcer is. This is important, because large stomach ulcers (greater than one inch or so in diameter) are more often malignant than are smaller ones. With X-rays of the stomach, a visual inspection by gastroscopy (which involves pushing a tube into the stomach via the mouth) and a biopsy, we can distinguish between benign and malignant ulcers with a 95 percent confidence rate.

Some 14,000 Americans die of gastric cancer every year, and the early signs of stomach cancer can be mistaken for an ulcer. That's one reason it is important to quickly diagnose stomach problems. Once the diagnosis of an ulcer has been made, there are several steps that can help most people:

1. Adopt a healthful diet. Although many medical authorities say that diet is not important for the healing of peptic ulcer disease, I believe it is very important to adopt a diet high in fiber and complex carbohydrates, low in fat and with moderate amounts of protein.
2. Avoid hot and spicy foods, as well as any others that cause you problems.
3. Stop smoking immediately and stay away from smoky areas, as second-hand smoke is also harmful. Cigarette smoke can interfere with healing and possibly encourage the return of ulcers.
4. Avoid alcohol and caffeine.
5. Learn how to recognize and relieve the signs of stress. When I'm faced with a stressful situation, I ask myself, "Is this worth dying for?" If the answer is no, I walk away.
6. Use medications, as necessary, to relieve the symptoms and help the ulcer heal.
7. Adopt preventive measures to help ward off future ulcers.
8. Have your physician perform a careful follow-up to make sure that any recurring malignancies or ulcers are caught immediately.

Let's take a closer look at items 6 and 7, medications and preventive measures.

Ulcer medications

Twenty years ago, we treated ulcers with diet, antacids and anticholinergic drugs (used to reduce acid and relax the intestine). Today there is more emphasis on the latest medications, but I believe that antacids are not outmoded. They still relieve pain and may still be used. (Take at least two hours after meals, at bedtime and when ulcer pain strikes.)

For ulcer pain, a number of drugs called "H-2 Antagonists" can help by reducing the secretion of acid. One of these H-2 Antagonists, cimetidine (Tagamet) was, I believe, the first drug to reach the billion-dollar sales mark. Since then, others such as Zantac, Pepsid and Axid have become available. If you are taking an H-2 Antagonist, discuss its use carefully with your physician. H-2s may affect the levels of other medications, such as theophylline (used in asthma), phenytoin (used to prevent convulsions) and warfarin (Coumadin, used to thin out the blood).

Another medication, sulcrafate (Carafate), has been shown to be as effective as the H-2 blockers in healing peptic ulcers. It is especially effective in duodenal ulcers. And there are newer and apparently more effective medications, such as omeprazole (Prilosec), which greatly reduce the amount of gastric acid made by the parietal cells of the stomach. This drug is only for short-term use.

Helping to prevent future ulcers

Ulcers can strike more than once. Duodenal ulcers, especially, seem to come back time and time again. That's why all peptic ulcer disease patients should adopt preventive measures. These include:

- An immune-boosting diet based on fresh vegetables and fruits, plus plenty of whole grains and smaller amounts of low-fat dairy products, lean meat and poultry. Take care, however, to avoid any foods that cause you pain or other problems. There's no hard-and-fast rule, so let your body be your guide. If the food bothers you, don't eat it.

  I may suggest to my patients that they try bananas, cabbage, cinnamon, figs, ginger, licorice, seaweed, green tea and other foods and drinks that have helped many other ulcer patients.

- Supplements, such as the 4 ACES. The 4 ACES are vitamin A as beta carotene, vitamin C, vitamin E (alpha tocopherol) and the mineral selenium. Along with the mineral zinc, the 4 ACES help to maintain general health. Depending upon the patient's condition, I may recommend 25,000 mg of beta carotene, 1,000 mg of vitamin C twice a day, 200 IU of vitamin E and 100 micrograms (mcg) of selenium.

- Lifestyle changes to reduce stress. Working together, my patients and I are often able to find ways to simplify their lives. Sometimes it's simple things, like not throwing the big dinner parties that make you a nervous wreck. Other times the changes are bigger and more daring, like finding a new job or passing up a promotion. Yes, money and career are important, but they pale in comparison to the terrible pain a little ulcer can produce.

- Exercise to reduce the effects of stress. Many of my patients have found that a regular exercise program seems to "dissolve" much of their stress (along with the extra pounds). And as they get into shape, they develop pride in their new physiques. Exercise can also increase the production of endorphins, the natural "morphine within" that can help to relieve certain types of pain and depression.

- Learn to look at life with optimism and serenity. No matter what the cause of an ulcer, its symptoms are undoubtedly made worse by anger and frustration. These and other negative feelings trigger the "stress response" that floods the body with high-voltage chemicals that weaken our resistance to a variety of diseases and make every existing problem seem worse.

Although studies have not yet proven that optimism and serenity can cure ulcers, many years of experience as a physician has taught me that overall, happy, optimistic people tend to do better than unhappy, angry patients. As far as I'm concerned, positive thoughts are a very good medicine.

---

[1]   Cortisone is a group of drugs used to treat allergies, inflammation and autoimmune diseases, such as Lupus Erythematosis. Prednisone is the most commonly used cortisone.

[2]   Patty, E., et al. Controlled trial of vitamin A in gastric ulcer. Letter. *Lancet,* 2:876, 1982.

[3]   Chernow, M.S., et al. Stress ulcer: A preventable disease. *J Trauma,* 12:831, 1972.

[4]   Riggs, H.E., et al. *JAMA,* 124:639, 1944.

[5]   Dubey, S.S., et al. Ascorbic acid, dehydroascorbic acid, glutathione and histamine in peptic ulcer. *Indian J Med Res,* 76:859-62, 1982. Russell, R.L., et al. Ascorbic acid levels in leukocytes of patients with gastrointestinal hemorrhage. *Lancet,* 2:603-6, 1968. Crescenzo, V.M., Cayer, D. Plasma vitamin C levels in patients with peptic ulcer. Response to oral load of ascorbic acid. *Gastroenterology,* 8:755-61, 1947.

[6]   Horwitt, M.K. *Fed Proc,* 18:530, 1959. Horwitt, M.K. *Fed Proc,* 17:245, 1958.

[7]   Frommer, D.J. The healing of gastric ulcers by zinc sulfate. *Med J Aust,* 2:793-6, 1975.

[8]   Welsh, J.D. Diet therapy of peptic ulcer disease. *Gastroenterology,* 72:740-45, 1977. Graham, D.Y., et al. Spicy food and the stomach: Evaluation by videoendoscopy. *JAMA,* 260(23):3473-75, 1988.

[9]   Cheney, G. *California Med,* January, 1956.

Conclusion

I'm a physician, an Internist and a Cardiologist trained in traditional Western medicine. I'm proud to say that medical science has made tremendous strides in the past century, developing medicines and treatments that have conquered many disabling conditions and killer diseases of the past. Emerging new techniques, such as gene therapy and imaging ("seeing into") the human body, will help us to do even more for our patients.

But proud as we doctors are of our accomplishments, we must remember that we hold only a part of the solution to the health puzzle. When I was in medical school back in the 1950s, it was considered "unethical" for physicians to refer patients to chiropractors. Believe it or not, a doctor could literally be thrown out of the local medical society for even socializing with chiropractors or other "frauds." Since that time, we've come to realize that not everyone who disagrees with traditional approaches is a fraud, and we are slowly recognizing the many helpful ideas that have been developed in the alternative realm. The proponents of nutritional therapy and the mind-body connection, to name just two alternative approaches, have made great strides, documenting successes and pushing themselves into the mainstream. Other alternatives, such as chiropractic, have proven themselves to be even better than traditional medicine in some aspects.

I look forward to the day when the successful ideas and tools of all disciplines—both traditional and alternative—will be used by health professionals, for then we will best serve our patients. I believe that day is coming soon.

Other conditions

Unfortunately, space limitations prevent me from taking an in-depth look at all of the many diseases and disorders that send people to their doctors' offices. So let's take a brief look at 20 common conditions, plus the standard and alternative treatments for each.

The following information is offered for educational purposes only and is not intended as a recommendation. If you are ill, see your physician immediately.

Acne

Also known as pimples and "zits," acne consists of bumps on the skin caused by blockages of the sebaceous glands, which are located at the base of each hair follicle. The glands keeps producing fluid, but the fluid cannot escape. Pressured, the glands expand, pushing on the skin above and causing a pimple. The gland may also become infected.

Acne is mostly seen in adolescents, although women in the pre-menstrual or mid-menstrual cycles may develop pimples related to hormones. Stress, oral contraceptives and some types of diets can also cause acne. Although acne itself is not usually dangerous, in some cases it may become severely infected, leaving scars and pits, and require a great deal of medical attention. In addition, the psychological consequences of acne may be great.

Physicians offer a slew of oral medications, creams, lotions and ointments. Some people with severe scaring may undergo a surgical treatment called *dermabrasion*. Alternative therapies used include:

- Aromatherapy: Bergamot (Monarda didyma), cedarwood (Juniperus virginiana), juniper (Juniperus communis), lavender (Lavandula officinalis).
- *Herbology:* Garlic *(Allium sativum)*, Echinacea *(Echinacea angustifolia)*, myrrh *(Commiphora myrrha)*, nettles *(Urtica urens)*, thyme *(Thymus vulgaris)*.
- *Homeopathic remedies*: *Antimonium crudum, Ledum palustre,* sulfur.

• *Nutrition:* Vitamins B6 and B12; selenium; zinc; a low-fat, high-fiber diet. Good sources of these vitamins and minerals are: B6—barley, salmon and whole grains; B12—fish, cheese and eggs; selenium—carrots, cabbage and onions; zinc—oysters, whole grains and split peas.

I recommend antioxidants, especially vitamin A. One of the medicines commonly used for acne, Retin-A, is derived from vitamin A. *Warning:* Since this vitamin can be toxic, vitamin A therapy should be undertaken only under the supervision of a physician. Women who are pregnant or plan to get pregnant should not use Retin-A without checking with their physicians, because it may cause birth defects. Food sources of vitamin A include beef and chicken livers, milk and cheese.

In addition, vitamin E , folic acid, zinc and high chromium yeast can be helpful. For acne flareups that come during PMS, vitamin B6 seems to help. Do not, however, expect acne that comes at other times to be helped by B6. Although current thinking tends to discount the role of diet, I have had cases in which acne cleared up when patients stopped eating chocolate, milk and other foods, and switched to a low-fat, high complex carbohydrate diet. Vitamin E can be found in wheat germ, nuts and green beans.

Finally, a gel containing 5 percent benzoyl peroxide, put on the face nightly after washing with a nonmedicated soap, can be helpful.

Alcoholism

The simple definition of alcoholism is excessive drinking of alcohol, leading to physiological and psychological dependence on the drug. This, in turn, may prompt chronic diseases, such as stomach inflammations, ulcers, brain problems, fatty liver and, later, cirrhosis of the liver. Alcoholism can also disrupt a person's family life, interpersonal relationships and ability to work.

In the early stages of alcoholism, people become anxious easily, miss days at work and suffer from insomnia and nightmares. They suffer from Monday morning hangovers, start drinking early in the day, hide their alcohol from family and friends, and feel upset and guilty when told that they are drinking too much. As alcoholism progresses, problem drinkers may suffer from "blackouts," have abnormal liver tests, numbness and tingling of the hands, a loss of sexual interest and a decreased ability to have an erection (alcohol "feminizes" men by harming the testicles and reducing male hormones). Problems associated with later stages of alcoholism include cardiomyopathy (a disease of the heart muscle), enlargement of the liver, a fullness of the upper abdomen, swelling of the feet, sweats, tremors, rapid heart beats and confusion. They may even hallucinate if they don't get their alcohol for a day or so. I remember, as a young physician at the Los

Angeles County Hospital, entire floors filled with end-stage (terminal) alcoholism patients tied down to their beds, with bloated bellies and terribly thin arms and legs.

Doctors sometimes use medicines, such as Antabuse, that will make alcoholics very sick if they start drinking again. However, I have not found this to be of any value. Doctors may also give injections of various vitamins and prescribe a nutritious diet. Standard medical treatment also includes counseling, such as Alcoholics Anonymous. Many alternative therapies used for alcoholism include:

- *Aromatherapy:* Fennel *(Foeniculum vulgare)*, rose *(Rosa damascena)*, myrrh *(Commiphora myrrha)*, rosemary *(Rosmarinus officinalis)*.
- *Ayurveda:* Drinking excess alcohol "heats" the body by increasing the Pitta (fire), leading to various Pitta disorders and liver damage. Aloe, gotu kola *(Centella asiatica)*, turmeric *(Curcuma longa)*, barberry *(Berberis spp.)*, passion flower *(Passiflora incarnata)*, hops *(Humulus lupulus)* and other herbs are used to detoxify and balance the liver and blood and to reduce the body's fire.
- *Nutrition:* Vitamin A, B-complex, vitamin C, vitamin E, calcium, magnesium, phosphorus, selenium and choline.

I recommend the B-complex, including folic acid, vitamins C and E, magnesium, potassium, zinc and calcium. (Good nutrition is vital, because many alcoholics eat very poor diets.) An amino acid called glutamine is also useful. So is another amino acid named L-carnitine, which helps to slow the fattening of the liver. The mineral selenium, used for the enzyme glutathione peroxidase, also helps to protect the liver against damage. DLPA (dl-phenylalanine) is very helpful to raise endorphin levels. Finally, the low-fat, low-cholesterol diet based on fresh vegetables, fruits and whole grains is important to make sure that the person is getting plenty of nutrients.

For acute alcoholism, an intravenous treatment including vitamins C and B-complex, calcium and magnesium, can detoxify people quickly.

Alzheimer's disease

Alzheimer's disease is a terrible, devastating condition in which the brain cells degenerate much more rapidly than normal. We all lose brain cells as we age and can afford to lose a great many before we have any difficulties. But with Alzheimer's, the loss is too great and the mind fails. (Although commonly associated with aging, an aggressive, rapidly developing form may strike people ages 35 to 45.)

Alzheimer's causes memory problems and intellectual and emotional dysfunction. It leads to complete physical breakdown, difficulty in swallowing, loss of weight and many other problems. Symptoms often begin with an inability to remember events, difficulty in performing common chores, poor judgment and impulsivity. In later stages, victims may have difficulty recognizing family members, feeding themselves and so on. They suffer from insomnia, anxiety and irritability. In advanced stages, Alzheimer's patients cannot care for themselves, control their bladders or bowels or recognize anybody.

I may recommend alpha-lipoic acid, one of the strongest known antioxidants, for its ability to prevent the degeneration of neurons (brains cells). To help keep the brain sharp and increase the flow of blood, I may suggest pycnogenol, coenzyme Q10, ginkgo biloba and the 4 ACES (vitamin A in the form of beta carotene, vitamins C and E and the mineral selenium). In addition, DLPA (dl-phenylalanine) helps to delay the progression into the more serious symptoms.

There are some newer brain medications that appear to slow the progression of the disease, including piracetam (Nootropil) and Deprenyl (sold as Eldepryl in the United States).

Anorexia

Anorexia nervosa is a psychologically based eating disorder driven by the victims' conviction that they are fat and must lose weight. They eat very little, lose weight and keep on dieting, no matter how slim they become. Twenty years ago, a five-foot-two woman weighing 95 pounds came to my office asking me to put her on a weight loss diet. She had the typical "doll" look, with arms and legs that looked like match sticks. Besides not eating, she was taking 100 laxative tablets a day to help keep her weight down.

More women than men are anorexic, especially adolescents and young adults. Usually they lose about 25 percent of their body weight, but they have no specific illness. They are depressed but often don't realize it. Although anorexics are very thin and eat little, they tend to have a great deal of energy. If not treated, up to 25 percent of those with anorexia nervosa will die. That's why it's important to pull out all the stops, apply all therapies, do whatever it takes to help them realize that they are not fat and they must eat. Standard treatment for anorexics includes antidepressants, "refeeding" programs and psychological counseling. Alternative therapies used for anorexia include:

- *Ayurveda:* Anorexia is believed to be an emotional disease that damages the digestive fire, making it difficult or impossible to retain food in the stomach. Fear, insomnia and chest pain indicate that the problem is manifesting in the Vata (air) humor, while severe weight loss suggests the problem is in the Kapha (water) humor. A mild diet is used along with herbs and spices to calm the nerves and encourage digestion. These include cardamom *(Elettaria cardamomum)*, fresh ginger *(Zingiber officinale)*, nutmeg *(Myristica fragrans)*, valerian *(Valeriana officinalis)* and sandalwood *(Santalum album)*. Massage oils applied to the head and feet are also helpful.

- *Homeopathic remedies: Antimonium crudum, Bryonia alba, Carbo vegetabilis, Ipecacuanha, Phosphorus, Sepia.*

I believe that psychological counseling is a must. DLPA (dl-phenylalanine) is often indicated, since so many anorexics are depressed. All-around good nutrition is important, but since the victims are reluctant to eat, I give them intravenous (IV) or intramuscular injections of vitamins and other nutrients.

Anxiety

Anxiety and depression are perhaps the most common thing doctors deal with in primary and internal medicine, and the most common mental health problem.

Anxiety is a nonspecific feeling of discomfort, dread, danger or fear. There are two types of anxiety. *Situational* anxiety is caused by fear of a situation, such as a test or performance review. Situational anxiety tends to dissipate when the situation has passed. *Generalized* anxiety is not tied to specific situations and may last six months or more.

Some of the symptoms of anxiety that send people to their doctors include headaches, neck aches, backaches, muscle tension, irritability, sleeplessness, palpitations, rapid heart action, difficulty breathing, hoarseness, difficulty in swallowing, dry mouth, sexual problems, memory problems and difficulty in concentration. The most common symptom of anxiety is fatigue. The standard medical treatment (high-power medicines such as Xanax) should be used only for a short while because of the possible side effects. Alternative therapies include:

- *Aromatherapy:* Benzoin *(Styrax benzoin)*, chamomile *(Matricaria chamomilla)*, camphor *(Cinnamomum camphora)*, cypress *(Cupressus sempervirens)*, jasmine *(Jasminum officinale)*, lavender *(Lavandula officinalis)*, melissa *(Melissa officinalis)*, patchouli *(Pogostemon patchouli)* and ylang-ylang *(Cananga odorata)*.
- *Herbology:* Pasque flower *(Anemone pulsatilla)*, skullcap *(Scutellaria lateriflora)* and vervain *(Verbena officinalis)*.
- *Homeopathic remedies:* Borax, lachesis, *Natrum muriaticum*, phosphorus and pulsatilla.

I prefer "talk" therapy and cognitive therapy (which helps them to understand that there is actually little reason to worry). To relieve the anxiety, I often suggest a homeopathic remedy called L.72 Anti-Anxiety remedy and the herbs Kava kava and valerian.

Carpal tunnel syndrome

A "modern" problem related to the use of computers, automatic scanners and other modern machinery and jobs, carpal tunnel syndrome is a nerve disorder related to the repetitive use of the wrist and fingers. Typically, activities that cause the problem force the fingers to move while the wrist is held bent. The median nerve that runs through the center of the wrist (on the palm side) becomes irritated, inflamed or swollen, producing pain or tingling of the hands (especially the thumb and first three fingers). A broken bone or dislocated wrist can cause similar problems. I've seen carpal tunnel associated with obesity, hypothyroidism, diabetes and pregnancy. Symptoms include weakness, stiffness and cramping of the hands, difficulty making a fist, a burning sensation in the involved fingers, shooting pains, numbness and tingling that goes from the wrist down to the involved fingers.

Standard medical treatment includes anti-inflammatory medications, a splint, surgery and physical therapy. I always look for an underlying cause. If the problem is due to hypothyroidism, I treat it with thyroid medication. If the patient is obese, I help him or her lose weight. Vitamin B6 (50 mg) twice a day works well. (Use no more than 50 mg of B6, two to three times a day.)

Cataracts

A cataract is a "clouding" or "crystallization" of the lens of the eye. The lens may be damaged by free radicals, which are caused by solar radiation, smog, infrared light, various chemicals, certain medications, eye injury, the high blood sugar found in diabetes and other factors. Cataracts, which may form in one or both eyes, can occur at any age but are more common as we get older, because the lens has had more time to be exposed to free radicals and oxidative stress. Symptoms include poor, blurred and sometimes double vision. If your vision is blurred when exposed to bright light (which often happens when driving at night), think about having your eyes checked for cataracts.

The standard treatment is surgical removal of the lens and replacement with an implant.

As with other diseases, I believe that prevention is the best cure. To help guard against free radicals and oxidative damage to the eyes, I may recommend folic acid, vitamins B1, C and E, selenium, zinc, bioflavonoids, coenzyme Q10, proanthocyanidins, carotenoids and taurine to my patients, along with a low-sugar diet based on fresh vegetables and fruit. I may also suggest alpha lipoic acid (Alpha Lipotene), one of the most powerful antioxidants known.

Colds

The throat, nose, wind pipe, sinuses and voice box are usually affected by this viral infection of the upper respiratory tract. The most common symptoms are a stuffy nose with a white or watery discharge, hoarseness of the voice and a scratchy or sore throat. There may be a mild fever along with fatigue, loss of appetite and a general "blah" feeling. A couple hundred viruses can cause a cold. It's easily spread from person to person by hands and by droplets from the mouth or nose. Standard medical treatment for colds consists of drops or sprays for the nose, antihistamines, aspirin and bed rest. Many alternative therapies are used, including:

- *Aromatherapy:* Black pepper *(Piper nigrum)*, eucalyptus *(Eucalyptus globulus)*, marjoram *(Origanum marjorana)*, peppermint *(Mentha piperita)*, rosemary *(Rosmarinus officinalis).*
- *Herbology:* Yarrow *(Achillea millefolium)*, ginger *(Zingiber officinale)*, peppermint *(Mentha piperata)*, elder flower *(Sambucus nigra).*
- *Homeopathic remedies: Aconitum napellus, Dulcamara, Gelsemium, Pulsatilla.*

I may recommend Sambucol as soon as the first symptoms strike. Sambucol is an herbal product made from extracts of black elderberries *(Sambucus nigra)* and raspberries *(Rubus idaeus)*. (See the section on "Influenza" for more on Sambucol.) I may also suggest drinking about a quart of orange juice a day as well as two quarts of regular water. Several thousand mg of vitamin C, two to three times a day, and herbs such as echinacea and golden seal help to keep the body's defenses strong.

Constipation

Many of us have had the infrequent but difficult and painful bowel movements characteristic of constipation. Symptoms include straining to move the bowels, inability to move the bowels for a prolonged period of time and possibly pain and bleeding. Constipation can be a mild problem that resolves on its own, or it can progress, possibly causing a bowel obstruction.

The problem is usually caused by a low-fiber, low-fluid diet. It often occurs in older people who are inactive and depressed and who eat poorly. There are other causes, including diseases such as hypercalcemia (too much calcium in the blood) and hypothyroidism. A sore in the anus that discourages bowel movements by making them painful can bring on constipation. Many prescription drugs, such as Norpace for the heart and Prozac for depression, can bring on constipation.

Treatment and prevention involves a high-fiber diet, including four or more vegetables per day, at least three pieces of fruit, peas, beans and lentils and at least eight glasses of water. Alternative therapies include:

- *Aromatherapy:* Black pepper *(Piper nigrum)*, fennel *(Foeniculum vulgare)*, marjoram *(Origanum marjorana)*.

- *Herbology:* Psylium *(Plantago psyllium)*, rhubarb.

- *Homeopathic remedies*: *Alumina, Bryonia alba, Graphites, Silicea,* sulfur.

- *Nutrition:* Folic acid, pantothenic acid, magnesium, a high-fiber diet. Food sources of these vitamins and minerals are: folic acid—apricots and leafy green vegetables; pantothenic acid—liver, eggs and avocado; magnesium—dried beans, garlic and collard greens.

Depression

A very serious problem that may afflict at least one of 10 Americans at some point in their lives, depression is a feeling of unhappiness, lack of hope and loss of interest in normal activities, in others and perhaps in life itself.

Symptoms of depression include fatigue, headaches, chest pains, loss of interest in sex, loss of erectile ability in males, loss of appetite or overeating, constipation, listlessness, boredom, insomnia, hypersomnia (sleeping more than usual but still feeling tired) and various aches and pains. Depressed people may feel that they're not needed or appreciated, and so they isolate themselves from others.

Standard treatment for depression has improved quite a bit. The newest drugs, such as Zoloft, Paxil and Prozac, work well. Alternative therapies include:

- *Aromatherapy:* Bergamot *(Monarda didyma)*, chamomile *(Matricaria chamomilla)*, clary *(Salvia sclarea)*, jasmine *(Jasminum officinale)*, lavender *(Lavandula officinalis)*, neroli *(Citrus aurantium)*, sandalwood *(Santalum album)*, ylang-ylang *(Cananga odorata)*.

- *Herbology:* Basil *(Ocimum basilicum)*, borage *(Borago officinalis)*, damiana *(Turnera diffusa)*, lavender *(Lavandula officinalis)*, lemon balm *(Melissa officinalis)*, St. John's Wort *(Hypericum perforatum)*, skullcap *(Scutellaria laterifolia)*.

- *Homeopathic remedies: Aconitum napellus, Aurum metallicum, Ignatia, Pulsatilla, Rhus toxicodendrom, Sepia.*

I believe that a compassionate, understanding therapist is very important. For severe depression, psychotherapy is also helpful and hospitalization may be required in some cases.

Most depression is treated by general doctors. The key is to gain the patients' trust and get them to improve their diet, exercise, take helpful herbs (such as St. John's Wort) and do other things that improve their general health while giving them a sense of control over their lives. I've also had success using the amino acid DLPA (dl-phenylalanine) as part of the treatment for many cases of depression.

Diabetes

Diabetes mellitus Type I, also called insulin dependent diabetes, is a metabolic disease in which the body does not produce enough insulin. The condition, which used to be called juvenile diabetes, generally begins before the age of 30.

With diabetes mellitus Type II, also called noninsulin dependent, the body can make insulin, but the body cells become resistant to the insulin due to obesity, age, pregnancy, certain drugs (such as contraceptives or cortisone) and other factors.

The most common symptoms of diabetes are extreme thirst and urination, fatigue and overeating coupled with weight loss. The patient may suffer from an increased tendency toward infections, especially of the urinary tract. Diabetic women may suffer from more yeast infections of the vagina. Long-term complications include ulcers and gangrene of the feet (possibly leading to amputation) and an increased risk of heart attack, stroke, kidney failure, blindness and other problems.

The standard medical treatment for Type I is a life-long series of self-administered insulin shots, careful adherence to a special diet, exercise and very strict medical control. For Type II, diet, weight loss, exercise and possibly oral medicines lower the blood sugar. In advanced Type II cases, insulin "pushes" the sugar into the cells. Diabetics must give special care to their feet, because they are at risk of ulceration, gangrene and amputation. Alternative therapies include:

- *Aromatherapy.* Eucalyptus *(Eucalyptus globulus)*, juniper *(Juniperus communis)*.
- *Ayurveda.* Diabetes is believed to be caused by an imbalance in the body's water system. In the early stages, it may be a Kapha (water) disorder, related to obesity. Excess Pitta (fire) can also prompt diabetes by disturbing the functions of the liver and pancreas. Chronic diabetes is often a Vata (air) disturbance in which excess Vata has damaged the pancreas. The general treatment for diabetes includes diet, herbs, spices, exercise and meditation, as well as wearing rings made from stones such as yellow sapphire or yellow topaz.

• *Nutrition.* Pectin, niacin, thiamin, vitamin B6, vitamin C, calcium, chromium, copper, magnesium, manganese, phosphorus, potassium, zinc, bioflavonoids, biotin, coenzyme Q10 and inositol. Also, remain at ideal weight and eat a low-fat, high-plant fiber diet. A few food sources for these nutrients are: Pectin—apples and grapefruit; niacin—almonds, chicken, fish and whole grains; vitamin B6—bananas, cantaloupe, beans and sweet potatoes; vitamin C—broccoli, Brussels sprouts, grapefruit and parsley; calcium—cantaloupe, carrots, garlic and green beans; chromium—apples, oranges and spinach; copper—beans and peas; magnesium—barley, carrots and onions; manganese—blueberries, pineapples and whole-grain rice; phosphorus—fish, nuts and seeds; potassium—bananas, carrots, tomatoes and green leafy vegetables; zinc—oysters, cinnamon and milk; bioflavonoids—oranges, grapefruit and tangerines; biotin—beans, corn and peas; coenzyme Q10—sardines and mackerel; inositol—bananas, corn, peas and peanuts.

I believe that antioxidants are helpful for both types of the disease in order to prevent the breakdown of body tissue that occurs as a result of high blood sugar.

Alpha-lipoic acid is one of the most powerful of the antioxidants. It helps to normalize blood sugar and protects the body against the damage caused by high blood sugar. Alpha-lipoic acid "quenches" the free radicals that cause the oxidative stress that, in diabetics, can damage the pancreas (which makes insulin), eyes and other parts of the body. One of alpha-lipoic's great benefits for diabetes is its ability to reduce glycation (the combination of sugar with proteins of the arteries that damages the tiny blood vessels of the heart, eyes, kidneys and other parts of the body). Alpha-lipoic acid increases sugar transport, "moving" it so that it doesn't "stick" and cause damage. It also improves the nerve function caused by diabetic neuropathy.

In addition, I often put my diabetic patients on a low-fat, low-sugar diet based on fresh vegetables and whole grains, and I recommend beta carotene, vitamins C and E, selenium and other supplements. I suggest that they exercise often and learn how to recognize and defuse stress.

Diarrhea

Diarrhea produces frequent, watery, loose, unformed bowel movements. It is not a disease. Rather, it is a symptom of one or more diseases. Most common causes are food allergies, food poisoning, bacterial or viral infections of the intestine, and diseases such as influenza, Crohn's Disease, ulcerative colitis and Irritable Bowel Syndrome. A less common cause of diarrhea is cancer. Radiation treatment for cancer can cause diarrhea, as can laxatives, antacids, antibiotics and other medications. In many cases, the diarrhea is uncomfortable but clears up by itself or with minor treatment.

Standard medical treatment includes medication such as Immodium, Lomotil and antispasmodics such as Bentyl. Alternative therapies include:

- *Aromatherapy.* Black pepper *(Piper nigrum)*, camphor *(Cinnamomum camphora)*, neroli *(Citrus aurantium)*, peppermint *(Mentha piperita)*, sandalwood *(Santalum album)*.
- *Herbology.* Cranesbill *(Geranium maculatum)*, bayberry *(Myrica cerifera)*, oak bark *(Quercus robur)*, meadowsweet *(Filipendula ulmaria)*.
- *Homeopathic remedies. Chamomilla, China officinalis, Colocynthis, Podorphyllum.*
- *Nutrition.* Folic acid, niacin, vitamins A, B12, C and K, magnesium, potassium and zinc. You'll find the nutrients in these and other foods: Folic acid—beans, spinach and walnuts; niacin—almonds, chicken, fish and whole grains; vitamin A—milk, cheese and beef and chicken liver; vitamin B12—brook trout, salmon, eggs and yogurt; vitamin C—broccoli, Brussels sprouts, grapefruit and parsley; vitamin K—broccoli, lettuce and turnip greens; magnesium—barley, carrots and onions; potassium—bananas, carrots, tomatoes and green leafy vegetables; zinc—oysters, cinnamon and milk.

I explain to my patients that it is important to look for and treat the underlying cause of the problem. As for the diarrhea itself, you want to replace the fluids, sodium, potassium, magnesium and electrolytes lost with the watery bowel movements. For acute diarrhea, I may recommend drinking a sugary water solution containing sodium chloride (salt), sodium bicarbonate, potassium and magnesium. Rest is helpful, as is avoiding milk and dairy products, junk foods, high-fat foods, caffeine, alcohol and highly seasoned foods. In many cases, bismuth subsalicylate (Pepto Bismol) takes care of the problem.

Eczema

Eczema is a chronic, allergic skin disorder involving many parts of the body, especially the hands, face and back of the neck. Symptoms include itching, blistering and oozing from the blisters. At a later stage, the skin gets thickened and scaly from the ongoing irritation. Homemakers and others who work with harsh chemicals, soaps, detergents and cleansers have a greater risk of developing eczema.

Sometimes we can identify the cause of the problem. (When I was young, my mother often had scaly, itching skin on her hands due to the harsh soaps used back then.) Certain foods may cause eczema, including milk, seafood, wheat and eggs. Ironically, some lotions sold for skin problems can produce the symptoms, as can various medicines doctors prescribe for skin care. Dyes and other chemicals may be the culprits. In some people, very hot or cold weather can worsen the symptoms. Stress, in my opinion, always seems to make it worse.

Standard medical treatment includes a variety of ointments, antihistamines to cut down on itching, sedatives or tranquilizers if itching and pain are too bad, cortisone ointments that reduce inflammation and antibiotics for secondary infections. Alternative therapies include:

- *Aromatherapy.* Bergamot *(Monarda didyma)*, hyssop *(Hyssopus officinalis)*, juniper *(Juniperus communis)*, lavender *(Lavandula officinalis)*.
- *Herbology.* Burdock *(Arctium lappa)*, evening primrose *(Oenothera lamarkiana)*, chickweed *(Stellaria media)*, marigold *(Tagetes erecta)*, St. John's Wort *(Hypericum perforatum)*, marshmallow root *(Althaea officinalis)*. Also chamomile *(Matricaria chamomilla)* and skullcap *(Scutellaria laterifolia)* as an infusion.
- *Homeopathic remedies.* Antimonium crudum, Calcarea carbonica-ostrearum, Mezereum, Psorinum.
- *Nutrition.* Vitamin A, vitamin C, selenium, zinc and omega-3 fatty acids. These nutrients are in many foods, including: Vitamin A—milk, cheese and chicken liver; vitamin C—okra, raspberries, strawberries and green peas; selenium—chicken, garlic, whole-grain rice and wheat; omega-3 fatty acids— salmon, sardines, mackerel and other fish.

It's important to examine the diet, possibly removing the wheat, cow's products, corn and other items that may provoke symptoms. In some people, fruit may be the culprit. The family history should also be checked for allergies.

Zinc is one of the most helpful substances for eczema. Vitamins E, A and B6, magnesium, alpha-lipoic acid and essential fatty acids, such as evening primrose oil, are also useful. For cracked hands, I often suggest a marigold gel called Alpine Herb or Propolis Ointment, which is based on an antibiotic produced by bees. Both are available through BioHealth in Irvine, Calif.

Hemorrhoids

Also known as piles, hemorrhoids are caused by blood clots that form in the small veins either outside or just inside the anal opening.

The ones on the outside of the opening are called external hemorrhoids, while the others are referred to as internal hemorrhoids. There are also hemorrhoids that prolapse, that is, they form on the inside but "hang" down to the outside of the anus.

Hemorrhoids may be caused by constipation, hard bowel movements or not enough fiber in the diet. They're more common in taxi and truck drivers, who sit a lot, and in pregnant women. Rarer, but more ominous, is a hemorrhoid caused by a cancerous tumor higher up in the colon that is blocking a vein. The most common symptoms of hemorrhoids are pain and difficulty in moving the bowels. You may also see red or bright red blood in the toilet or on the toilet tissue.

Standard therapy includes rectal suppositories to relive pain, hot sitz baths, surgery, laser ablation of hemorrhoids and analgesics for pain (but pain pills with narcotics or codeine may worsen the problem by causing constipation). High-fiber preparations, such as Metamucil, are also used. Alternative therapies for hemorrhoids include:

- *Herbology.* Pilewort *(Ranunculus ficaria)*, horse chestnut *(Aesculus hippocastanum)*, witch hazel *(Hamamelis virginiana)*.
- *Homeopathic remedies. Aesculus hippocastanum, Aloe, Graphites, Ignatia, Lycopodium clavatum.*
- *Nutrition.* High-fiber diet based on fresh vegetables, whole grains and fruit.

I recommend eating a high-fiber diet, including three to four servings of fruit a day, three to five servings of vegetables and two servings of legumes (peas, beans and lentils). Vitamin C, the B-complex, beta carotene, zinc for healing and a teaspoon full of linseed oil to help soften the stools are all helpful. Zinc oxide is an old remedy that can be applied to the external or prolapsed hemorrhoids for healing and prevention.

Impotence (erectile dysfunction)

Impotence is characterized by a gradually increasing problem in achieving or maintaining an erection sufficient to have sexual intercourse. The most common causes are psychological difficulties, an insufficient supply of the male hormone testosterone, a nerve problem associated with diabetes and hardening of the arteries that supply blood to the penis. Many medicines may be to blame, including the beta blockers for hypertension, various psychiatric medications, antihistamines, sedatives and a number of drugs used to treat ulcers. Certain spinal cord injuries, strokes, syphilis and multiple sclerosis may cause erectile dysfunction. Many men who have undergone prostate surgery also have difficulties. Long-term use of alcohol causes problems for some men because it is a "feminizing" substance that shrinks the testicles. And in the short term, as Shakespeare pointed out, alcohol provokes the desire but can ruin the performance.

The standard medical treatment for erectile dysfunction is pretty good. If a hormonal imbalance lies at the root of the difficulty, testosterone replacement therapy works well. Bypass surgery will often bring blood flow to the penis, if lack of circulation is the cause. Other men can be taught to self-administer injections of PGE1 into the base of the penis, producing erections that last three to four hours. There are also penile implants, which need more refining, and a hand-held vacuum device that "manually" produces an erection.

Many alternative therapies are used for impotence, including:

- *Aromatherapy.* Clary *(Salvia sclarea)*, geranium *(Pelargonium odorantissimum)*, jasmine *(Jasminum officinale)*, rose *(Rosa spp.)*, melissa *(Melissa officinalis)*.

- *Homeopathic remedies.* For impotence, *Baryta carbonica*, *Lycopodium clavatum*, sulfur.

- *Oriental medicine.* Both impotence and infertility are usually treated by stimulating the energy stored in the lower abdomen and with proper eating, exercise and good living. Because the kidney is associated with sexual energy, acupuncture points corresponding to the kidney will be stimulated. These points include Kidney 3 (between the inner ankle and the Achilles tendon) and Spleen 6 (three finger breadths up from the inside ankle bone). Herbal formulas for infertility include *Tai Pan Tang Yi Pian* and *Lu Wei Ba Jing*. Herbal formulas for impotence include *Tai Pan Tang Yi Pian* and *Kwei Ling Chi.*

I believe that it is very important to search for and treat the underlying cause, if any. Sometimes, simply examining the many medications patients are taking and reducing the doses, exchanging them for others or eliminating them altogether, solves the problem. I also recommend a low-fat, low-cholesterol diet to prevent arteriosclerosis of the blood vessels of the penis. The healthful diet, along with exercise and supplements, if necessary, help to maintain overall good health. And of course, psychological counseling may be helpful.

Influenza

Commonly known as the flu, influenza is a very common viral infection of the upper respiratory tract. Symptoms include headache, fatigue, a runny nose, sore throat, cough and muscle aches.

Not too long ago, the flu was greatly feared. During the great influenza epidemic following World War I, millions of people died. My mother, who was a girl in Philadelphia at the time, was sent out to "the countryside" of New Jersey in order to get away from the danger. Fortunately, it presents much less of a problem today.

There is no cure for the flu, although we do have flu vaccines that help to prevent it from striking. The vaccines work, but we don't know which strain of virus is going to sweep through the country each year. The companies making vaccines get together with the Centers For Disease Control (CDC) to decide which one(s) will be appropriate. If the vaccine manufacturers make the right one(s), we're fine, otherwise we only get marginal protection.

Standard medical treatment for the flu includes rest, drinking lots of fluids and taking medications for the symptoms. Alternative therapies used for influenza include:

- *Aromatherapy.* Cypress *(Cupressus sempervirens)*, eucalyptus *(Eucalyptus globulus)*, juniper *(Juniperus communis)*, peppermint *(Mentha piperata)*, rosemary *(Rosmarinus officinalis)*.
- *Ayurveda.* The flu generally manifests itself in the Kapha (water) humor, so an anti-Kapha diet is prescribed. Dairy products, oily foods, heavy and damp foods are eliminated. Many herbs are used, including ginger *(Zingiber officinale)*, sage *(Salvia officinalis)*, hyssop *(Hyssopus officinalis)*, basil *(Ocimum basilicum)*, as well as lemon and ginger juice.
- *Herbology.* Elder flower, ginger, peppermint, yarrow.
- *Homeopathic remedies.* Aconitum napellus, Dulcamara, Gelsemium, Nux vomica, Pulsatilla.

I may recommend Sambucol, an herbal product made from extracts of black elderberries *(Sambucus nigra)* and raspberries *(Rubus idaeus)*. In order for the virus to multiply and cause the flu, it must enter the cell of an animal or human. Laboratory studies have shown that Sambucol prevents the virus from entering the cells and multiplying. To me this is extraordinary, because despite many years of research, traditional medicine has not found an effective treatment for the flu. Sambucol provides a much higher success rate. In a double-blind study, flu patients were given either black elderberry extract or a placebo. About 90 percent of the patients who received the elderberry were symptom-free within two to three days. But those who received the placebo had to wait a least six days to enjoy the same relief.

Insomnia

Insomnia is the "nighttime" condition involving difficulty falling and/or staying asleep. Sufferers may wake up frequently during the night or get up sooner than they want to. Although insomnia can strike at any age, it is more common among the older population.

Many cases of insomnia may be related to the age-associated falling levels of melatonin, the "sleep hormone" secreted by the brain.

Many people have transient difficulty sleeping, especially if they're excited or stressed. That's why doctors don't label an occasional difficulty, or one obviously related to a specific problem, as insomnia.

Some of the symptoms include taking longer than normal to fall asleep, feeling nervous or restless while trying to fall asleep, waking up after a short period of sleep and waking up in the middle of the night (sometimes with unhappy thoughts). Many factors can bring on insomnia, including depression, anxiety, hyperthyroidism (overactive thyroid), heart conditions, asthma, lung conditions, chronic pain, prostate enlargement, gastrointestinal problems, drinking coffee or other fluids containing caffeine too soon before bedtime, daytime napping, certain drugs, crazy work hours, shift changes and alcoholism.

Standard medical treatment includes a checkup to look for underlying problems. (Sometimes a study conducted in a sleep-study laboratory may find a specific physical problem, such as the lack of oxygen during sleep, called sleep apnea.) For most cases where there is no underlying problem, sleeping pills are prescribed. Many alternative therapies are used for insomnia, including:

- *Aromatherapy.* Chamomile *(Matricaria chamomilla)*, lavender *(Lavandula officinalis)*, neroli *(Citrus aurantium)*, rose *(Rosa spp.)*, sandalwood *(Santalum album)*.
- *Herbology.* Hops *(Humulus lupulus)*, passion flower *(Passiflora incarnata)*, wild lettuce *(Lactuca virosa)*, Jamaican dogwood *(Piscidia erythrina)*, valerian *(Valeriana officinalis)*.
- *Homeopathic remedies. Aconitum napellus, Coffea cruda, Lycopodium clavatum.*

I may recommend losing weight if a patient is overweight. Chronic pain may need a multidisciplinary team of healers to relieve the pain and its underlying cause. For many of my patients, however, taking a hormone called melatonin 30 to 40 minutes before bedtime solves the problem. Melatonin, which is made in the pineal gland of the brain, is "nature's sleeping pill." The body's levels of melatonin fall as we age.

Other simple measures include drinking a glass of warm skim milk before bed, meditating before bedtime, making sure the bedroom is neither too hot nor too cold, using a comfortable pillow, not arguing with your spouse before going to bed, avoiding alcohol and caffeine, having your physician review your medications to make sure none is keeping you awake, using heavy curtains in the bedroom to block out light and using a fan or "white noise" machine to block out distractions.

It also helps to examine your life for unnecessary stress. The amino acid DLPA (dl-phenylalanine) helps if depression is causing your insomnia. If the problem is due to anxiety, I may recommend a homeopathic remedy called L.72 Anti-Anxiety or an herb called Kava kava, both made by Enzymatic Therapies. The herb valerian is also helpful.

Irritable bowel syndrome

Irritable bowel syndrome (IBS) is an inflammatory, irritable condition of the intestine, which doctors call a functional disorder. This means that there is no infection or cancer, and it's not contagious. The problem has to do with functioning, not germs or disease. Muscles that normally push things through the intestine aren't working properly. They may go into severe contraction, causing spastic colitis. Or they may contract at odd times, causing pain and other discomfort.

The symptoms of IBS include pain in the lower abdomen, which is often relieved by bowel movements. There may also be rectal pain, back pain, bloating, noise in the abdomen, diarrhea and excessive passing of gas. Fatigue, anxiety and depression may grow as the problem continues. And with spastic colitis, there may be constipation.

IBS may resolve itself, especially if it was caused by a situational problem, such as stress or overwork. However, it often becomes a chronic problem, incapacitating the victim, who cannot go far from a bathroom. As the IBS patient ages, it can interfere with nutrient absorption, leading to osteoporosis and numerous nutrient deficiencies.

Warning: If your stool is black, tarry or red, if you get a fever, if you vomit or if you unexpectedly lose more than five pounds, see your doctor. These signs and symptoms might indicate a more serious problem, such as gastrointestinal bleeding, intestinal infection, autoimmune disease or cancer of the bowel.

Standard treatment for IBS includes medicines to prevent spasms, relieve cramps and cut down on gas, tranquilizers and high-fiber powders. Among the alternative therapies for IBS are:

- *Herbology.* Chamomile *(Matricaria chamomilla)*, hops *(Humulus lupulus)*, Mexican wild yam *(Dioscorea villosa)*, fennel *(Foeniculum vulgare)*, peppermint *(Mentha piperata)*.
- *Nutrition.* Eliminate spicy and other irritating foods, avoid refined carbohydrates and eat a low-fat, high-fiber diet.

I have found that a high-fiber diet is an excellent aid in the treatment of IBS. In addition, I recommend experimenting with the diet and keeping a log of everything eaten and bowel habits in order to discover which foods trigger problems. Eliminate alcohol and hot spicy foods and eat four to five small meals a day.

Beta carotene, vitamins C and E, the mineral selenium, alpha-lipoic acid and other antioxidants are important to prevent the free radical damage that I believe plays a role in this condition. It's also very important to develop a healthy frame of mind. Optimistically looking forward to a cure is, in itself, a strong medicine.

Stroke ("brain attack")

One of the leading causes of death in this country, a stroke is damage to brain cells caused by a sudden drop in the flow of blood to the brain. In a sense, a stroke resembles a heart attack except it is brain cells—not heart muscles—that suffer from the lack of blood.

Also known as cerebrovascular accidents (CVA) and "brain attacks," strokes tend to afflict people over the age of 50. They're also more common in alcoholics. Symptoms include headaches, confusion, dizziness, slurred speech or an inability to speak, lack of coordination, loss of consciousness and a "droopiness" on one side of the face. Which symptoms strike depend on what part of the brain is damaged.

Strokes are usually caused by high blood pressure, hardening or thickening of the arteries in or leading to the brain, a blood clot or a ruptured blood vessel. A commonly overlooked cause is what we call "embolisation," in which a blood clot forms in the heart and travels to the brain, where it blocks a blood vessel. Transient ischemic attacks (called "TIAs") are "small" strokes that cause what appear to be relatively minor problems, such as slurred speech, visual disturbances or a weakening of an arm or leg on one side. However, they are warnings of greater problems to come. *Warning: If you have any of these symptoms, see your physician immediately. The earlier treatment begins, the better the odds of recovery or prevention of permanent damage.*

Stroke-induced symptoms may resolve themselves, may be corrected with physical therapy and/or medication, may produce long-term or permanent disability (such as inability to move one side of the body) or may be fatal.

Standard medical treatment for strokes includes drugs to reduce blood pressure, prevent blood clots and relieve pain. There is also surgery to remove blockages in the neck (carotid) arteries leading to the brain. Stroke treatment is almost always after-the-fact. A large amount of time and resources are spent in rehabilitation of stroke victims. The many alternative therapies for stroke include:

- *Homeopathic remedies. Aconitum napellus, Arnica montana.*
- *Nutrition.* Vitamin B6, calcium, magnesium, potassium and omega-3 fatty acids. Some sources of these nutrients are:
  Vitamin B6—albacore, chestnuts, navy beans and tuna;
  calcium—cabbage, cantaloupes, barley and spinach;

magnesium—bananas, beets, spinach and onions; potassium—leafy green vegetables, winter squash and orange juice; omega-3 fatty acids—salmon, sardines, sablefish and other fish. Also, reduce alcohol and cholesterol, in addition to eating plenty of fresh vegetables and fruits.

It's very important to prevent strokes by keeping the arteries clean and open. The most important step is to control blood pressure. If a patient's pressure is very high, I believe it is important to use medications to bring the pressure down immediately. Then, as the pressure falls, I work to reduce medications as lifestyle changes take hold.

The lifestyle changes include adopting a low-fat, low-cholesterol, high-complex-carbohydrate, moderate-protein, low-sodium diet. Keep your cholesterol levels at the total level of approximately 100 plus your age, the LDL ("bad") cholesterol below 100 and the HDL ("good") cholesterol at 55 or above. Also, abstain from alcohol or limit yourself to one glass of red wine per day with a meal. Get at least 30 minutes of light exercise daily, such as walking.

Antioxidants, such as beta carotene, vitamins C and E and alpha-lipoic acid, should be used to prevent atherosclerotic plaques from forming and blocking the arteries. Taking ginkgo biloba helps to increase the flow of blood to the brain and improves cognition. Studies have shown that aspirin is helpful in preventing platelets from sticking together and forming unwanted clots. Your physician will tell you how much to take. Finally, learn how to recognize and avoid the effects of stress. When you feel yourself getting upset, ask yourself if it is worth dying over. If not, forget it.

Yeast infections (candidiasis)

Candidiasis comes about when a yeast called *candida* attacks the gastrointestinal tract, vagina or other parts of the body, or gets into the blood stream. Candida is a yeast found in the intestines, vagina and skin. Ordinarily, it is balanced by "good" bacteria such as acidophilus and bifidebacteria, which produce natural, anticandida and antibacterial substances. However, if the good bacteria is killed off by excess antibiotics or other factors, the yeast may get the "upper hand," growing rapidly and spreading. No longer checked by the good bacteria and a strong immune system, it can cause a variety of problems.

In women, candida may cause an inflammation of the vagina and cervix, producing a characteristic, odoriferous discharge associated with itching and irritation. Candida is a major cause of vaginal discharge. In children, if it attacks the mouth or throat, it's called "thrush mouth," causing pain and difficulty in eating and swallowing. It may also get into the kidney, bladder, brain and other parts of the body. If it strikes in an HIV-positive person, the immune system is severely compromised.

Other symptoms of candidiasis include rectal itching, "jock itch," prostatitis, recurrent urinary tract infections and a wide variety of allergies. It can also cause asthma-like symptoms and gastrointestinal symptoms, such as diarrhea, cramping and gas. Chronic fatigue and depression have been associated with candidiasis.

Standard medical treatment for candidiasis is often not offered, because many traditional Western physicians do not believe that it is a problem, except for vaginal candidiasis. There is a new, one-dose drug for vaginal candidiasis, and various antifungal agents are available. Nysatin is the most popular antifungal being used today, but candida can avoid the medicine by mutating into other forms.

Although there is some controversy concerning the incidence and severity, I believe it is important that the patient be given a careful history and physical examination, and that laboratory studies be performed. It is worthwhile to follow a comprehensive program that includes:

1. A low-sugar diet, since yeast grows well in the presence of sugar. (The high-sugar American diet should be considered a causative factor in this condition.) This means avoiding fruit juices, honey, molasses, table sugar, candy bars and lactose (the sugar found in milk). Foods containing yeast, such as baked goods and vinegar, should also be avoided until food-sensitivity tests are performed. Molds found in cheese and various fermented foods, such as sauerkraut, can produce similar symptoms and should be avoided.
2. Giving up all forms of alcohol, which contains fermented sugars and harms the immune system. Observations suggest that drinking alcohol aggravates the symptoms of candidiasis.
3. Telling your physician that you don't want to take antibiotics unless they are absolutely necessary, because they upset the balance between the good bacteria and the candida.
4. Strengthening the immune system with a healthful diet and supplements. The B-vitamins are important because some of these are made by the intestinal bacteria that are killed off by antibiotics. Also, beta carotene, vitamins C and E, zinc and other nutrients are very helpful.
5. Using herbs, such as goldenseal, caprylic acid, garlic and Pau d'Arco, to further strengthen the immune system

Many people who have candidiasis are not able to get treatment for their symptoms. I believe that every patient should be given a full examination and all the appropriate treatment.

Alternative health organizations

The Academy for Guided Imagery
P.O. Box 2070
Mill Valley, CA 94942
800-726-2070

American Association of
  Acupuncture and Oriental
  Medicine
4101 Lake Boone Trail
Suite 201
Raleigh, NC 27607
919-787-5181

American Association of
  Acupuncture and Oriental
  Medicine
433 First St.
Catasauqua, PA 18032
610-433-2448

American Association of
  Naturopathic Physicians
2366 Eastlake Ave. East
Suite 322
Seattle, WA 98102
206-323-7610

American Chiropractic Association
1701 Clarendon Blvd.
Arlington, VA 22209
703-276-8800

American College of Advancement
  in Medicine
P.O. Box 3427
Laguna Hills, CA 92654
714-583-7666
800-532-3688

American Holistic Medical
  Association
4101 Lake Boone Trail
Suite 201
Raleigh, NC 27607
919-787-5146

American Massage Therapy Assn.
820 Davis St.
Suite 100
Evanston, IL 60201
312-761-2682

The American Society of Clinical
  Hypnosis
2200 East Devon Ave.
Suite 291
Des Plaines, IL 60018
847-297-3317

Homeopathic Educational Services
2124 Kittredge St.
Berkeley, CA 94704
800-359-9051

International Chiropractors Assn.
1110 N. Glebe Rd.
Suite 1000
Arlington, VA 22201
703-528-5000

International Foundation for
  Homeopathy
2366 Eastlake Ave. East
Suite 301
Seattle, WA 98201
206-776-4147

International Institute of Reflexology
P.O. Box 12462
St. Petersburg, FL 33733
813-343-4811

International Medical and Dental
  Hypnotherapy Association
4110 Edgeland
Suite 800
Royal Oak, MI 48073
313-549-5594
800-257-5467

National Center for Homeopathy
801 N. Fairfax
Suite 306
Alexandria, VA 22314
703-548-7790

National College of Naturopathic
  Medicine
11231 Southeast Market St.
Portland, OR 97216
503-255-4860

The National Guild of Hypnotists
P.O. Box 308
Merrimack, NH 03054
603-429-9438

The Pacific Institute of
  Aromatherapy
P.O. Box 6842
San Rafael, CA 94903
415-479-9121

Glossary

Acupuncture part of the larger system of Oriental medicine, acupuncture uses needles to restore the body's energy balance in order to treat pain and disease.

Affirmations brief, positive statements that one already has what one desires. Reciting and believing in the affirmations helps to alter body chemistry and improve health.

AIDS (Acquired Immunodeficiency Syndrome) a breakdown of the immune system caused by HIV (Human Immunodeficiency Virus). AIDS victims typically succumb to diseases that otherwise healthy people could fight off. Having HIV is not the same as having AIDS, but the HIV often progresses to the clinical state of AIDS.

Alpha lipoic acid a powerful antioxidant that helps to slow or prevent the ravages of aging and has been used to treat certain forms of heart disease, diabetes, AIDS and other diseases. Known by the trade name Alpha-Lipotene.

Alzheimer's disease a rapid deterioration of the brain that typically afflicts older people, eventually leaving them unable to care for themselves, and leading to death.

Analgesia pain relief.

Antioxidant substances that prevent oxidants from harming the body. There are natural antioxidants produced by the body, such as SOD (superoxide dismutase), and other antioxidants found in foods and supplements, including beta carotene and vitamins C and E.

Aromatherapy a healing art that utilizes the aromatic essences of flowers and plants to influence the mind and body.

Arthritis an inflammation of one or more joints. Osteoarthritis and rheumatoid arthritis are the most common forms of this disease.

Ayurveda a 5,000-year-old healing art developed in India, which is part of the larger system of Vedic science that interprets the working of the universe. Ayurvedic healing utilizes nutrition, spirituality, herbs, massage, psychology, meditation, gems and other means to heal the body and mind.

Benign tumor a slow-growing tumor that does not spread to other parts of the body (metastasize). It may obstruct, interfere with or pressure other body tissue, but it is not cancerous.

Beta carotene the "plant form" of vitamin A found in dark orange and dark green leafy vegetables, such as carrots, spinach, collard greens, mangoes, broccoli and other foods. Although the body converts beta carotene to vitamin A as necessary, beta carotene in and of itself has anti-cancer and free-radical quenching abilities.

Bioflavonoids a group of compounds, such as quercetin and catechin, that have antioxidant properties. Found in orange and yellow citrus fruits, green tea and other foods.

Carcinoma cancer, although the term is usually applied to the group of cancers that develop from coverings and linings in the body (such as the lining of the stomach).

Chiropractic a healing art that utilizes spinal manipulation, massage and other techniques to treat disease.

Cholesterol a waxy sterol produced by the body and taken in when we eat meat and other foods of animal origin. Eating saturated fats causes the liver to produce excessive amounts of cholesterol. Although some cholesterol is necessary, excesses have been linked to coronary heart disease. To help ensure good heart health, the total cholesterol should be 100 plus your age, and no more than 180.

Coenzyme Q10 also known as ubiquinone, an antioxidant that helps to "disarm" the harmful LDL cholesterol. Q10 is found in many fish and nuts, soybeans and other foods.

Color therapy a healing art that uses colors to diagnose and treat disease. Bacteria, viruses and other germs, as well as diseases, are believed to give off light of particular wave lengths. Applying light of the same wave length will combat the disease.

Coronary heart disease (CHD) the most common form of heart disease, also known as coronary artery disease or "clogged arteries." Blockages in the coronary arteries that supply fresh blood to the heart muscle become blocked, blood flow stops and heart muscle dies as the victim suffers a heart attack.

DHEA (dehydroepiandrosterone) a hormone made by the adrenal glands (which sit atop each of the kidneys). Considered by some to be the best "biomarker" (indicator) of age, DHEA is believed to protect against heart disease, cancer, diabetes, mental deterioration and many autoimmune diseases (such as rheumatoid arthritis). The hormone also increases one's resistance to the viral and bacterial infections that are so often associated with AIDS.

Diabetes a metabolic disease in which the body is either unable to produce enough insulin to control blood sugar or is unable to properly respond to the insulin it does produce.

DLPA (dl-phenylalanine) an amino acid that protects the endorphins, which are natural anti-pain and mood-elevating substances made by the body. DLPA is used to treat many chronic pain conditions and other mental and physical ailments.

Duodenal ulcers ulcers that occur in the part of the small intestine called the duodenum.

Ellagic acid a substance found in strawberries, grapes and other foods that helps protect the body against cancer-causing substances.

Free radicals unstable molecules that "steal" electrons in order to stabilize themselves. In doing so they can destroy other molecules, damage cellular DNA, injure the lining of the coronary arteries and otherwise damage the body. Free radical damage is believed to cause or contribute to heart disease, cancer, premature aging and many other ailments.

Gastric ulcers ulcers that arise in the stomach.

Ginkgo biloba an herb that stimulates the immune system, increases blood circulation to the brain and has other positive effects on health.

Glutathione an antioxidant found in watermelon, asparagus, avocado, strawberries, oranges, squash, broccoli and other foods.

Gouty arthritis the arthritis associated with gout. Gout is caused by elevated levels of uric acid. Some of the uric acid crystallizes ("hardens") in the joints, leading to pain and joint damage. Largely a disease of adult males, it may strike women. Although mostly due to diet and genetics, it may also be caused by certain drugs, kidney problems, high blood pressure and other factors.

HDL high density lipoprotein, the "good" cholesterol that helps to clear cholesterol off the artery walls. Your HDL should be 50 or more.

HIV (Human Immunodeficiency Virus the virus said to be responsible for AIDS.

Herbal healing the use of herbs to treat disease.

Homeopathy a healing art based on the principle that "like cures like." In other words, symptoms of a disease can be cured with substances that cause the same symptoms in a healthy person.

Hypnosis a healing art in which the practitioner uses an artificially induced state of increased suggestibility to influence the unconscious mind, and through the mind, the body.

Hypertension elevated blood pressure.

Indoles substances with powerful anti-cancer properties found in cabbage, cauliflower, broccoli and other "cruciferous" vegetables.

Isoflavones hormone-like substances, found in peas, beans and lentils, that may help prevent the growth of estrogen-driven tumors.

LDL low-density lipoprotein, the "bad" cholesterol that helps to increase blockages in the arteries. Your LDL should be 100 or less.

Life expectancy the actual number of years the average person lives. (The life expectancy was about 50 years in 1900. It's roughly 75 years now.)

Lifespan the maximum number of years that some humans have been able to live. (The lifespan is estimated to be 115 to 120 years.)

Lignans anti-cancer substances found in flax and lignans.

Lycopene an antioxidant that may help prevent cancer of the cervix, bladder and pancreas. It is found in tomatoes, red peppers and other foods.

Malignant tumor a fast-growing, cancerous tumor that invades other parts of the body, either directly or by metastasis.

Melatonin a natural hormone produced by a part of the brain, which helps us sleep at night. Melatonin is also believed to improve the memory, increase longevity, decrease breast cancer, enhance the immune system, prevent jet lag and increase energy.

Monoterpenes antioxidants found in various vegetables and fruits.

Music healing a healing art using music, imagery and suggestion to stimulate the body's natural defenses against disease.

Naturopathy a multifaceted healing art that suggests disease can be cured by simulating the body's natural healing powers. Naturopathy uses nutritional therapy, water therapy and other techniques to encourage the body to heal itself.

Neoplasm a cancerous new growth, an abnormal mass that serves no useful purpose and grows at the expense of other cells.

Nonsteroidal anti-inflammatory drugs also called NSAIDs, these are drugs used to reduce the pain and inflammation of arthritis and other conditions. Some common NSAIDs are Indocin, Naprosyn and Feldene.

Nutritional healing the use of foods, vitamins, minerals and other supplements to treat disease.

Ojas in Ayurvedic healing, ojas is the body's vigor, the nontangible essential energy of the body's vital secretions and reproductive system. Centered in the heart but spread throughout the body, ojas keeps us alive. When the ojas drops to low levels, the body is susceptible to infections, nervous disorders and degenerative diseases. When the ojas is gone, life is gone.

Omega-3 fatty acids fats found in fish, especially cold-water fish (such as salmon), that help to protect against heart disease, arthritis and other diseases.

Oriental medicine an ancient and comprehensive system of healing that uses acupuncture, herbs, nutrition and other disciplines to help the body heal itself.

Osteoarthritis a form of arthritis in which the cartilage that normally cushions the ends of joints breaks down. It is the most common form of arthritis.

Osteoporosis a "thinning" of the bones often associated with aging, especially with postmenopausal women. There may be symptoms of pain or no symptoms at all until a bone breaks.

Oxidation and free radical theory of aging argues that accumulated cellular damage due to free radicals and oxidation causes aging. In other words, our mental and physical abilities are buried under piles of metabolic trash.

Oxidation a naturally occurring but dangerous reaction between oxygen and certain substances in the body. Oxygen is supposed to interact with very specific substances, such as red blood cells. The problem arises when oxygen interacts with other substances, "rusting" them and making them unable to work properly. Although each single piece of oxidation damage is small, over time the accumulated damage can damage cells, organs and entire body systems. The body has natural antioxidants to control oxidation.

Parkinson's disease a central nervous system disease that leads to rigidity of the muscles, tremors and other problems, including mental deterioration in the advanced stages.

Pectin a fiber found in grapefruit, apples and other fruits and vegetables that helps to reduce cholesterol and protect against heart disease.

Proanthocyanidins powerful antioxidants derived from grape seed extracts and/or the bark of a maritime tree.

Protease inhibitors substances that help to prevent breast, colon and other cancers. Found in whole grain oats, rice, potatoes, chick peas, soybeans, kidney beans and other foods.

Psychoneuroimmunology a relatively new branch of medical science that utilizes the "mind-body" connection to strengthen the body's natural defenses against current and future diseases. It is based on the theory that all thoughts are "translated" by the brain into chemical or other "messengers" that can affect every part of the body, for better or worse. Brief, positive statements called affirmations are used to fill the mind with positive thoughts.

Quercetin an antioxidant and member of the bioflavonoid family found in many fruits and vegetables.

Reflexology a healing art that applies pressure to specific parts of the feet in order to relieve tension, improve the circulation, stimulate the nerves and normalize the functioning of the organs and glands.

Remedies homeopathic "medicines" used to treat disease.

Rheumatoid arthritis a chronic autoimmune disease that involves the joints, muscles, ligaments, tendons, coverings of the muscles (fascia) and even the bones. It may be very mild and brief, or may become a severe, progressively crippling disease.

Saponins anti-cancer substances found in sunflower seeds, soybeans and other foods.

Shiatsu a Japanese system of bodywork designed to improve the flow of energy and blood throughout the body.

Subluxation a term used by chiropractors to describe imbalances or dislocations that interfere with the nerves. They may be caused by injury, stress, inherited spinal problems, poor posture and other problems, and may cause a variety of diseases and disorders.

Sulfides natural substances found in cruciferous vegetables, such as broccoli and cauliflower, as well as in garlic, that help protect healthy cells from carcinogens.

Tumor an abnormal, new growth that serves no useful purpose, does not work with other cells for the good of the body and grows at the expense of other cells.

Ubiquinone see coenzyme Q10.

Water therapy a healing art based on the theory that the body's energies can be changed when one is stimulated in specific ways by hot water, cold water, ice and steam.

Index